KV-638-588

John W. McLean

The Science and Art of Dental Ceramics

Volume I: The Nature of Dental Ceramics
and their Clinical Use

EDINBURGH'S TELFORD COLLEGE

0001360

WITHDRAWN

This bc

to be returned on or before
t date stamped below.

The Science and Art of Dental Ceramics

Volume I: The Nature of Dental Ceramics and their Clinical Use

John W. McLean, O.B.E.
D.Sc., M.D.S. (University of London)
L.D.S. R.C.S. (England)

Consulting Professor
in Fixed Prosthodontics and Biomaterials

Louisiana State University Medical Centre School
of Dentistry

Quintessence Publishing Co., Inc.   1979
Chicago, Berlin, Rio de Janeiro, Tokyo

CAT NO: 2579

Telford College
Library

617·675 545

160997

© 1979 by Quintessence Publishing Co., Inc., Chicago, Illinois.
All rights reserved.

This book or any part thereof must not be reproduced by any means or in any
form without the written permission of the publisher.

Lithography: Industrie- und Presseklischee, Berlin.
Composition: Westkreuz-Druckerei Berlin/Bonn.
Printing and binding: North Central Publishing Co., St. Paul.
Printed in the U.S.A.

ISBN 0 931386 04 7

Foreword

Dr. *John McLean's* practice of aesthetic dentistry goes back many years. In 1963 he initiated a programme of research with the Warren Spring Government Laboratory in England with the object of developing stronger dental porcelains without sacrificing aesthetics. This programme led to the development of the Aluminous Porcelains which have largely supplanted regular dental porcelain for the construction of jacket crowns.

Dr. *McLean* is one of a handful of individuals endowed with exceptional clinical talent and the scientific ability to produce an aesthetic restoration from the basic raw ingredients.

This series of monographs is a new endeavour to present, in detail, the finer points of ceramic art in dentistry. It is our intention at Louisiana State University School of Dentistry to use this work as the basis for a continuing education programme in dental ceramics which we hope will encourage younger men to specialise in this rapidly expanding field.

Edmund Jeansonne
November 1974   Dean

5

Preface

This series of monographs on "The Science and Art of Dental Ceramics" has been written principally for the serious student or researcher in dental ceramics. They may also assist the dental technician in a better understanding of his craft and will explain why failures may occur during the firing of dental ceramic work.

Each monograph attempts to penetrate, in some depth, the present state of the art, and some of the material is not available in current textbooks or research papers in the dental field. The research student might find the gathering together of the newer research in dental porcelain of some assistance if he is preparing a thesis. It is for this reason that the Monographs were originally published by Louisiana State University as two separate books.

The increasing demand for information on dental ceramics has continued since the publication of the Monographs in 1974 and the Quintessence Publishing Company considered it an opportune moment to revise the text and publish it in one volume.

The scientific section has been updated particularly with regard to the latest developments in the metal-ceramic field. Two major symposia have been held in the United States of America in 1977 on dental porcelain and alternatives to gold alloys. The proceedings were published by the University of Southern California and the National Institute of Health.

Reference is made to these symposia in the text and the clinical section of the book has been enhanced by the inclusion of colour photographs which do so much for the beauty of porcelain work.

The first two monographs are concerned with the nature of dental ceramics and glasses and how these brittle materials may be strengthened or prevented from fracturing. Further monographs deal with the problems of colour, occlusion in dental porcelain, and the preparation of teeth for ceramic crown and bridgework. The building of ceramics with a brush and methods of obtaining colour and translucency are also dealt with in detail. The importance of obtaining this natural enamel effect cannot be over-emphasized since much of the ceramic work today lacks the natural depth of translucency of human teeth. Without depth of translucency, ceramic crowns will never become submerged in the mouth and be undetectable from their human counterparts.

The increasing use of metal-ceramics has brought with it the problems of maintaining the health of the periodontium. In addition, the problems of dealing with highly reflective opaque backgrounds on metal surfaces is one that has yet to be completely mastered. The maintenance of original tooth contour, together with the provision of correct colour values, is an area which is given great prominence in this series of monographs; this work forming part of the continuing education programme at Louisiana State University.

No attempt has been made in this volume to cover all aspects of fixed prosthodontics and the reader is advised to consult other works in

7

this field. For a basic understanding of crown and bridgework the text by Shillingburg, Hobo and Whitsett "Fundamentals of Fixed Prosthodontics" is recommended. Other works that provide additional instruction are Johnston, Phillips and Dykema's "Modern Practice in Crown and Bridge Prosthodontics" and Tylman's "Theory and Practice of Crown and Bridge Prosthodontics".

The design and construction of metal ceramic bridgework and developing occlusion in dental porcelain will be covered in the second volume of "The Science and Art of Dental Ceramics" entitled "Laboratory Procedures in Dental Ceramics". In this volume a critical look is taken of obtaining maximum light tranmission through the anterior crown. Many students are being instructed only in the metal-ceramic techniques and therefore tend to accept the aesthetics of these materials without question. This has resulted in many commercial laboratories eliminating the porcelain jacket crown from their armamentarium. The "metal-ceramic smile" is more common than we perhaps would care to admit.

The cast metal-ceramic restoration is of enormous value in dentistry and is deservedly the most widely used porcelain restoration. However, a plea is made in these monographs for more selectivity in the use of porcelain materials. To adopt one system or brand of porcelain and use it indiscriminately and without appreciation of its aesthetic or mechanical limitations can result in unsightly dentistry. There is a place for all our materials – the full porcelain veneer crown, the bonded alumina crown, and the metal ceramic crown. Each should be used where its properties can be developed to maximum advantage.

It should be noted that throughout the text, the new Système International d'Unités (SI) is used. The SI derives all the quantities needed in all technologies from only six basic and arbitrarily defined units. This contrasts with the metric systems currently used, in which additional quantities (for instance, 'calorie' and 'horsepower') are arbitrarily and, indeed, differently defined in different metric countries. Relationships between units are thus greatly simplified in the SI, the introduction of which offers existing metric countries a unique opportunity to harmonize their measuring practices. It is likely that most countries will eventually adopt this international system of measurement and, for convenience, a conversion table is inserted at the end of each volume.

The Harvard System of references has been chosen quite deliberately since it requires the insertion in the text of the name of the author quoted as a reference. The reader is then able to identify the person quickly and realise who had developed the original thought.

Acknowledgements

In preparing this series of monographs on the "Science and Art of Dental Ceramics" I have had considerable help from experts in the fields of ceramics, metallurgy, and silicate chemistry.

In particular I would like to thank Mr. *David Binns* of the British Ceramic Research Association, Dr *Alan Wilson* of the Laboratory of the Government Chemist, Mr. *R. Batchelor* of Harrison Meyer Ltd., and Dr. *Ian Sced* of the National Physical Laboratory, for assisting me with the sections on the nature of glasses, ceramics and metals.

I have had the good fortune of working with Mr. *T. H. Hughes* of the Warren Spring Laboratory, Stevenage, on the development of the aluminous porcelains. Without his help these monographs would not have been possible.

A great deal of my knowledge on porcelain has been gained during the production of the aluminous porcelains and I am greatly in debt to Mr. *Clifford Hall* of Harrison Meyer Ltd., Stoke-upon-Trent, who has always allowed me free access to his laboratories and technical staff. I am also indebted to Dr. *H. Rauter*, K. G., of Vita Zahnfabrik, West Germany, for his co-operation in producing alumina reinforced porcelains, and to Dr. *Pralow*, his chief chemist, with whom I have worked for a number of years.

The late Mr. *Jan Adriaansen* of Amsterdam taught me how to build porcelain and he has given considerable inspiration to my technicians.

Mr. *Richard Gale*, Mr. *John Seviour*, Mr. *Michael Kempton*, Mr. *John Hubbard* and Mr. *Michael Kedge* have performed much of the work on the aluminous porcelains and their willing assistance materially improved the techniques of construction.

Mrs. *K. Wilder* has given invaluable service during the preparation of my manuscripts and my daughter, *Diana*, has prepared all the line drawings. Mr. *James Morgan* and his staff of the photographic department at the Institute of Dental Surgery, Eastman Dental Hospital, have prepared most of the other illustrations and I am greatly indebted to all of them for their years of painstaking work.

The production of this work has been possible only with the help and encouragement of Dean *Jeansonne* and his staff at Louisiana State University Dental School. In particular, the advice of Dr. *Howard Bruggers* on the format of the monographs and his editorial help is greatly appreciated. I would also like to thank Mr. *Raymond Calvert*, Mrs. *Mary U. Fontenot*, Mrs. *Linda S. Garner*, Mr. *William Stallworth*, Mr. *Barry Morgan*, Mr. *Alex Barkoff*, Mrs. *Christine Taylor*, Mrs. *Areme Kavanaugh* and Miss *Michelle Jilek*, of the Learning Resources Department who have been responsible for the production of these monographs.

John W. McLean
38 Devonshire street
London, WIN 1LD

Contents

Contents

Monograph III:

Aesthetics of Dental Porcelain

Contents

Monograph IV:

Porcelain as a Restorative Material   183

WITHDRAWN

TELFORD COLLEGE LIBRARY

Contents

Introduction

Ceramics are the earliest group of inorganic materials to be structurally modified by man, and his early history is principally traced through these materials. The origin of glazing techniques is probably the most interesting advance that was later to be so significant from a dental standpoint. Glazed porcelain is our only restorative material from which bacterial plaque can be easily removed, and increasing attention is now being paid to research into the significance of plaque formation on dental restorations.

The earliest glazing technique was a Sumerian invention made famous about 4000 B.C. as Egyptian blue faïence. This glaze was not, like later ones, a melted premix of glass-forming materials but was made by a type of cementation process. Potash was drawn by capillarity to react with the surface of a preformed body of siliceous particles to form a glassy coat of copper-coloured eutectic silicate. The process is still in use today in Iran.

From this early work stemmed all the developments in ceramic technology, and the remarkable fact is that the early ceramists were exploiting almost all the properties of solids that are the concern of the modern solid-state physicists. With the exception of electrical and magnetic effects the ceramist was, sometimes inadvertently, using such properties as moisture-dependent plasticity and thixotrophy in his shaping techniques. Decorative textures were derived from vitrification and devitrification, the nucleation of various crystalline phases, and local variations of viscosity, surface tension and expansivity. Colours depended on various states of oxidation, on abnormal ionic states, on excitons and on structural imperfections in crystals. The understanding of these processes came later when crystal structures could be analysed by means of X-ray diffraction. Their complexity is such that even today much of our decorative ceramic technique remains an art rather than a science. Equally the building of a porcelain jacket crown requires artistic skill; however, with an understanding of the science of ceramics, the technician is better placed to improve his art.

The European development of porcelain came about in the 18th century, and the originator of the first porcelain paste used for denture work was a French apothecary, *Alexis Duchâteau.* His early dentures were ill-fitting because of the uncontrolled firing shrinkage, and after several fruitless experiments, he sought the help of a dentist, *Dubois de Chemant,* who had all the qualities of the tireless clinician. In 1788, *de Chemant* published his book on artificial teeth and the subsequent action brought against him by Parisian dentists who accused him of stealing *Duchâteau's* invention led to his emigration to England.

John Woodforde in his book "The Strange Story of False Teeth" describes how de Chemant set up in London in 1792 and continued to manufacture dentures of porcelain paste supplied by the famous Wedgwood porcelain factory.

The first single porcelain teeth were launched

in 1808 by an Italian dentist, *Guiseppangelo Fonzi,* who worked in Paris, but they never met with great approval because of their brittleness and opacity. It was not until the 1850's that *Samuel Stockton* of Philadelphia, his nephew *S. S. White,* and *Claudius Ash,* in England, placed the porcelain tooth on a successful commercial basis. Then with the advent of vulcanite rubber at this time, dentures for the masses became a reality.

The dental profession did not really master the art of ceramics until the end of the nineteenth century when fixed restorations were realised. Dr. *Charles H. Land* of Detroit was a pioneer in this field and he filed the first patent in 1889 for the construction of the porcelain jacket crown. An ever-growing list of clinicians followed in his footsteps, and the refinement of the shoulder preparation in 1903 has been attributed to Dr. *E. B. Spaulding.* Dr. *W. A. Capon* of Philadelphia and Dr. *Hugh Avery* of San Francisco, did much to enhance the porcelain inlay technique and indeed some of the concepts advanced at that time still find a place in text-books today.

The old trick of baking a porcelain jacket crown to fit a nail was reported in 1908 and Dr. *A. E. Schneider* was impressing audiences as he hammered the crown into a block of wood. *Schneider,* at that time, also made the observation that the crown shoulder should be at a right angle to the force of occlusion. With the publication of Dr. *Albert Le Gro's* book on "Ceramics in Dentistry" in 1925, the use of porcelain had become firmly established. About this time in Europe, the high fusing porcelains were developed to a high degree of aesthetics and *Jan Adriaansen* of Amsterdam pioneered the technique of building up porcelain with a brush. He also developed "Prisma" high fusing porcelain with *Harrison's,* the glaze manufacturers at Stoke-upon-Trent in England, many of these crowns being in use today.

During this period, several attempts were made to use metal reinforcement in the porcelain. Iridioplatinum was used in various forms by Doctor *Swann, Felcher, Hovestad, Johnson,*

Lakermance, Gonod and *Granger,* and their pioneering of the reinforced porcelain bridge led to the development of the current metal-ceramic materials.

It was not until 1962, when *M. Weinstein, S. Katz* and *A. B. Weinstein* filed their first patent in the U.S.A. on the use of gold alloys for porcelain bonding that the universal use of metal-ceramics became a real possibility. Other methods of reinforcing porcelain were also being explored at this time, and the first viable technique for making alumina reinforced crowns was developed in 1963 by *McLean* and *Hughes* in England. This work has been taken a stage further by *McLean* and *Sced* in 1976 in the development of a stronger platinum bonded alumina crown. Attachment of aluminous porcelain to the platinum being achieved by surface coating of the metal with a thin layer of tin. This new system of porcelain attachment using electroplating techniques does not require base metals to be incorporated in the alloy as in the previous metal-ceramic systems.

Other major advances were made in firing dental ceramics and *Vines, Semmelman, Lee* and *Fonvielle* developed the use of vacuum firing techniques at the Dentists' Supply Company in the U.S.A. This method opened up a whole new field in aesthetic dentistry.

With the introduction of all these new porcelains and techniques, the current interest in dental ceramics is growing even faster. Dental porcelain has now reached a stage of development where it seems highly unlikely to be replaced by plastics within the foreseeable future. Materials science is expanding quickly and new methods of strengthening glasses, including techniques such as nucleation, ion-exchange and dispersion strengthening of glasses have yet to be fully exploited in dentistry.

It is very probable that the dental profession will be using glasses or ceramics well into the next century for the replacement of lost tooth enamel. Even assuming that the problem of caries is conquered, we must be ever mindful of the effects of natural abrasion on tooth structure and it is likely that this problem could become of major concern to a longer-living populace demanding retention of its teeth.

References

Avery, H. (1916). Present Status of Porcelain in Dentistry. Paper to the Annual Session N.D.A. July.

Felcher, F. R. (1937). Platinum Reinforced Porcelain Restorations, D. Digest 43:24.

Granger, E. R. (1940). Platinum-iridium Castings; a new Concept of the Dental Casting Process. J.A.D.A. 27:1718.

Hovestad, J. F. (1936). Porcelain Bridges. D. Items Int. 58:239, 330, 418, 509, 615.

Lakermance, R., and *Gonod, P.* Bridges in Reinforced Porcelain. J. Am. D. Club Paris 2:1.

Le Gro, A. L. (1921). Present Status of Porcelain in Dentistry. Paper to the Michigan State Dental Society. April.

Le Gro, A. L. (1925). Ceramics in Dentistry, Dental Items of Interest Publishing Co. Brooklyn, N. Y.

McLean, J. W., and *Hughes, T. H.* (1965). The Reinforcement of Dental Porcelain with Ceramic Oxides. Brit. dent. J. 119:251.

McLean, J. W., and *Sced, I. R.* (1976). The Bonded Alumina Crown I. The bonding of platinum to aluminous dental porcelain using tin-oxide coatings. Austr. Dent. J. 21, 119.

McLean, J. W., and *Sced, I, R.* (1977). Production of Metal-Ceramic Dental Restorations. British Pat. No. 1,483,362.

McLean, J. W., and *Hughes, T. H.* (1968). Improvements in Dental Materials. British Pat. No. 1,105,111.

Schneider, A. E. (1908). Paper Presented to the Illinois State Dental Society.

Smith, C. S. (1967). Materials. Scient. Amer. Sept. 217:69.

Swann, H. (1931). Torque Resisting Porcelain Bridge, Chicago.

Tylman, S. D. (1970). Theory and Practice of Crown and Fixed Partial Prosthodontics (bridge). C. V. Mosby Co., St. Louis.

Vines, R. F., Semmelman, J. O., Lee, P. W., and *Fonvielle, F. D.* (1958). Mechanisms Involved in Securing Dense Vitrified Ceramics from Preshaped Partly Crystalline Bodies. J. Amer. Ceram. Soc., 41:304.

Weinstein, M., Katz, S., and *Weinstein, A. B.* (1962). U.S. Pat. No. 3,052,982.

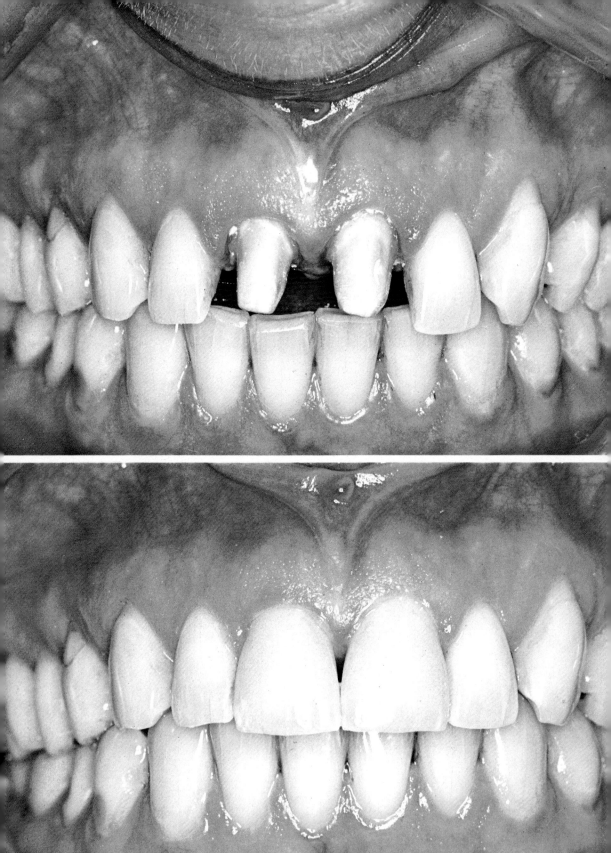

The Nature of Dental Ceramics

The word "ceramic" is derived from the Greek "keramikos" which means "earthen". A ceramic is therefore an earthy material, usually of a silicate nature and may be defined as a combination of one or more metals with a non-metallic element, usually oxygen (*Gilman,* 1967). The larger oxygen atoms serve as a matrix, with the smaller metal atoms (or semi-metal atoms such as silicon) tucked into the spaces between the oxygens (Fig. 1-1).

The atomic bonds in a ceramic crystal have both a covalent and ionic character. These strong bonds are responsible for the great stability of ceramics and impart very useful properties, such as hardness, high modulus of elasticity and resistance to heat and chemical attack. On the other hand, the nature of this bonding creates difficulties for the dental ceramist since all ceramic materials are brittle.

Crystalline Ceramics

Regular dental porcelain, being of a glassy nature, is largely non-crystalline, and exhibits only a short range order in atomic arrangement. It is therefore more appropriate to consider this material in the second part of this chapter, "The Nature of Glasses".

The only true crystalline ceramic used at present in restorative dentistry is Alumina (Al_2O_3) which is the hardest and probably the strongest oxide known. The hardness and strength of alumina makes it difficult to cleave because of the "interlocking" nature of the structure. *Binns* (1970) considers that when a plane intersects a crystal, the force holding the two halves of the crystal together depends upon the number of chemical bonds cut and the strength of the individual bonds. The number of bonds is dependent upon the packing of the solid and is given by the number of gram-atoms per unit volume. The bond strength is less easy to assess, but probably the most important feature is the extent to which bonding is covalent. Ionic potential is defined as charge/ionic radius and *Pauling* (1945) has reported values. The greater the ionic potential of a cation the greater its polarizing power on the anion. According to *Fajans* (*Weyl* and *Marboe,* 1962) the more the anion is polarized by the cation the greater is the degree of covalency of the bond. Thus the degree of covalency, and hence the bond strength, increases with the valency. In the series of oxides Na_2O, MgO, Al_2O_3, SiO_2, where the ionic potential of the cation increases, the bonding becomes increasingly covalent. In the case of Na_2O the bonding is almost completely ionic, whereas SiO_2 would have about 50 percent covalent bonding. If the number of gram-atoms is multiplied by the valency of the metal, a quantity is obtained which, for some of the harder materials, compares reasonably well with the hardness. This is a simplified explanation which applies only to perfect single crystals; in practice, the conclusions are modified

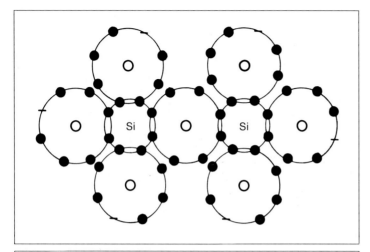

Fig. 1-1a Diagram of a silicate unit with each SiO tetrahedra sharing an oxygen atom.

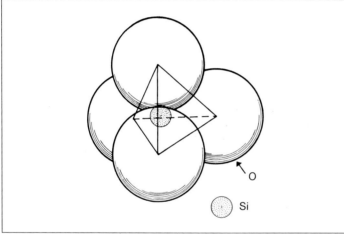

Fig. 1-1b Three dimensional drawing of a silicate unit in which the silicon atom Si is surrounded by four oxygen atoms.

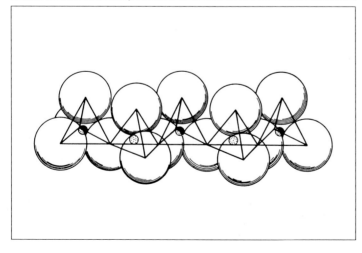

Fig. 1-1c Three dimensional drawing of linked silicate units which form the continuous network in glass.

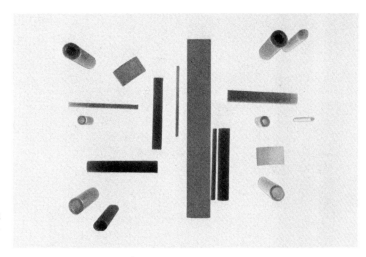

Fig. 1-2 Sintered high alumina profiles used in restorative dentistry.

by dislocations, slip, grain boundary effects, and flaws.

Extraction of Alumina

Alumina is the oxide of aluminium (Al_2O_3), commonly extracted from the mineral bauxite, which is mainly a hydrated aluminium oxide. According to normal practice, the ore is crushed and ground to -10 mesh and is digested in a concentrated solution of caustic soda. The aluminium-bearing liquor recovered from this process is clarified, and the alumina is precipitated in the form of alumina trihydrate crystals which are then washed and dried without removal of the chemically combined water. The alumina trihydrate is converted to alumina by calcination, usually in a rotary kiln at a temperature of 600 °C which drives off the chemically combined water in the hydrate to form gamma-alumina. Further calcination at 1250 °C converts it to alpha-alumina (gamma-alumina is predominently required by American metal producers while European users mainly require the alpha-form). For ceramic applications the alpha-form is employed and is generally ball milled and commercially supplied as a fine powder, usually below 10 to 20 microns in size.

Fabrication of Alumina Components

Sintered alumina is used in restorative dentistry in the form of prefabricated profiles or reinforcements for the construction of crowns, bridges, or individual pontics (*McLean* and *Hughes,* 1965).

These reinforcements are made by mixing the fine calcined alumina powder with a binder such as methyl cellulose and a release agent. The plastic alumina mass is then extruded through tungsten carbide nozzles to the desired shape or form; for dental purposes rods, tubes or sheets are most commonly used (Fig. 1-2).

The moulded profiles are then placed on refractory trays and fired in a standard industrial tunnel kiln. Very slow oven drying is used to prevent warping and the alumina is finally sintered or recrystallised at temperatures of up to 1650 °C. The resulting product is a hard, impermeable ceramic of very high strength and chemical resistance.

Sintering of Alumina

Many theories exist as to the exact processes which occur during the firing cycle of alumina, although none are entirely certain; the terms

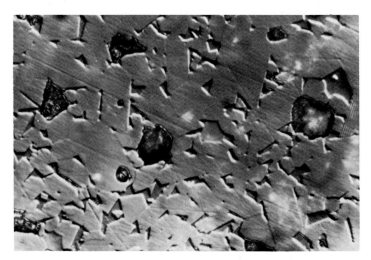

Fig. 1-3 Photomicrograph showing the surface of sintered alumina (95 percent Al$_2$O$_3$). Relief polished. *Normaski* interference contrast. Mag × 850. Courtesy of *D. B. Binns*. British Ceramic Research Association.

sintered, fused and recrystallised are widely used to describe the alumina end-product.

Burke (1958) defined the term "recrystallisation" as changes in microstructure that occur in crystalline or largely crystalline bodies when atoms move to positions of greater stability. By contrast metallurgists use the term recrystallisation in a much more restricted sense: the nucleation and subsequent growth of a new generation of strain-free grains into the deformed matrix of a cold-worked material.

It appears that during the firing of alumina, the following steps occur. Firstly, a welding occurs at points of contact between adjacent oxide particles, giving rise to a lensing effect as normally occurs in sintering processes, i.e. partial fusion. Migration of atoms then leads to growth of the lens areas, movement of grain boundaries and reduction in porosity. During sintering, the shift in grain boundaries results in the formation of a closely interlocking crystalline structure of considerable strength (Fig. 1-3). This improved packing of the oxide particles results in shrinkage of the ceramic body and compensatory mould design is required similar to the oversize tooth moulds used in a tooth factory.

The driving force for the shrinkage in alumina ceramics is surface tension. The surface tension of free surfaces (pores etc.) in a porous ceramic body will always try to make the piece shrink to reduce surface energy. It has been suggested by *Nabarro* (1948) and *Herring* (1950) that the lattice vacancies formed at the surface of a pore can be discharged at grain boundaries as well as at the free surface of the piece, and this might explain the relative independence of sintering rates upon specimen size. Sintered alumina will exhibit this phenomenon and it can be shown that pores near the grain boundaries have disappeared, whereas pores near the centre of the grains remain (Fig. 1-4). The latter pores account for the opacity of alumina where only 2 to 10 percent light transmission is obtainable on 1 mm thick discs (*McLean,* 1966). This opacity will therefore make alumina suitable for use only in the anchorage areas of artificial teeth or crowns.

Translucent Alumina

More recently methods of firing high purity aluminas containing up to 0.2 percent MgO have been devised in which a spinel is formed at the

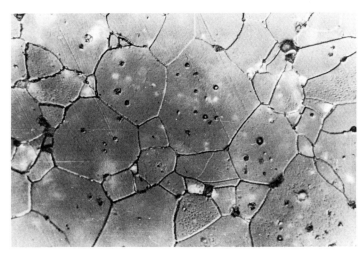

Fig. 1-4 Photomicrograph of pores trapped in the centre of sintered alumina crystals (99.5 percent Al_2O_3). Thermal etch. *Normaski* interference contrast. Mag $\times$ 775. Courtesy of *D. B. Binns*. British Ceramic Research Association.

grain boundaries, slowing down grain growth and allowing the diffusion of porosity along grain boundaries. These aluminas (G.E.C. Lucalox) are probably fired in hydrogen or oxygen atmosphere at high temperature (1800 °C) which increases rate of diffusion of porosity. The resultant materials are almost pore-free which in turn produces a highly translucent body, through which it is possible to read newsprint. It is conceivable that these materials might have possibilities in a veneer crown technique where the alumina is used as the main reinforcing shell.

Effect of Debasing Alumina

The function of a debasing or fluxing agent, added to high purity alumina, is to lower the sintering temperature. It may do this either by forming a liquid phase, or by going into solid solution in the alumina lattice and increasing the diffusion rate.

Debasing agents must be selected so that they do not appreciably affect the mechanical properties of the fired specimens; for example, by causing excessive grain growth which weakens the ceramic body.

A wide range of compositions has been used in the past, but the chief oxides used are CaO, MgO, SiO_2, TiO_2, MnO_2. The function of the first three is almost entirely that of forming a glass phase to bond the structure together. The last two, although also taking part in glass formation, are generally added to increase atomic diffusion in the alumina itself. The proportions of the different oxides used has varied over quite a wide range, but it is probably most common for the SiO_2 content to be at least half of the added oxide content and for the CaO content to be larger than that of MgO. Useful ways of adding these oxides are as wollastonite (Ca Si O_3) and talc ($Mg_3Si_4O_{10}(OH)_2$).

A high purity alumina of 97 to 99 percent requires a firing temperature of 1600 °C to 1650 °C, for a mixture which has been debased to 85 percent purity of alumina, the balance being at least half SiO_2; sintering occurs at 1500 °C, whilst a mixture comprising 75 percent alumina may be fired at 1300 °C to 1350 °C. This enables cheaper and simpler furnaces to be used for the firing process. A typical composition for an 85 percent alumina refractory mixture would be as follows:

		Weight percent
Alumina	Al_2O_3	87.70
Silica	SiO_2	7.10
Calcium Oxide	CaO	1.61
Magnesium Oxide	MgO	1.32
Chromium Sesquioxide	Cr_2O_3	1.13
Ferric Oxide	Fe_2O_3	0.25
Titanium Dioxide	TiO_2	0.13
Sodium Oxide	Na_2O	0.40
Potassium Oxide	K_2O	0.36

Colouring Alumina

The colour of sintered alumina is white or cream. However, in order to use this material in restorative dentistry, a range of suitable background colours is necessary when enamel veneers are applied. Dental alumina is therefore coloured with high temperature resistant pigments. These pigments may consist of up to 2 percent of manganese-alumina pink, vanadium-zircon blue, or praesodymium-zircon yellow (*McLean,* 1966).

Dental Alumina

Composition. Alumina ceramics used in dentistry are of high purity and generally consist of at least 95 percent Al_2O_3. Minor quantities of debasing agents are added to aid sintering, and pigments of the type just mentioned are added to produce a natural dentine colour. Sintered alumina ceramics of high purity are conveniently referred to as high alumina.

Physical Properties

The physical properties and characteristics of a dental high alumina are illustrated in Table 1-1. These high purity aluminas have excellent resistance to abrasion and chemical attack and are suitable for use up to a working temperature of 1500 °C. The significance of this is that at normal firing temperatures used in dental furnaces (900 °C to 1150 °C) the alumina is completely stable and will not creep or flow. For purposes of comparison the mechanical properties of dental porcelain have been included in Table 1-1 and it may be seen that high alumina is markedly stronger in all essential properties. The high tensile strength is perhaps of greatest significance since tensile failure of dental ceramics is the commonest cause of fracture.

Although the strength of high alumina is quite remarkable for a ceramic material, it still does not match its theoretical strength.

The prime causes of weakening in crystalline ceramics has been well summarized by *Gilman* (1967).

1. Local separation, or voids, may occur between crystals, with the result that atoms can wander through the spaces, gases can permeate the material, and the crystals can slide past one another.
2. Weakness at boundaries may be caused if one crystal is out of line or twisted with respect to its neighbour; the bonds between them may be stretched or otherwise distorted.
3. Ions with the same charge (positive or negative) may be in juxtaposition in the crystal lattice; the consequent electrostatic repulsion may produce stress in that region of the material and generate cracks.

It is clear that all high strength ceramics suffer more from crystal boundary defects than metals, and current research is concentrating on eliminating internal boundaries or minimising their effects.

The use of ceramics in fixed bridgework is limited by these inherent physical defects and in addition shrinkage control still remains one of the main problems with crystalline ceramics. The versatility of metals both in casting accuracy and the nature of the metallic bond leaves them unrivalled in restorative dentistry.

Table 1-1 Physical Properties and Characteristics of a Dental High Alumina and Dental Porcelain

	High Alumina		Dental Porcelain
Tensile Strength	138 N/mm²	(20,000 p.s.i.)	34.4 N/mm²
			(5,000 p.s.i.)
Compressive Strength	2,180 N/mm²	(316,000 p.s.i.)	344 N/mm²
			(50,000 p.s.i.)
Modulus of Rupture	379 N/mm²	(55,000 p.s.i.)	68.9 N/mm²
			(10,000 p.s.i.)
Hardness Moh Scale	9		
Coefficient of Linear Expansion			
Parts/million/°C			
20°C− 400°C	6.6		
20°C− 600°C	7.2		
20°C−1,000°C	8.2		
Porosity Fuchsine dye penetration	Nil		
Water absorption	Nil		
Specific gravity	3.85		
Working temperature maximum °C	1,500		
Colour	Ivory		

The Nature of Glasses

Dental porcelains are, in part, glassy materials and in order to understand their formulation, a knowledge of glass formation is essential.

Glasses may be regarded as supercooled liquids or as non-crystalline solids. This lack of crystallinity distinguishes them from other solids, and their atomic structures and resultant properties depend, not only on composition, but also on thermal history. The glass-maker selects complex or impure solutions in order to modify the physical properties of the glass both in the molten and solid form. These properties would include viscosity, melting temperature, chemical durability, thermal expansion and resistance to devitrification. Frictional forces inhibiting the formation of new molecular configurations in the liquid glass should also be as high as possible. This can be achieved by rapid cooling or preferably, for dental purposes, by using materials that produce high viscosity in the melt, e.g. Aluminium oxide Al_2O_3.

Glass Formation

The principal anion present in all glasses is O_2^- ion which forms very stable bonds with small multivalent cations such as silicon, boron, germanium, or phosphorous, giving rise to structural units, such as the SiO_4 tetrahedra illustrated in Fig. 1-1, which form a random network in glass. These ions are thus termed **glass formers.**

Zachariasen (1932) examined the characteristics of these glass-forming oxides and proposed his random network theory of glass structure. He considered that the interatomic forces in glasses and crystals must be essentially similar and that the atoms in glass oscillate about definite equilibrium positions. He deduced that the atoms must be linked in the form of a three-dimensional network in glass as in crystals, and because glasses do not give a sharp X-ray diffraction spectra they could not be periodic (in an ordered arrangement). *Zachariasen* considered that although the units of structure in the glass, (i.e. SiO_4 tetrahedra) and in the crys-

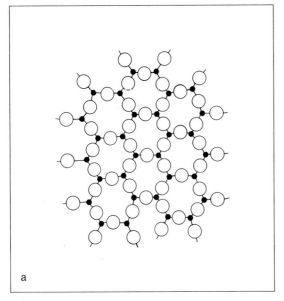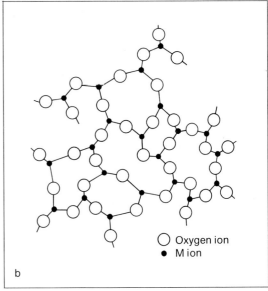

a   b

Oxygen ion
M ion

Fig. 1-5a and b   Two-dimensional representation of an oxide M_2O_3 in (a) the crystalline form (b) the glass form. Adapted from *McMillan, P. W.* Glass-Ceramics (1964) Academic Press.

tals are practically identical, in the crystal these structural units are built up to give a regular lattice. By contrast, in the glass there is sufficient distortion of bond angles to permit the structural units to be arranged in a random network (Fig. 1-5). *Zachariasen* proposed certain conditions for glass formation:

1. An oxygen atom must not be linked to more than two M atoms.
2. The number of oxygen atoms surrounding M must be small.
3. These oxygen polyhedra must share corners only and not edges or faces.

For dental purposes, only two glass-forming oxides are used – silicon and boron oxide – and they form the principal network around which a dental glass can be built. Alumina, under certain circumstances, may be regarded as a glass-forming oxide when in combination with other oxides as will be explained.

Formulation of Dental Porcelain

Dental porcelains use the basic silicon-oxygen network as the glass-forming matrix but additional properties, such as low-fusing temperature, high viscosity, and resistance to devitrification, are built in by the addition of other oxides to the glass-forming lattice SiO_4. These oxides generally consist of Potassium, Sodium, Calcium, Aluminium and Boric oxides.

The Role of Fluxes

Potassium, Sodium and Calcium oxide are used as glass modifiers, and act as fluxes by interrupting the integrity of the SiO_4 network. The purpose of a flux is principally to lower the softening temperature of a glass by reducing the amount of cross-linking between the oxygen and glass-forming elements, e.g. silicon. For example, if soda (Na_2O) is introduced into

30

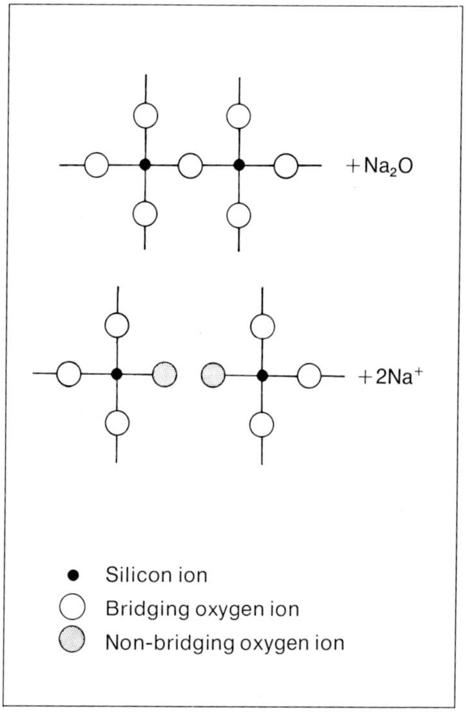

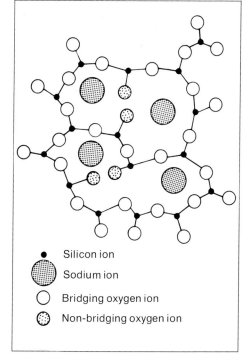

Fig. 1-6 Reaction between sodium oxide and silica tetrahedra. The sodium oxide contributes one of the non-bridging oxygen ions which interrupt the continuity of the silica network. (For simplicity, only a two-dimensional representation of the SiO_4 groups is given; in the actual glass structure these groups take the form of tetrahedra as illustrated in Fig. 1-1). Adapted from *McMillan, P. W.* Glass-Ceramics (1964) Academic Press.

Fig. 1-7 Two-dimensional representation of the structure of sodium silicate glass. (The structure is shown in a simplified form since only three of the four oxygen ions surrounding each silicon ion are depicted.) Adapted from *McMillan, P. W.* Glass-Ceramics (1964) Academic Press.

a silicate melt to produce sodium silicate glasses, structural changes occur as in Fig. 1-6. Instead of the bridging oxygen ions which formed the link between the two SiO_4 tetrahedra, there are now two non-bridging oxygens, one of which has been contributed by the sodium oxide. A gap is therefore produced in the SiO_4 network and the sodium ions are accommodated in the interstices or holes in the random network structure as shown in Fig. 1-7. The greater the number of Na^+ ions added, the more $Si-O-Si$ bridges are broken. The O:Si ratio in a glass is of the greatest importance and will affect both the viscosity of the glass and its thermal expansion. For example, in dental porcelain used for bonding to metal, it is usual practice to increase the soda content in order to raise the thermal expansion of the porcelain near to that of the gold alloys. Other alkali metal oxides, such as lithium or potassium oxides, take part in the glass structure in a similar manner. Lithium ions will be accommodated in smaller structural interstices and the sodium ions and the potassium ions in larger ones. Magnesium, calcium and barium oxides may also act as modifying oxides.

The use of these alkali metal oxides must be very carefully controlled to preserve the original glass-forming network, otherwise problems of devitrification may occur. Potassium, sodium or calcium oxides are introduced into a glass melt via their respective carbonates which revert to oxides on heating.

Intermediate Oxides

The addition of glass modifiers or fluxes to the basic glass-forming network SiO_4 in dental porcelain will not only lower the softening point but also decreases the viscosity. Dental porcelains require a high resistance to slump or pyroplastic flow and it is therefore necessary to produce glasses with a high viscosity as well as low firing temperatures. This can be done by using intermediate oxides which although not usually capable of forming a glass can take part in the glass network.

The hardness and viscosity of a glass can be increased by the use of an intermediate oxide such as aluminium oxide (Al_2O_3). The role of Al_2O_3 in glass formation is complicated. It cannot be considered as a true glass former by itself because the dimensions of the ion excludes the possibility of AlO_3 triangles being formed and the O:Al ratio precludes the formation of AlO_4 tetrahedra. In crystals, the aluminium ion can be four or six coordinated with oxygen giving rise to tetrahedral AlO_4 or octahedral AlO_6 groups. The tetrahedral groups can replace SiO_4 tetrahedra in silicate lattices to give the arrangement shown in Fig. 1-8. Since each aluminium ion has a charge of $+3$ as compared with a charge of $+4$ for each silicon ion, an additional unit positive charge must be present to ensure electroneutrality. When metallic oxides, such as sodium oxide, are present, one alkali metal ion per AlO_4 tetrahedron would satisfy this requirement and the alkali metal ions could be accommodated in the interstices between tetrahedral groups. In this way, as each Al^{3+} ion replaces a Si^{4+} ion in the network, one Na^+ ion is taken in to preserve neutrality. This type of structural arrangement is found for many aluminosilicates such as felspars and zeolites, where the crystals are built up of linked SiO_4 and AlO_4 groups (*McMillan,* 1964). Large univalent or divalent cations are present in these structures to the extent of one alkali ion or "half" an alkaline earth ion per AlO_4 tetrahedron. A similar situation probably exists in a glass network where the electroneutrality requirement imposes the condition that each gram-molecule of aluminium oxide present in the glass requires the presence also of one gram-molecule of an alkali oxide or alkaline earth oxide. This rule is obeyed for many types of aluminosilicate glass (*McMillan,* 1964).

In the case of the aluminous porcelains, the enamel veneers are made from glasses containing a high combined alumina content of up to 20 percent or by further addition of alu-

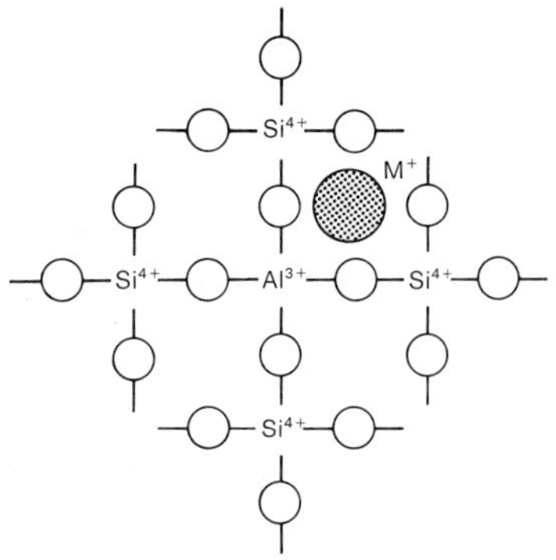

Fig. 1-8 Aluminium in a silicate network. (The structure is shown in a simplified form; the true structure is three-dimensional, the AlO$_4$ and SiO$_4$ groups having tetrahedral configurations.) The alkali metal ion (M$^+$) such as sodium maintains electroneutrality. Adapted from *McMillan, P. W.* Glass Ceramics (1964) Academic Press.

minium oxide to a felspar frit. Aluminium oxide is usually added to the melt in the form of its hydroxide.

Boric Oxide Fluxes

Boric oxide (B$_2$O$_3$) is also a powerful flux but at the same time can act as a glass former. In vitreous B$_2$O$_3$ the boron, being three co-ordinated, forms a continuous three-dimensional network of BO$_3$ triangles. Because the bonds extend in only three directions, as opposed to four in SiO$_4$, the stability of the B$_2$O$_3$ structure is weaker, i.e. lower softening point, lower viscosity and higher expansion. If B$_2$O$_3$ is added to a glass it acts as a flux and the structure is a three-dimensional continuous network of SiO$_4$ tetrahedra and BO$_3$ triangles. The cation:O ratio changes affect B$_2$O$_3$ glasses in a different way from silica glasses. The addition of extra oxygen atoms can change the boron co-ordination from three to four, thus forming strong BO$_4$ tetrahedra and producing a more stable glass. This explains the "Boron Anomaly" where at ratios of about 12 percent B$_2$O$_3$ the physical properties of the glass change quite markedly. Initial additions of B$_2$O$_3$ to alkali-silicate glasses, such as

dental porcelain, form BO$_4$ tetrahedra giving low expansion and good chemical resistance. Above the critical B$_2$O$_3$ value of 12 percent, no more BO$_4$ tetrahedra are formed and the less stable form BO$_3$ takes over. Boric oxide is therefore used in quantities below the critical 12 percent value and the BO$_4$ network is predominant. A twin lattice is formed with SiO$_4$ in which the BO$_4$ tetrahedra still act as a flux by interrupting the SiO$_4$ network, but at the same time a gross weakening of the glass is not produced by formation of the less stable BO$_3$ triangles.

Chemical Composition of Dental Porcelain

It is now possible to see how a modern aluminosilicate dental glass is formed (Fig. 1-9).
The stability of the glass is highly dependent on the silicon-oxygen lattice and the covalent bonds must not be reduced too much, otherwise problems of hydrolytic stability and devitrification may arise. The average dental porcelain will therefore contain a minimum content of about 60 percent SiO$_2$. The balancing oxides or fluxes are carefully controlled to provide the requisite properties such as resistance to pyroplastic flow (slump), hardness, hydrolytic sta-

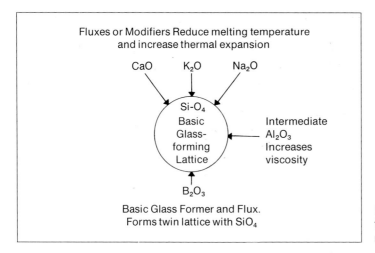

Fluxes or Modifiers Reduce melting temperature and increase thermal expansion

CaO   K$_2$O   Na$_2$O

Si-O$_4$
Basic Glass-forming Lattice

Intermediate
Al$_2$O$_3$
Increases viscosity

B$_2$O$_3$

Basic Glass Former and Flux.
Forms twin lattice with SiO$_4$

Fig. 1-9 Diagram of the formation of a glass used in making medium or low fusion porcelains.

bility, low melting temperature, and resistance to devitrification.

A typical low fusion dental porcelain should really be referred to as dental glass and would have a composition as follows:

Oxide	Weight per cent	
SiO$_2$	69.36	Glass formers
B$_2$O$_3$	7.53	
CaO	1.85	
K$_2$O	8.33	Glass modifiers
Na$_2$O	4.81	
Al$_2$O$_3$	8.11	Intermediate

Such a fluxed glass would have a maturing temperature of 900 °C to 930 °C.

Devitrification and Thermal Expansion

"Vitrification" in ceramic terms is the development of a liquid phase, by reaction or melting which, on cooling, provides the glassy phase. The structure is termed "vitreous".

When too many of the glass forming SiO$_4$ tetrahedra are disrupted in dental porcelain, the glass may crystallise or "devitrify". Devitrification is often associated with high expansion glasses since the usual way of increasing the thermal expansion of a glass is to introduce more alkalis, particularly soda (Na$_2$O). High expansion glasses are used in the metal-ceramic techniques and the increase in sodium and potassium ions can cause too much disruption of the SiO$_4$ tetrahedra. These porcelains are therefore more subject to problems of devitrification than regular porcelain and the manufacturers generally find themselves on the borderline of stable glass formation when manufacturing porcelains for bonding to metal.

Devitrification of high expansion porcelains may be seen when a cloudiness develops in the porcelain and this can be accentuated by repeated firings. Once a porcelain has devitrified, it becomes increasingly difficult to form a glaze surface.

By contrast the regular or aluminous porcelains are much less susceptible to devitrification due to their higher silica to alkali ratio. The aluminous porcelains contain much less soda (Na$_2$O), and their thermal expansions are lower. In addition, their high combined alumina content tends to neutralise the effect of excessive quantities of Na$^+$ ions which, as explained on page 32 are required to preserve electroneutrality in an aluminium silicate network.

Very low thermal expansion porcelains, giving high thermal shock resistance such as the "Vycor" type silica glasses, have never become popular. However, high resistance to thermal shock is a very desirable feature and the ceramic industry in general will continue to take great interest in zero or negative expansion ceramics.

Fritting

The term "frit" is used to describe the final glass product. The raw mineral powders (oxides or carbonates) are mixed together in a refractory crucible and heated to a temperature well above their ultimate maturing temperature when used in the dental laboratory. The oxides melt together to form a molten glass, gases are allowed to escape and the melt is then quenched in water. The red hot glass striking the cold water immediately breaks up into fragments and this is termed the "frit". The process of blending, melting and quenching the glass components is termed "fritting". A similar process is used in making felspathic porcelain. The natural felspar and glass fluxes are mixed together in powder form before the fritting process is commenced.

Alternative Additives to Dental Porcelain

Small quantities of alternative modifying agents can be added to the dental porcelain during fritting. Lithium oxide (Li_2O) may be added as an additional fluxing agent. However, this oxide does tend to induce rather more pyroplastic flow than is often desirable in a dental porcelain. Lithium oxide may also increase the risk of devitrification, since it has a higher field strength than either sodium or potassium and therefore exerts the greatest ordering effect on

surrounding oxygen ions. The conversion to a regular crystalline arrangement will therefore occur more readily in lithium silicates than in potassium or sodium silicates.

Magnesium oxide (MgO) may also be present, but usually in minute quantities. This oxide can replace CaO.

Phosphorous pentoxide (P_2O_5) is sometimes added to induce opalescence, and is also a glass-forming oxide.

A current medium fusion porcelain containing these additives is listed below.

Oxide	Weight per cent
SiO_2	64.2
B_2O_3	2.8
K_2O	8.2
Na_2O	1.9
Al_2O_3	19.0
Li_2O	2.1
MgO	0.5
P_2O_5	0.7

Maturing temperature $1060-1080\,°C$.

Felspathic Porcelain

The principal elements in natural clays are oxygen, silicon and aluminium, forming the compounds known as aluminosilicates. The precursor of common clay is felspar, a mineral found in many parts of the world.

Natural felspars are mixtures of albite $Na_2Al_2Si_6O_{16}$ and orthoclase or microcline $K_2Al_2Si_6O_{16}$ with free crystalline quartz. These felspars are never pure and the ratio of soda (Na_2O) to potash (K_2O) may vary quite considerably. However, for dental purposes, a high potash content felspar is generally selected because of its increased resistance to pyroplastic flow. Potash felspars have an extremely high viscosity and this viscosity decreases only relatively slowly with rising temperature.

When felspar is melted at about 1250 °C to 1300 °C, the alkalis (Na_2O and K_2O) unite with the alumina and silica to form sodium or potassium aluminium silicates. A glassy phase is formed with a free crystalline silica phase.

Felspar has been used to make dental porcelain for a number of decades due to the ease with which it can be fritted and coloured to produce high fusing dental porcelain (1250-1350 °C). For a long time manufacturers used natural felspar mixed with quartz in the proportion of 85 percent felspar to 15 percent quartz as their standard dental porcelain. However, the demand for lower fusion temperatures in dental porcelain and the abandonment of expensive platinum wound furnaces for nickel-chrome muffles produced an increasing interest in fluxed glasses. Felspar was therefore modified by the addition of glass modifiers or glass formers of the fluxing type, such as B_2O_3.

As can be seen from the following chemical analysis of natural felspar most of the elements necessary for glass making are already present in this mineral.

Felspar analysis

Potash Spar

SiO_2	66.80		CaO	0.45
Na_2O	3.01		MgO	0.13
K_2O	10.55		Fe_2O_3	0.30
Al_2O_3	17.58		TiO_2	trace

Loss on ignition 0.99

Soda spar

SiO_2	71.90		CaO	1.14
Na_2O	8.19		MgO	0.02
K_2O	0.64		Fe_2O_3	0.13
Al_2O_3	15.67		TiO_2	0.10

Loss on ignition 1.47

A low or medium fusion dental porcelain or glass can therefore be made by the appropriate addition of balancing oxides. The mixed felspar-glass flux mixture can then be fritted at specific temperatures according to how much felspar is required in solution. The mixture could be fritted until a completely homogeneous glass is formed, i.e. all the felspar constituents are dissolved. This would produce a lower firing temperature porcelain. Alternatively part of the felspar could be left undissolved and remain as discrete particles in the glassy matrix. This probably accounts for the term "dental porcelain" but it is not really accurate since the material contains very little free crystalline phase with the possible exception of crystalline quartz.

The glasses used in the manufacture of Aluminous Porcelain described in Monograph II are sometimes made from the raw oxides as outlined in the previous section on the formulation of dental porcelain. This results in much closer batch control with less risk of devitrification problems arising.

Nepheline Syenite

The use of nepheline syenite has been tried as a replacement for felspar (*Orlowski, 1944*). It exhibits less variation in composition than natural felspar and is an igneous rock, a syenite, somewhat resembling granite in texture, hardness, and general appearance. The essential mineral of this syenite is nepheline, and other principal minerals are potash felspar, and soda felspar. There is little or no free quartz; the molar composition of a Canadian nepheline syenite is:

Na_2O	0.75
K_2O	0.25
Al_2O_3	1.1
SiO_2	4.5

Nepheline syenite has never become popular for making dental porcelain and probably the major criticism levelled against it has been its greater pyroplasticity when compared with felspar.

Colouring and Opacifying Dental Porcelain

The basic dental porcelain frit will vary in colour depending upon whether the frit is a single phase or multi-phase glass (mixture of glasses).

In general, it may be stated that if the porcelain is manufactured as a single phase glass, in which all the oxide constituents are completely taken into solution, the resultant product should be as transparent as a good window glass. As described previously, in the case of fluxed felspathic porcelains some manufacturers may limit the degree of fusion and pyrochemical reaction in the frit to the extent that a proportion of the felspar remains undissolved in the glass flux. These felspar grains remain discreetly in the glass matrix, and because of the difference in refractive indices the final glass frit may appear opalescent or assume a grey-blue translucency similar to natural incisal enamel.

A further technique of developing translucent grey or opalescent characteristics is to use a mixture of two single phase glass frits of slightly different refractive indices. Such glasses can give translucencies similar to the mixed felspar porcelains.

Whatever the method of preparation of the glass used in dental porcelain the greatest colour problem encountered is the slightly greenish hue exhibited by all glasses. This can be seen when viewing plate glass along its edge.

In order to dampen down this effect and to produce life-like dentine and enamel colours the basic dental porcelain frit must be coloured.

Colour Pigments

The dental porcelain frit is usually coloured by the addition of a concentrated colour frit. These coloured glasses are prepared by fritting high temperature resistant pigments, generally metallic oxides, into the basic glass used in porcelain manufacture. The glass will then be highly colour saturated and when ground to a fine powder can be used to modify the uncoloured porcelain powder. Only small amounts of modifying colour frit are used and in addition opacifying agents would be added at the same time.

The colour pigments used in dental porcelain may consist of the following:

Pink – Chromium-tin or chrome-alumina. These pigments are stable up to a firing temperature of 1350 °C and are particularly useful in eliminating the greenish hue in the glass and giving a warm tone to the porcelain.

Yellow – Indium or praesodymium (lemon) are probably the most stable pigments for producing an ivory shade. Vanadium-zirconium or Tin oxide plus chromium can be used but are not so stable.

Blue – Cobalt salts are used to produce this colour and are particularly useful for producing some of the enamel shades.

Green – Chromium oxide is the main pigment for producing a greenish colour but it should be avoided in dental porcelain wherever possible since green is the characteristic colour of glass. In addition the main complaint from technicians is that some porcelains assume a greenish hue after baking and the inherent greeness of the basic dental porcelain can be accentuated by over-firing (over-vitrification).

Grey – Iron oxide (black) or Platinum grey are useful pigments for producing enamels or for addition to the greyer section of the dentine colours. Incorporation of grey colours can also give an effect ot translucency.

Opacifying Agents

The addition of concentrated colour frits to dental porcelain is insufficient to produce a life-like tooth effect since the translucency of the porcelain is too high. In particular the dentine colours require greater opacity if they are to simulate natural dentine overlaid by enamel. The addition of opacifying agents is therefore a delicate procedure, particularly when determining shades for the metal-ceramic materials.

An opacifying agent generally consists of a metal oxide ground to a very fine particle size (<5 μm) to prevent a speckled appearance in the porcelain.

Common oxides used are:

Cerium oxide
Titanium oxide
Zirconium oxide

Zirconium oxide is the most popular opacifying agent and is usually added with the concentrated colour frit to the uncoloured porcelain during final preparation.

The actual amounts used are often determined initially by trial and error until a thin fired porcelain blank assumes just the right degree of translucency and the colour saturation is correctly balanced.

In the case of the enamel porcelain very little opacifyer is used and the manufacturer will rely more on the addition of small quantities of colour frit. In addition the enamel porcelain may already have natural enamel characteristics derived from the use of glass mixtures. It will be seen that an opacifying agent behaves in the same way and relies on the use of differences in refractive indices to produce the degree of translucency required.

Various wave lengths of visible light are scattered differently by opacifying particles. This effect depends upon the size of the particles and also upon their volume distribution in the glass matrix. The difference in refractive indices between the glass and the opacifier also play an important role. The Dentists' Supply Company have used opacifying agents of a size range close to the magnitude of the wave-length of (visible) light and it is claimed that particles between the size of 0.4 to 0.8 μm produce a blue tinge in reflected light but turn yellowish-red in transmitted light, thus more closely resembling the natural tooth. During fritting these opacifiers can be made to crystallise out, more particularly if cooling is stopped temporarily on existing seeds (*Abbey*, 1962). SiO_2, Al_2O_3, ZrO_2, or their compounds aluminium or zirconium silicates have been used in these experiments.

Stains and Colour Modifiers

The stains and colour modifiers supplied in a kit of dental porcelain are made in the same way as the concentrated colour frits used for colouring basic dental porcelain frits. A stain is more concentrated than a colour modifier, the latter are used to obtain gingival effects or to high-light body colours, whereas the former are more generally used as surface colourants or to provide enamel check lines, de-calcification spots, etc., in the body of a porcelain jacket crown. Stains can be supplied as pure metal oxides but are sometimes made from lower fusion point glasses so that they can be applied at temperatures below the maturing temperature of the enamel and dentine porcelains. Colour modifiers are better used at the same temperature as the dental porcelain.

Fluorescence

The significance of fluorescence in porcelain restorations will be discussed in Monograph III under principles of colour. The production of fluorescence in dental porcelain has assumed greater prominence in recent years due to the use of lamps which emit the blue end of the spectrum in addition to some ultra-violet radiation. These lamps, when used in discotheques or dance halls, cause human teeth to fluoresce a bluish-white colour.

The manufacturers of dental porcelain have made great strides in duplicating this type of fluorescence, and some of the modern dental porcelain will fluoresce bluish-white under ultra-violet radiation.

The usual procedure for producing this fluorescence is by the addition of the uranium salt, sodium di-uranate. This salt produces a strong greenish-yellow colour and when small additions of cerium oxide are made, a bluish-white fluorescence can be achieved very similar to a human tooth.

Samarium, a rare earth (5 parts per million) or spinels (Magnesia alumina compounds) can be used but are not so effective as the powerful uranium salt. It should be noted that uranium is highly radio-active and has recently been banned from use in dental procelain. New non-radioactive porcelains are now becoming available containing rare earth oxides.

Glazes and Add-on Porcelain

One purpose of an industrial glaze is to seal the open pores in the surface of a fired porcelain. Dental glazes consist of uncoloured glass powders which can be applied to the surface of a fired crown to produce a glossy surface. A glaze should normally mature at a temperature below that of the restoration and the thermal expansion of the glaze should be fractionally lower than the ceramic body to which it is applied. In this way the glaze surface is placed under compression, and crazing or peeling of the surface is avoided.

It is important to recognize that a glazing porcelain must never be applied directly to a glazed restoration. The surface must be roughened slightly to prevent glaze peeling.

In the author's opinion porcelain crowns are better made without the use of glazes, since a modern felspathic or single-phase glass can be lightly ground and self-glazed far more satisfactorily. Glazes are difficult to apply evenly and are often used to seal off a poorly baked restoration. In addition detailed surface characterisation is almost impossible to obtain when separate glazes are used since they tend either to produce too high a gloss or a rough surface and do not reproduce the satin-like finish of human enamel.

The so called Add-on-Porcelains are of definite use and are generally made from similar materials to the glaze porcelain except for the addition of opacifiers and colouring pigments. An Add-on-Porcelain can be made from the same frit as used for the manufacture of regular porcelain and the glazing temperature can then be reduced by finer grinding of the powder, the latter procedure always making a porcelain powder more re-active. Add-on-Porcelains should be used sparingly for simple corrections to tooth contour or contact points.

Classification of Dental Porcelains

The standard classification of dental porcelain is only used for convenience and divides them into three temperature ranges, British Standard 5612.

Temperature	Maturing
High	1,200-1,400 °C
Medium	1,050-1,700 °C
Low	800-1,050 °C

It will be seen from this section on the "Nature of Glasses" that all dental porcelains are based upon the silicon-oxygen glass forming network. In the case of the high temperature maturing porcelain the glass network is formed by using natural felspar reinforced or stiffened by up to 15 percent free quartz.

The glass forming elements in natural felspar can be modified by the addition of glass fluxes containing boric oxide (B_2O_3) or lithium oxide (Li_2O) to produce medium or low temperature maturing porcelain. Alternatively, a completely synthetic low temperature maturing glass can be manufactured by the combination of the raw oxides as in industrial glass manufacture.

All these porcelains may then be modified by the introduction of pigments, crystalline inclusions or opacifying agents to produce the final dental product.

Porcelains Used in Tooth Manufacture

Porcelain teeth are generally made from felspathic glasses and are in the high temperature maturing range. Some manufacturers still use a high potash content felspar mixed with approximately 15 percent quartz, and suitable opacifiers and pigments. However, more sophisticated techniques have been developed both in the use of fluxed felspathic glasses and the dispersion of fluorescent and crystalline material to achieve natural enamel effects. This has resulted in a very high standard of aesthetics in the modern vacuum fired porcelain denture tooth.

Other materials such as the pure silica glass "Vycor", have been used in proportions of about 53 to 58 percent, the balance being a felspar flux, (Lee and Dietz, 1948). These teeth have a very low thermal expansion and can be ground without fracturing due to thermal shock. However, "Vycor" glass teeth have never become very popular, probably due to their great hardness and the fact that regular ceramic glazes and stains cannot be applied to them.

Condensation of Dental Porcelain

Volume Porosity of Powders

The shrinkage of dental porcelain, sintered to high densities, is largely controlled by the porosity of the powder bed after condensation and shaping of the tooth form.

The voids between the particles in dental porcelain are determined not only by the condensation technique but also by the original packing density of the powder.

The science of particle packing can be defined as the selection of proper sizes and proportions of particulate material, so that larger voids are filled with smaller particles, and so on. No plastic deformation of the particles occurs, and it is possible to pour the material out of a container after packing (McGeary, 1961).

In order to obtain high densities in an irregular particle system, it is usual to obtain a threefold difference between grain sizes (Binns, 1970). This type of system is known as gap-grading in which at least three sizes of powder are used. Such a powder would only be suitable for vacuum firing, and in general these powders are more easily compacted than the coarser air-fired powders due to the lack of fine particles in the latter (McLean, 1966). In addition the shape of the particle will also have an effect on packing density. Rounded particles (Fig. 1-10), produced by dry grinding will pack better than a wet ground powder (Fig. 1-11). The angular grains of the latter tend to cause interferences and will not settle to position so easily.

The volume porosity of regular air or vacuum firing powders is in the region of 40 to 49 percent. Table 1-2. Even if techniques were used to hydraulically compress dental porcelain powders onto a platinum matrix, the porosity of high pressure compacts would still be in the region of 30 per cent. Table 1-2.

At the present time, the densest vacuum firing powders reveal a volume porosity of around 40 per cent (McLean and Hughes, 1965) and with our current powder technology this probably represents the limit achievable with irregular shaped particles.

The volume shrinkage of dental porcelain powders when sintered to full maturity is directly related to the volume porosity of the condensed powder bed. Vacuum firing powders generally have less shrinkage than the coarser air-firing powders.

Table 1-2 Porosity of Porcelain when Compacted at Low and High Pressures

Type of Porcelain		Volume Porosity of Compacts per cent		
		Low Pressure Wet	High Pressure Dry 14.5 ton/in² (224 N/mm²)	Specific Surface (cm²/gm)
Low fusion air-firing	930 °C	41.9	30.1	3,410
Medium fusion air-firing	1,150 °C	49.8	34.6	2,059
Medium fusion	1,130 °C	41.0	31.0	3,889
Low Pressure – wet vibration in a mould		High Pressure – hydraulically pressed in steel die		

(From *McLean* and *Hughes,* Brit. Dent. J., [1965] 119,251)

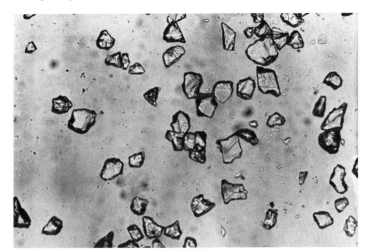

Fig. 1-10 Rounded angles on dental porcelain grains produced by dry grinding techniques.

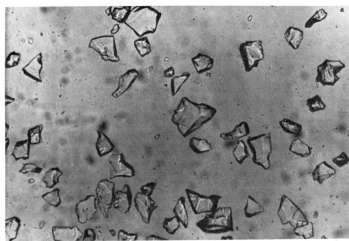

Fig. 1-11 Sharp angles on dental porcelain grains produced by wet grinding techniques.

Condensation

Porcelain powder is built to shape using a liquid binder to hold the particles together. The process of packing the particles together and of removing the liquid binder is known as condensation.

Distilled water is the most common and probably the most useful liquid binder to use, but additions of glycerine, propylene glycol or alcohol have been tried by some manufacturers. Starch can also be incorporated in the powder but is generally confined to use in the coarser air-fired powders.

The usual procedure of shaping dental porcelain is to mix the dry porcelain powder with distilled water to a thick and creamy consistency and then apply it to the platinum matrix using either brushes or metal instruments.

Methods of condensing dental porcelain powder are numerous, confusing and often misinterpreted. Terms such as gravitation, spatulation, whipping, vibration, are used to describe these procedures.

Surface Tension

It is more important for the ceramist to appreciate the factors involved in achieving high densities in a powder bed and once these factors are recognised, the condensing of dental porcelain can be better appreciated. The main driving force involved in condensing dental porcelain, is surface tension. The withdrawal of water from the porcelain powder will always cause the powder particles to pack more closely. Surface tension will therefore be working for the ceramist, and he must use this surface tension effect to the best advantage. A simple analogy can be made in comparing the way the bristles of a fine paint brush will bind tightly together once the brush is moistened. The bristles will pack even more closely if the brush is touched with a paper tissue and more water is withdrawn. Once the brush dries out, the bristles will spring apart

again and the surface tension effect created by the water disappears. The ceramist can only use surface tension effects to advantage if the porcelain is always kept moist during build-up. High room temperatures and dry atmospheres are to be avoided since porcelain powder can rapidly dry out and further placement of even wet porcelain powder on a dry surface will never allow the undersurface to be condensed properly. This is due to air spaces being created in the powder bed which will resist the further ingress of water. Crowns which are baked from such a build-up will inevitably be more subject to the entrapment of large air bubbles and areas of blotchy opacity may appear.

The so-called "Brush Application Method" in which dry powder is sprinkled over the wet porcelain surface is also not recommended since the control of this powder can be very difficult and time consuming. This will enhance the risk of the porcelain drying out.

The Wet Brush Technique

The final density of a porcelain crown build-up is also dependent upon the packing density of the porcelain powder, and, as explained on page 40 the vacuum-firing powders are generally more dense due to the incorporation of a larger number of very fine particles. However, whatever the nature of the particle size distribution the ceramist must decide what method of application will utilize surface tension effects to the best advantage. A "wet technique" must be the most logical approach and the consistency of the porcelain mix has a marked effect on the handling properties of porcelain. The mix should be creamy and capable of being transferred in small increments to the platinum matrix with an instrument or brush, so that the porcelain does not drip off the end of the instrument. The mix should not be over-stirred, otherwise incorporation of large air bubbles is more likely to occur. Finally the mix must not

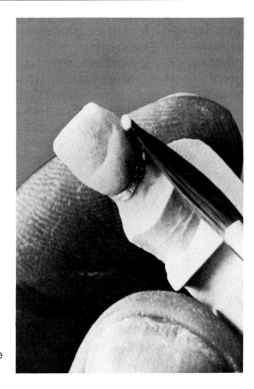

Fig. 1-12 Application of porcelain slurry with a fine sable brush.

dry out rapidly and temperature and humidity control are essential in maintaining the water content of the mix.

The instruments for applying the porcelain can be quite varied. Metal instruments, such as spatulas or the *Le Cron* carver can be used but the author favours the use of high quality sable hair brushes. It is possible to transfer small increments of wet porcelain to the platinum matrix very rapidly using the fine point of a sable brush (Fig. 1-12). It is important to note that this method, which might be called "The Brush-additive Technique" should not be confused with the so-called "Brush Application Method" using dry powder.

The condensation of porcelain can be started by using the brush to flow the wet porcelain around the matrix. A gentle pushing or tapping motion will agitate the porcelain particles into position and the brush will keep this porcelain moist. If water is now withdrawn with a paper tissue, surface tension will automatically cause the particles to settle closer together. When the motions are repeated a crown can be built up rapidly and it will be found that vibration of the porcelain can be kept to the minimum. Light tapping of the model base on the bench, or vibration with a serrated instrument, can often prove sufficient to remove excess water and allow the particles to take up their maximum packing density. Excessive vibration will only cause the porcelain build-up to slump and flow and all detailed surface contour will be lost; in addition, any built-in concentrated colours or enamel blend lines may alter in position and the ceramists efforts are wasted.

Whipping the surface of the wet porcelain with a large soft hair brush can also be detrimental. Although this may cause more water to rise to the surface, once again detailed characterisation will be lost. Such brushes can be used to smooth-off the crown surface and remove any excess water but the action must be gentle and the term "Brush Smoothing" gives a more accurate description of the correct technique. No attempt should be made to beat the surface of the porcelain with the brush, but a light dusting action will remove any coarse surface particles together with any remaining water.

Condensing of dental porcelain must not disturb the position of the veneer porcelains and concentrated stains or colours. By using the correct consistency of mix, a wet technique, and harnessing the power of surface tension, dense crowns may be built up rapidly and accurately.

Sintering of Dental Porcelains

Dental porcelain, being of a glassy nature, relies on its densification by a sintering process. The initial rate of sintering a compact of glass powder is inversely proportional to the particle size and viscosity and directly proportional to the surface tension. We are therefore concerned, when firing dental porcelain, in using surface tension as the driving force to eliminate porosity. The manufacturer has the responsibility of ensuring that the particle size of the powder is adjusted to give maximum density in the powder bed, and allow rapid fusion of the glass grains. The viscosity of the melt should also be high and resist pyroplastic deformation which causes loss of contour of the crown surfaces.

Air Firing Porcelain

All porcelain powders reveal a volume porosity in the dry powder bed of 40 to 49 per cent depending upon the packing ratio of the powder particles (*McLean* and *Hughes,* 1965). When these porcelains enter the hot zone of the furnace, each grain will be contacting its neighbour and furnace atmosphere will be present in the void spaces. The grains of porcelain will "lense" at their contact points and weld together once the softening point of the glass is reached (Fig. 1-13). Surface tension will cause some of this porosity to be swept out via the grain boundaries but if air-firing techniques are used a point is reached in all vitrified products where flow of the ceramic (glass grains) around the air spaces traps the air remaining in the ceramic body. (*Vines* et al, 1958). With rising temperature, the spaces containing entrapped air become sphere-shaped under the influence of surface tension (Fig. 1-14). Heating to higher temperatures, increases the pressure of the entrapped air and the bubbles enlarge to reach pressure equilibrium with the outside atmosphere. Cooling decreases the pressure in the bubbles and the bubble size decreases to reach equilibrium (Fig. 1-15). The surface of air-fired porcelain is generally free of bubbles because interstitial air nearest the actual surface cannot be trapped and escape easily. However, internally, due to the rapid firing techniques employed in dentistry, air bubbles remain entrapped and cannot escape.

The ideal time/temperature cycles for firing porcelain are employed by the industrial ceramist where the majority of his work must be air-fired. The "green ware" is placed on trays which enter a tunnel kiln and the ceramic ware is gradually moved along the tunnel until it reaches the hot zone of the furnace. This process can often exceed 24 hours. Gases or air entrapped in the ceramic can escape and very high densities are obtainable in the fired body.

If air-firing methods are employed by the dental ceramist, a very slow maturation period is the ideal for which to aim in order to allow the maximum amount of entrapped air bubbles to escape. During this slow heating the porcelain must not be raised to its full maturing temperature and as a general guide, the ceramist is advised to stay within a range of at least 30 °C to 50 °C below the maximum firing temperature recommended by the manufacturer. Such a temperature will mature the porcelain without caus-

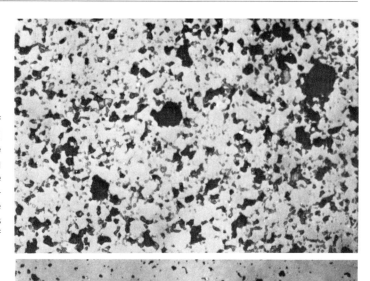

Fig. 1-13 Photomicrograph of the surface of an air-fired dental porcelain (maturing temperature 920 °C) showing initial sintering process at 800 °C. Lensing of the grains has occurred at their contact points but the air spaces are still irregular. The porcelain has reached a "low bisque" stage of maturity.

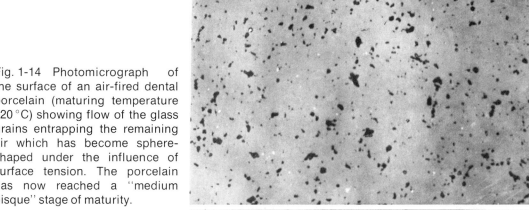

Fig. 1-14 Photomicrograph of the surface of an air-fired dental porcelain (maturing temperature 920 °C) showing flow of the glass grains entrapping the remaining air which has become sphere-shaped under the influence of surface tension. The porcelain has now reached a "medium bisque" stage of maturity.

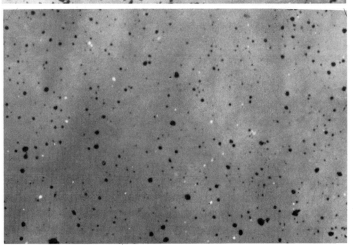

Fig. 1-15 Photomicrograph of the surface of an air-fired porcelain which has reached full maturity prior to glazing. Entrapped air bubbles constitute approximately 6 per cent by volume of the total fired body. The porcelain has now reached a "high bisque" stage of maturity.

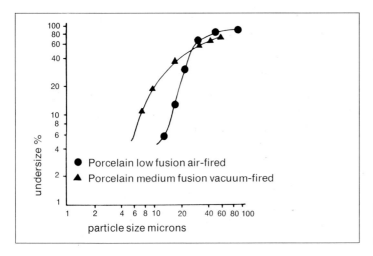

undersize %

● Porcelain low fusion air-fired

▲ Porcelain medium fusion vacuum-fired

particle size microns

Fig. 1-16 Particle size distribution of air and vacuum-firing porcelain powders.

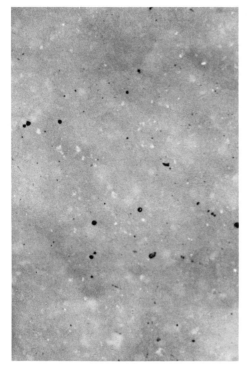

Fig. 1-17 Photomicrograph of the surface of a vacuum-fired porcelain sintered to full maturity. The remaining entrapped air bubbles constitute approximately 0.1 per cent of the total volume of the fired body.

ing loss of colour and high densities will be achieved. A heat soak of up to half-an-hour can often be safely contemplated with a reduced temperature/longer time cycle and the crown should only have matured to a high bisque (*Adriaansen,* 1966). It is important that this method is not used with the high expansion metal-ceramic porcelains where prolonged firing can induce devitrification.

Particle Size and Translucency

There is often no difference in the chemical composition of porcelains prepared for vacuum or air-firing and a manufacturer can prepare both materials from the same glass frit. The only difference between the materials is in the particle size of the powders and the amount of pigment, opacifiers, or crystalline material used to obtain the dentine or enamel colour. Vacuum powders require greater concentrations of opacifying agents.

The particle size distribution of a dental porcelain has a marked influence on the translucency of the final product. Translucency is affected both by the number and size of the entrapped air bubbles. Large particle sizes will have fewer but much larger interstitial voids in the powder bed than a fine powder. As a result, on firing a coarse powder, the entrapped air bubbles will be larger but fewer in number than a corresponding fine powder. Fewer bubbles, even of a large size, give improved translucency, and it is clear that air-fired porcelain powders must, of necessity, be of a comparatively coarse nature. The normal size distribution is given in Fig. 1-16, where the top size is around 70 μm and all fines below 7 μm are removed. By contrast, it is well known that if a fine powder prepared for vacuum firing, Fig. 1-16 is fired in air the final product will be cloudy and very opaque. This is due to the inclusion of a high percentage of fine particles in the region of 5 to 20 microns in size. These tiny particles will have large numbers of small spaces between them and resultantly

produce very many more fine air bubbles than the coarser powders.

Vacuum-firing-Porcelains

The demand by the dental ceramist for improved aesthetics led to the development of finer powders which are fired in vacuo (*Vines* et al, 1958).

Vacuum-fired porcelains were introduced primarily to give improved aesthetics in the enamel porcelains. In addition, other useful properties such as ease of handling, and the production of dense surfaces that could be ground and repolished, must also be taken into account. Vacuum firing techniques were therefore a major step forward in the dental ceramic field.

Vines et al (1958), have explained the densification of porcelain by vacuum firing very simply: Air or atmosphere is removed from the interstitial spaces before sealing of the surface occurs and hence there is nothing to hinder the porcelain from shrinking to a dense, pore-free mass. The actual mechanism is somewhat more involved since the vacuum used in a dental furnace (760 Torr [101-3 k Pa]) is really air at reduced pressure. Although the vacuum removes most of the air from the interstitial spaces, it does not remove it all. This remaining air becomes sphere-shaped under the influence of surface tension and increased furnace temperature. When air, at normal atmospheric pressure, is once again allowed to enter the furnace muffle, it exercises a strong compression effect on the dense surface skin, which hydraulically compresses the low pressure internal bubbles. This results in a relatively dense pore-free porcelain since the remaining bubbles are very few in number and of an extremely small size (Fig. 1-17). Due to the rapid action of vacuum sintering, the firing schedule for these porcelains can be reduced in comparison with the longer period recommended for air-fired porcelain. A comparison of the internal porosity of air-fired and vacuum-fired porcelain is given in Table 1-3.

Table 1-3 Comparison of Porosity of Air and Vacuum Fired Porcelain

Porcelain	Porosity per Cent	
	Air-fired	Vacuum-fired
Medium fusion	6.7	0.1
Low fusion	6.0	0.08

Porosity determined by point counting on fully matured specimen bars.

The ceramist may learn three important lessons from an understanding of the processes involved in vacuum-firing.

1. Porcelain powder must be dried slowly to eliminate all water vapour and vacuum must be applied before the porcelain enters the hot zone of the furnace. In this way the internal pores are reduced before the surface skin seals off the interior too rapidly.
2. Vacuum-firing should never be prolonged once the porcelain has matured and the surface skin is sealed. Further application of vacuum can cause surface blistering since residual air bubbles will try to rise to the surface through the molten porcelain. Firing at too high a temperature can be even more dangerous and can cause "bloating" or swelling. All glazing must be done in normal atmosphere.
3. The vacuum should be broken whilst the work is still in the hot zone of the furnace. This allows the dense surface skin of porcelain to hydraulically compress the low pressure internal air bubbles. Fortunately, modern vacuum-firing furnaces are designed to achieve this object.

Vacuum-firing also has its limitations. If large bubbles are trapped in the porcelain by poor condensation techniques, these bubbles cannot be reduced in size to any significant degree. Vacuum-firing is not a panacea for poor technique and the blistering often experienced by some ceramists can be due to entrapment of large air bubbles and not to faults in the materials. In particular bulk placement of dental porcelain with a spatula is a common way of trapping air. Additions of porcelain to a matured crown can sometimes cause slight blistering. If any major bubbles have been entrapped in the matured crown, the second bake of additional porcelain can produce an effect similar to prolonging the vacuum after maturity has been reached. Additions of porcelain should therefore be made when the crown is at a medium bisque, i.e. when the porcelain has commenced to fuse and shrink but is still slightly porous.

Diffusible Gas Firing Process

An alternative technique for producing high densities in dental porcelain is by the substitution of a diffusible gas for the ordinary furnace atmosphere. Air is driven out of the porcelain powder bed and the diffusible gas is substituted. If the new furnace atmosphere is helium, hydrogen, or steam, then these gases will be sealed in the interstitial spaces of the powder bed. With these gases, the interstitial spaces do not enlarge under the influence of increasing temperature, but decrease in size or disappear. This occurs because these gases diffuse outward through the porcelain or actually dissolve in the porcelain (*Vines* et al, 1958).

Pressure Cooling Process

After a dental porcelain has been fired conventionally and is still in a semimolten, fluxible condition, the remaining entrapped air may be compressed by extra pressure into a small fraction of its original volume using the molten porcelain as a hydraulic medium. Pressure in the furnace is generally raised to about 10 atmospheres after the porcelain has fully matured and this pressure is maintained during cooling. Pressure firing suffers from the disadvantage that the compressed air bubbles will return to pressure equilibrium at normal atmosphere if the porcelain tooth or crown is refired. This results in the bubbles returning to their original size. Pressure firing is used by some tooth manufacturers but cannot be considered a viable system for use in the dental laboratory.

Classification of Stages of Maturity

Ceramists have found it convenient to classify the various stages of sintering or "firing" dental porcelain. The common expression used for describing the surface appearance of un-glazed porcelain is "bisque" or "biscuit" since this gives a fairly accurate picture of surface texture.

Low bisque – The surface of the porcelain is very porous and will easily absorb a water soluble die. At this stage the grains of porcelain will have started to soften and "lense" at their contact points. Shrinkage will be minimal and the fired body is extremely weak and friable (Fig. 1-13).

Medium Bisque – The surface of the porcelain is still porous but the flow of the glass grains will have increased and any entrapped furnace atmosphere that has not escaped via the grain boundaries will be trapped and become sphere-shaped. A definite shrinkage will have taken place (Fig. 1-14).

High bisque – The surface of the porcelain will be completely sealed and present a much smoother surface (Fig. 1-15). In the case of the non-felspathic glasses a slight shine will appear and at this stage the porcelain is strong and any corrections by grinding can be made prior to final glazing.

It should be noted that additions of porcelain can be made at any of the bisque firing stages, but it is usual to do this at either a medium or high bisque.

Glazing and Thermal Shock Prevention

The glazing of dental porcelain is probably the most important step in the whole procedure of baking a crown, since it is at this stage that many crowns are irretrievably ruined. An over-glazed crown will appear glassy and often take on the classical greenish tinge of natural glass. Colour values will deteriorate and the surface will no longer have the texture of human enamel.

As explained on page 39 the author does not favour the application of separate glazes but prefers to use porcelains that are self-glazing.

Glazing is simply a further stage of advancement in vitrification from the bisque finish. This is quite obvious if one observes the effect of increasing the time of maturing a high bisque crown; it will become glazed. The essential object in glazing is to avoid loss of surface detail by markedly increasing the pyroplastic flow of the porcelain. The latter effect will always be caused by using too high a glaze temperature. Rounding of line angles and obliteration of the surface characteristics produced by grinding can be avoided if a crown is glazed slightly below its recommended maturing temperature. A lower temperature and longer time cycle should be the basic aim of the ceramist. In this way the pyroplasticity of the crown is controlled to a level where the surface will assume an enamel-like sheen but will not slump or flow at critical line angles. The ceramist must be aware that as the furnace temperature rises, the viscosity of dental glasses decreases. He must control this viscosity and use it to his advantage.

Thermal Shock

Stressing of a ceramic crown by thermal shock is not uncommon. Great emphasis has been placed in the literature on the need for slow cooling of a porcelain restoration and it is surprising that only this aspect has received attention.

Thermal shock is caused by uneven heating or cooling. A crown's surface may expand or contract more quickly than the interior and due to the differential thermal expansion, stresses will be set up.

All ceramics are stronger when placed under compression rather than under tension, and it should be the endeavour of the ceramist to ensure that his crown surfaces are placed under compression. When a crown is removed from the furnace and cooled in air, the surface will be losing heat more rapidly than the interior. The crown surface will contract faster than the interior, but generally will be placed in compression by the balancing tensile stresses developed either in the core porcelain or metal coping due to their higher thermal expansions. A crown that is moved into the furnace rapidly, prior to glazing, will receive the full force of the radiant heat from the muffle. The surface of the crown will tend to expand faster than the interior and the latter surface can be placed in such tension that the thermal cracks could develop from the inner surface and break through the outer skin.

At this stage it is often possible to induce thermal cracks which might disappear on cooling but can re-appear later on re-heating. These cracks can also open up in the mouth at a later date and this is not infrequent in some of the porcelain veneer gold crowns, particularly where soldering techniques have been used.

Thermal shock is more severe on re-heating or glazing a crown than when cooling it. The ceramist is therefore strongly advised to insert the mature crown very slowly into the hot zone of the furnace muffle so that all sections of the porcelain are evenly heated.

Very rapid cooling of crowns is also not advised since the balancing tensile stresses in the interior may rupture the outside layer or "skin" (*Skinner* and *Phillips,* 1967). However, this is not likely to occur if the crown is allowed to cool at the muffle entrance and then bench cooled in air. In this way the outside layer will be placed in compression, thus fulfilling the basic laws of ceramics.

Solubility

The solubility of dental porcelain is extremely low and it is probably the most resistant material to attack by oral fluids and bacterial plaque that is used in dentistry today.

Typical solubilities for dental porcelains are given below:

	Per cent Sol. K_2O	Per cent Sol. Na_2O
Vacuum Porcelain A	0.0006	0.0016
Vacuum Porcelain B	0.0005	0.0007
Vacuum Porcelain C	0.0014	0.0020
Manufactured Tooth	0.0010	0.0012

Soaked for 4 days in 0.25 % HCl at room temperature.

Washed and then tested in 0.25 % HCl for 24 hrs. at 30 °C.

It should be noted that the solubility of dental porcelain is very dependent upon the degree of vitrification and a glazed surface is more resistant to acid attack.

Monograph I

References

Abbey, A. (1962). Improvements in and Relating to Ceramic Artificial Teeth and a Process for the Preparation Thereof. British Patent No. 897, 686.

Adriaansen, J. (1966). A.T. Laboratories. The Netherlands. Personal communication.

Binns, D. B. (1970). British Ceramic Research Association. Personal communication.

Burke, J. E. (1958). Recrystallisation and Sintering in Ceramics. In: Ceramic Fabrication Processes. pp 120-131. John Wiley and Sons, Inc., New York. London.

Charles, R. J. (1967). The Nature of Glasses. Scientific American, 217:113.

Gilman, J. J. (1967). The Nature of Ceramics. Scientific American, 217:113.

Herring, Congers (1950). Diffusional Viscosities of a Polycrystalline Solid. J. Appl. Phys., 21:437.

Kingery, W. D. (1958). Ceramic Fabrication Processes pp 131-145. John Wiley and Sons, Inc., New York. London.

Lee, W., and Dietz, C. (1948). Porcelain Type Denture Composition and Method of Preparing the Same. U.S. Patent No. 2,443,318.

McGeary, R. K. (1961). Mechanical Packing of Spherical Particles. J. Amer. Ceram. Soc., 36:159.

McLean, J. W., and Hughes, T. H. (1965). The Reinforcement of Dental Porcelain with Ceramic Oxides. Brit. dent. J. 119:251.

McLean, J. W. (1966). The Development of Ceramic Oxide Reinforced Dental Porcelains with an Appraisal of their Physical and Clinical Properties. M.D.S. Thesis, University of London.

McMillan, P. W. (1964). Glass-Ceramics. Academic Press. London. New York.

Nabarro, F. R. N. (1948). Deformation of Crystals by Motion of Single Ions. Report of a Conference on Strength of Solids. p. 75. Phys. Soc. London.

Orlowski, H. J. (1944). Dental Porcelain. Ohio State University Studies: Engineering Series, Engineering Experimental Station, Bulletin No. 118, 13. No. 2.

Pauling, L. (1945). The Nature of the Chemical Bond. Cornel Univ. Press. 2nd Ed. Chapter X.

Skinner, E. W., and Phillips, R. W. (1967). The Science of Dental Materials. W. B. Saunders Co. Philadelphia and London.

Vines, R. F., Semmelman, J. O., Lee, P. W., and Fonvielle, F. D. (1958). Mechanisms Involved in Securing Dense, Vitrified Ceramics from Preshaped Partly-Crystalline Bodies. J. Amer. Ceram. Soc., 41:304.

Weyl, W. A., and Marboe, E. C. (1962). The Constitution of Glasses. A Dynamic Interpretation Vol. 1. Fundamentals of the Structure of Inorganic Liquids and Glasses. Interscience, New York and London Chapter III.

Zachariasen, W. H. (1932). The Atomic Arrangement in Glass. J. Amer. Chem. Soc. 54:3841.

Monograph II

The Strengthening of Dental Porcelain

The Strengthening of Dental Porcelain

In order to understand the methods employed to strengthen dental porcelain, it is important that the sources of weakness in this material are clearly outlined.

Crack Propagation in Dental Porcelain

Invariably, fractures in dental porcelain originate from microcracks, often less than 0.2 microns wide, which are present on the surface and act as stress concentrators (Figs. 2-1 and 2-2). Because of these small flaws, around which the stress reaches very high levels, the measured strength of dental porcelain is thus limited by the most highly stressed flaw in the area under load. This statement may appear to be of academic interest only, but it is also of direct clinical significance when considering occlusal forces. Patients who indulge in bruxism or parafunctional activities are much more likely to overload the flaw system in dental porcelain and produce a sudden fracture of the porcelain restoration.

The measure of a material's ability to retain its strength in the presence of cracks is determined by what is termed the work of fracture of the material, i.e. the energy required to break it.

Tough materials generally possess a high work of fracture, whereas dental porcelain being a brittle material has a very small work of fracture and will not tolerate cracks much deeper than .025 mm (1/10,000 inch) before fracture occurs. *Cook* and *Gordon* (1964) have shown that a characteristic of a brittle solid, such as dental porcelain, is that the tip radius of a crack of molecular dimensions in the material remains sensibly constant as the crack extends. It follows that the longer the crack the less the force required to propagate it, and so, in a brittle solid under tension, once a crack begins to extend, complete fracture will occur suddenly. It will be appreciated that the means of initiating cracks in dental porcelain will never be lacking. Surface porosity, abrasion, grinding effects, or thermal stressing are all ready means of introducing a flaw system.

A significant clinical factor in the weakening of glass surfaces is the effect of moisture contamination. Water plays a vital part in the static fatigue of glass and produces a time-dependent reduction in strength. *Wang* and *Tooley* (1958) have described this process as a replacement of the alkali ions in glass by hydrogen ions, which attract water molecules into the spaces originally occupied by the alkali. This water (saliva) could act as a type of network modifier in weakening the glass. Undamaged glass is weakened by wet storage and shows delayed fracture when stressed at constant load under wet con-

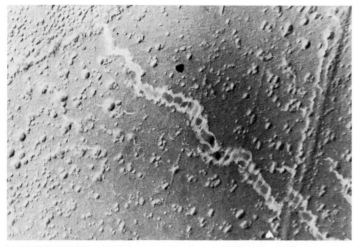

Fig. 2-1 Microcrack in the surface of glazed porcelain produced by thermal stress during cooling. (Mag x 10,000).

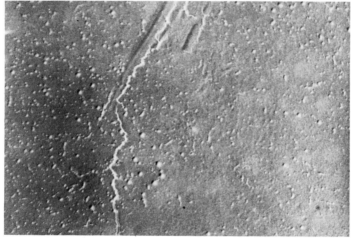

Fig. 2-2 Microcrack in the surface of dental porcelain showing a change in direction due to a fault in the glazed surface. This is typical of the flaw system which may be present in the surface of porcelain crowns. (Mag x 5,000).

ditions (*Gurney*, 1964). It is highly probable that surface weakening of dental porcelain may also occur in the mouth and occlusal loads that would not normally break the material might over-stress the flaw system once static fatigue sets in.

Cracks cannot easily propagate in porcelain when the material is under compression but any occlusal forces that produce tensile stresses which can overcome the surface compression will propagate a crack. When porcelain jacket crowns receive insufficient support from the underlying dentine, tension may build up on the internal surfaces to the point where sudden fracture will occur. It is for this reason that preparations with insufficient coronal length give little resistance against fracture of the porcelain crown (Fig. 2-3).

The most common faults in tooth preparation which can cause fracture of porcelain jacket crowns will be discussed in Monograph IV. In general, it may be stated that the two worst faults are failure to provide sufficient support or retention for the jacket crown against torsional or bending stresses produced in masticatory function.

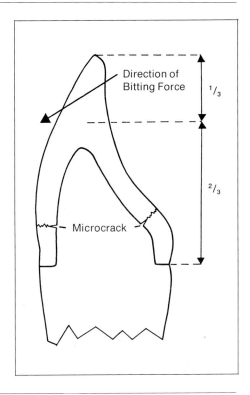

Fig. 2-3   Diagram illustrating tensile failure of a porcelain jacket crown. Fracture initiates from a microcrack as in Figs. 2-1 and 2-2 which opens up under tensile stress. Coronal length of preparation is insufficient to support the crown.

Mechanical Testing

Dental Porcelain is much stronger when loaded under compression than under tension. *Saachi* and *Paffenbarger* (1957) found that both low and high fusing porcelains had similar compressive strengths in the region of 340 N/mm² (48,000 p.s.i.). This strength would appear to be more than adequate to resist any forces experienced under clinical conditions.

Tensile failure of dental porcelain is the commonest cause of fracture and for this reason mechanical tests are usually devised to assess this property. The slow bend test (modulus of rupture) provides a measure of the tensile failure of a ceramic and will give very repeatable results (*Hodson*, 1959; *McLean* and *Hughes*, 1965; *Wilson* and *Whitehead*, 1967).

Impact testing has an appeal from a clinical viewpoint and dropping weight impact tests have been specially devised for testing dental porcelain (*Kulp* et al., 1961). However, the scatter of results can be very wide (*Binns*, 1964) and as yet no acceptable test has been devised which can produce consistent results.

Even when a slow bend test is used to determine the flexural strength of ceramic materials, *Shevlin* and *Lindenthal* (1959) have shown that the results may vary considerably, depending upon the conditions of testing. Among the factors affecting the breaking strength of ceramics are: the texture of the surface, e.g. surface flaws, etc., the gaseous or liquid environment of the specimen under test, the ratio of span to diameter (cross-sectional area) of the specimen, the shape of the cross-section, the configuration of the load, and the rate of application of load.

The fracture strength of various dental porcelains was measured by *Jones* et al. (1972) and was significantly influenced by strain rate. The

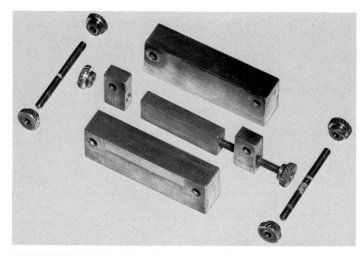

Fig. 2-4a Split steel mould for preparation of porcelain test bars; exploded view.

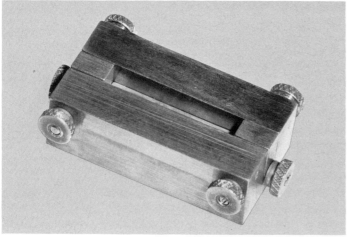

Fig. 2-4b Split steel mould for preparation of porcelain test bars; assembled.

modulus of rupture was higher when the rate of strain was increased from 0.01 cm per minute up to 800 cm per min (i.e. the speed of chewing). It follows, therefore, that the mechanical testing of dental porcelain presents formidable problems if meaningful results are to be obtained.

Testing Ground Porcelain Specimens

The most widely used method of mechanically testing dental porcelain has been by the preparation of rectangular test bars using a wet vibra-

tion compaction technique, similar to dental laboratory procedure. These bars are prepared in split steel moulds (Fig. 2-4), using distilled water to bind the porcelain together. After firing of the porcelain to a medium glaze, each bar is lapped on all surfaces with an abrasive slurry to produce accurate edges and flat surfaces. The modulus of rupture is then determined by supporting the bars at either end and loading them in the centre until fracture occurs. The modulus of rupture or flexural strength may be calculated from the formula:

$$M = \frac{3PL}{2BD^2}$$

where M = Modulus of rupture, P = Load required to break test piece, B = Breadth of bar, D = Depth of bar, L = Length of bar.

The depth of the bar is measured in the direction of application of load.

Jones et al. (1972) found that alterations in the span to depth ratio between 5:1 and 15:1 did not produce significant variation in the modulus of rupture when 2×2 mm specimens of aluminous core porcelain were used. However, variations in the geometry of the specimens did produce differences.

Testing Glazed Specimens

A more convenient way of testing the strength of glazed surfaces was found to be by the use of hydraulically-pressed rods of dry powder (*McLean* and *Hughes*, 1965). Although this does not represent actual laboratory methods of condensation, the surface integrity of fired rods of porcelain proved to be better than rectangular bars and there was less chance of surface flaws interfering with the results, and producing a wide scatter of modulus of rupture figures.

Strength of Glazed and Surface Ground Porcelain

Typical strengths of both air and vacuum-fired porcelains are depicted in Table 2-1.

The strength of dental porcelain is more influenced by composition and surface texture than by the type of atmosphere used during firing (*McLean* and *Hughes,* 1965). In particular, it should be noted that the high strength of glazed rods of porcelain is reduced by nearly 50 percent when the surface is ground. This illustrates the importance of the role that the surface integrity of the glaze plays in reducing the number of surface flaws. Providing the surface skin is undisturbed, minor porosities of 6 to 8 percent in the air-fired porcelains do not appear to weaken the material.

Other small differences in strength which are apparent on the lapped bar specimens can be accounted for more by differences in composition of the porcelain than by minor surface porosities. The medium-fusion felspathic porcelains are generally made by almost complete fusion of the felspar constituents and these porcelains behave more like the single-phase glasses which are made from the raw oxides and carbonates. Single-phase glasses are usually more abrasion resistant and harder than a felspathic porcelain containing undissolved felspar. This may account for the higher strengths listed in Table 2-1 in which the low fusion felspathic porcelain is slightly weaker in flexural strength.

The majority of current studies on the strength of dental porcelain indicate that vacuum-firing techniques do not significantly strengthen dental porcelain (*McLean* and *Hughes,* 1965; *Jones* et al. 1972). It was also found that heat treatment of specimens of porcelain at temperatures just above the strain point did not produce any significant strength variations in the materials examined. It is for this reason that alternative methods of strengthening dental porcelain are now being used.

Influence of Condensation Technique on Mechanical Strength

Different techniques for condensing regular dental porcelain appear to have very little influence on the final strength of the fired product. Experiments conducted during the course of developing the aluminous porcelains (*McLean* and *Hughes,* 1965) revealed that regular porcelains of the low and medium maturing types were not affected in mechanical strength by extremes of condensation pressure or no condensation at all. The modulus of rupture

Table-2-1 Transverse Strength of Dental Porcelains

Type of Porcelain	Method of Firing	Type of Specimen	Modulus of rupture N/mm²	p.s.i.
Low Fusion Felspathic	Air	Lapped bar	61.2	8,865
Low Fusion Single-phase glass	Air	Lapped bar	87.7	12,721
Medium Fusion Felspathic	Air	Lapped bar	78.2	11,376
High Fusion Felspathic	Air	Lapped bar	75.7	10,980
Low Fusion Felspathic	Vacuum	Lapped bar	61.8	8,970
Low Fusion Single-phase glass	Vacuum	Lapped bar	91.3	13,254
Medium Fusion Felspathic	Vacuum	Lapped bar	80.7	11.714
Low Fusion Felspathic	Air	Glazed rod	132.8	19,278
Low Fusion Single-phase glass	Air	Glazed rod	146.4	21,235
Medium Fusion Felspathic	Vacuum	Glazed rod	140.7	20,465
Low Fusion Felspathic	Air	Ground rod	82.8	12,032
Low Fusion Single-phase glass	Air	Ground rod	89.5	12,978
Medium Fusion Felspathic	Vacuum	Ground rod	79.7	11,547

Bars tested at 22.0 kg min⁻¹ (10 lb./min.). Rods tested at 462.0 kg min⁻¹ (210 lb./min.).

of two regular porcelains used for air and vacuum firing using different condensation techniques is illustrated in Table 2-2. High pressure compacts condensed at 224 N/mm² (14.5 ton/in²) differed very little in strength from those prepared in a steel mould using either the standard wet vibration technique or no vibration of the mould. There was a small increase in the strength of the low fusion air-fired porcelain when high pressure compaction was used and this might be expected from the nature of the particle size of the air-fired porcelain; high pressure compacts increase the "green" density by about 10 percent.

Inadequate condensation of dental porcelain will increase the shrinkage of the fired ceramic and may increase the number of included air bubbles. However, it should be noted that in the case of both the low and medium maturing porcelains, a non-vibratory compaction technique caused no change in the modulus of rupture. In this case the wet slurry of

Table 2-2 Influence of Condensation Methods on the Strength of Dental Porcelain

Type of Porcelain	Method of Condensation	Modulus of Rupture		Standard Deviation	Variance Coefficient
		N/mm²	p.s.i.		
Medium maturing vac. A	High pressure 224 N/mm² (14.5 ton/in²)	78.1	(11,547)	8.10	10.18
Low maturing air B	High pressure 224 N/mm² (14.5 ton/in²)	73.7	(10,893)	4.91	5.93
Medium maturing vac. A	Wet vibration	77.3	(11,426)	7.92	10.05
Low maturing air B	Wet vibration	61.2	(8,865)	8.52	13.94
Medium maturing vac. A	No vibration	76.8	(11,387)	4.07	4.35
Low maturing Air B	No vibration	57.2	(8,307)	5.48	5.68

porcelain was dried off with a paper tissue and even by this means, surface tension effects were created causing a drawing together of the particles. Working a porcelain powder which is drying out is much more likely to entrap excessive air, as explained on page 42, Monograph I. Condensation of dental porcelains in the wet state is essential in order to minimise shrinkage and avoid the inclusion of excessive numbers of air bubbles which could mar the aesthetics of the final crown. Mechanical strength is more affected by the time/temperature cycle used to obtain maximum sintered densities, by the composition of the porcelain and by the surface texture of the fired crown.

The crystalline aluminous porcelains are much more affected by poor condensation techniques and their strength can be lowered considerably with increased porosity in the fired body. These effects are discussed in the section dealing with dispersion strengthening of glasses.

Methods of Strengthening Dental Porcelain

It has already been shown that porcelain jacket crowns generally fracture when tensile stresses occur on the internal or fit surfaces (Fig. 2-3). Sometimes these stresses can be of a low order of magnitude and yet fracture may occur quite suddenly.

In order to strengthen dental porcelain, it is essential that a mechanism should exist to prevent crack propagation under low tensile stresses. In the case of a porcelain jacket crown, this can be achieved in several ways. The inner surface can be reinforced by a metal or a higher strength ceramic, or, alternatively, the surface of the porcelain can be treated to improve its strength (Fig. 2-5). Once a stronger material is used as an inner skin for the porcelain crown, then cracks can only develop when the stronger material is deformed or broken. This presupposes, of course, that the porcelain is firmly

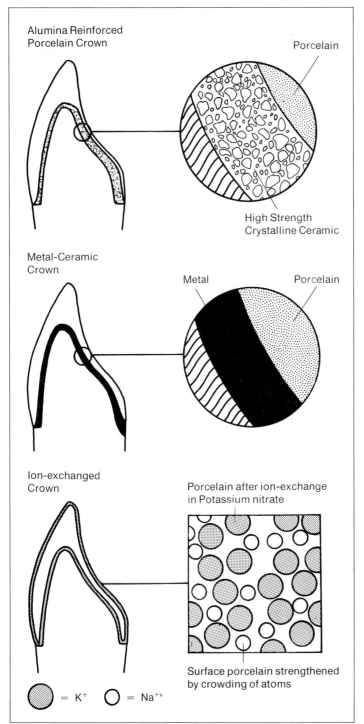

Alumina Reinforced
Porcelain Crown

Porcelain

High Strength
Crystalline Ceramic

Metal-Ceramic
Crown

Metal   Porcelain

Ion-exchanged
Crown

Porcelain after ion-exchange
in Potassium nitrate

Surface porcelain strengthened
by crowding of atoms

○ = K⁺   ○ = Na⁺ˢ

Fig. 2-5 Methods of Strengthening Dental Porcelain.

bonded to the reinforcing substrate. Other methods rely on strengthening the entire ceramic body by the growth of reinforcing crystals in situ.

Current and future research would appear to centre around five approaches to strengthening dental porcelain:

1. Enamelling of metals.
2. Dispersion strengthening of glasses.
3. Enamelling of high strength crystalline ceramics.
4. Controlled crystallisation of glasses.
5. Production of pre-stressed surface layers in dental porcelain via ion-exchange.

Enamelling of Metals

The term "fused-porcelain-to-gold" has been widely used to describe the bonding of porcelain to noble metal alloys. The term is not very accurate and this class of materials should really be described as metal-ceramics.

Metal-ceramic crowns are now widely used and have proved very successful under clinical conditions. Providing a strong bond is achieved between the porcelain enamel and the metal, there is no risk of leakage at the interface. In addition, the porcelain enamel is reinforced by the metal and is less likely to be placed under tensile forces which can cause brittle fracture.

Types of Metal-Ceramic Systems

A large number of metal-ceramic systems have now been developed for use in dentistry and they may be classified as follows:

Noble-Metal Alloy Systems

High gold	1. Gold-platinum-palladium alloys
	2. Gold-platinum-tantalum alloys
Low gold	3. Gold-palladium-silver alloys
Gold-free	4. Palladium-silver alloys

Base-Metal Alloy Systems

Nickel-chromium alloys
Cobalt-chromium alloys (rarely used in ceramic bonding)

Gold-Platinum-Palladium Alloys

The alloys used for the construction of metal-ceramic crowns and fixed bridgework must meet many more requirements than the traditional gold alloys used in dentistry. They must match the enamel in coefficient of thermal expansion, in order to minimise the stresses formed at the interface, and possess adequate mechanical properties such as strength, high modulus of elasticity, hardness and high-temperature strength. These requirements must be met without using metals such as copper or nickel that will discolour the enamel (*O'Brien* et al. 1964). Although it should be noted that small traces of copper can be tolerated and are used in some of the current alloys (*McLean* and *Sced,* 1973). To meet these requirements, a series of alloys have been formulated based on gold, platinum and palladium (table 2-3).

The main constituent of all these alloys is gold. Platinum and palladium are added to raise the melting temperature, reduce the coefficient of thermal expansion, and strengthen the alloys. The small proportions of base metals, indium, zinc, and tin are included to produce a thin oxide film on the surface of the gold alloy which

Table 2-3

Analysis of Typical Gold Alloys used in Metal-Ceramic Techniques

Weight per cent	Armator	Ceramco	Estaticor	Degudent	Herador
gold	82.6	87.7	84.0	84.8	83.2
platinum	12.4	6.1	7.9	7.9	15.6
palladium	0.8	4.6	4.6	4.6	—
silver	2.4	1.0	1.3	1.3	—
indium	—	0.6	1.1	1.25	0.9
iridium	—	—	0.2	0.15	0.3
zinc	1.8	—	—	—	—
tin	—	—	0.2	—	—
copper	—	—	0.2	—	—

Adapted from Nally, J. N. (1968) Int. Dent. J., 18:309-325, and McLean, J. W., and Sced, I. R., (1973) Trans. Brit. Ceram. Soc. 5:229-233.

may provide the means for chemical bonding between the metal and ceramic. It is essential that these oxides are chosen to be compatible with the porcelain, otherwise they may affect the thermal expansion of the interfacial porcelain (*McLean* and *Sced,* 1973). Base metals such as indium, zinc and tin will form oxides on the surface of the alloy by a process termed b u l k d i f f u s i o n.

These base metals, in addition to their role in oxide formation, may also harden the alloy and refine the grain structure (*O'Brien,* 1964; *Peyton,* 1968; *Vickery* and *Badinelli,* 1968; *Tuccillo,* 1977). It is interesting to note that the analyses of some of the more popular high-fusing alloys (table 2-3) do not reveal the presence of metals such as ruthenium, rhenium, or iron. The latter materials have been reported as

being useful ingredients in high-fusing gold alloys used in the metal-ceramic technique but their use appears to have been discontinued. However, it should be noted that the effect of iron age-hardening of gold alloys is receiving renewed attention (*Smith* et al., 1968).

Gold-Platinum-Palladium Alloys – Mechanical Strength and Heat Treatment

Considerable improvements in the strength of the current high-fusing gold-platinum alloys used in metal-ceramic techniques have been made in recent years. *Leinfelder* et al. (1969) have reported on the strengths of five commercial gold alloys and found that the hardness,

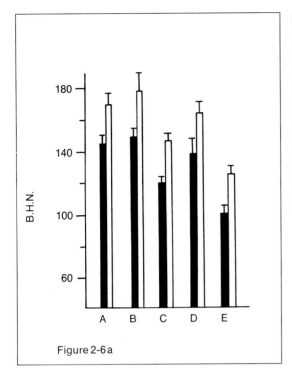

Figure 2-6 a

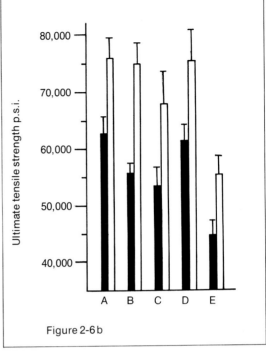

Figure 2-6 b

Fig. 2-6 a Mechanical properties of high-fusing gold alloys used in the metal-ceramic techniques. Treatment I. Thermal cycling to 1,000 °C followed by air cooling three times. Treatment II. Thermal cycling to 1,000 °C three times and then age-hardened at 538 °C for 30 minutes. Mean Brinell hardness values: black bars, Treatment I; white Bars, Treatment II. Adapted from *Lienfelder* et al. (1969) J. Pros. Dent., 21:523.

Fig. 2-6 b Mean ultimate tensile strength values: black bars, Treatment I; white bars, Treatment II.

Fig. 2-6 c Mean proportional limit values: black bars, Treatment I; white bars, Treatment II.

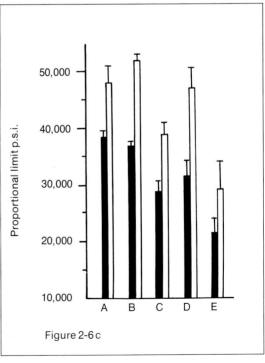

Figure 2-6 c

tensile strength and moduli of elasticity compared favourably with those of conventional crown and bridge alloys. However, ductility values were lower and the alloys exhibited greater brittleness.

When porcelain is fused to these high-fusing gold alloys at temperatures of about 930 °C to 960 °C, the alloys undergo a solution heat treatment and subsequently age-harden during a slow cooling in air (*O'Brien* et al., 1964; *Smith* et al., 1968). The result is that the alloys increase in hardness from the as-cast state. Further improvements can be made in the strength and hardness of these high-fusing gold alloys by ageing the metal at 538 °C. (1000 °F.) (*Leinfelder* et al., 1969). The effect of these two types of heat treatment is illustrated in Fig. 2-6 a-c.

Treatment I consisted of heating specimen test rods to 1000 °C (1832 °F) followed by air cooling three times. This thermal cycling is similar to the porcelain enamel baking procedures employed in the metal-ceramic techniques. Treatment II was the same as Treatment I with the addition of a constant temperature ageing upon completion of the cycling. This would be equivalent to giving a glazed metal-ceramic crown a further heat treatment. An ageing time of 30 minutes was used for each alloy tested at an ageing temperature of 538 °C (1000 °F).

The hardness and strength of four of the alloys appears to be adequate for clinical use without submitting them to a further ageing treatment as in Treatment II. The very considerable improvements obtained in physical properties after an ageing time of 30 minutes at 538 °C (1000 °F) Treatment II, would appear to be highly desirable, but might increase the risk of the veneer porcelain devitrifying.

Further heat treatment of a metal-ceramic restoration after the final glazing is not recommended at the present time since the porcelain may devitrify with constant annealing. Once devitrification is started, the effects are progressive and the porcelain will become cloudy and difficult to glaze.

Gold Bonding Agents

Certain types of bonding agents have become available for coating the metal surface prior to the application of the opaque porcelain. Two of these agents, "Britecote" and "Culver-Guard" pastes have been analysed by *Nally* (1969) and were composed of pure gold, probably in colloidal form, dispersed in a solid organic phase which becomes volatile during baking of the ceramic. Claims are made that improvements in the aesthetics of the porcelain can be obtained with the brighter gold surface. Even assuming some aesthetic advantages, the use of pure gold does not seem very logical since it will not form any attachment with dental porcelain and may even obscure the surface of the oxidised gold alloy and prevent bonding. The use of these materials has not been very widespread and with modern "paint-on-opaques", technicians find that coverage of the metal is very adequate.

Alternative Alloy Systems

The current gold-platinum-palladium alloys are well tried and clinically tested and set the standard for much of our future work. The only reasons, at the present time, for wishing to replace them are their high cost and also lack of fit after firing the porcelain due to metal creep, since alloys containing 84–85 % gold are too near the porcelain's firing temperature of 900 °C to 950 °C. The gold-platinum alloys are comparatively easy to cast and since the base metal additions can be carefully controlled, oxide production is not excessive and the tin and indium oxides appear to form a solid solution with the porcelain at the interface, bringing the metal into atomic contact with the porcelain, as will be described. The strength of the gold alloys is adequate for most clinical situations when used in correct section, but for bridges involving two or more pontics or in cases of multi-splinting of periodontally-involved teeth, improvements in yield strength and modulus of elasticity are desirable. Methods of improving the design of the preparation and the metal framework to resist creep have been well documented in recent years (*El-Ebrashi* et al., 1969, 1970; *Craig* and *Farah,* 1977; *Nally* et al., 1971; *Shillingburg* et al., 1973; *Warpeha* and *Goodkind,* 1976).

What improvements can be expected in the high gold content alloys? It is doubtful whether mechanical properties can be improved much further within the context of present knowledge. However, the aesthetic appearance of the ceramic type gold alloys has recently been improved.

Gold-Platinum-Tantalum Alloys

The high gold content alloys containing platinum and palladium are not ideal aesthetically; their rather dull grey and often black appearance does meet with criticism from the patient, particularly where thick gold collars are used. More recently, work in West Germany has concentrated on developing a more gold-coloured alloy* and this has been achieved by substituting tantalum for palladium in the alloy. Palladium is well-known as a hydrogen acceptor so that it is not ideal as a constituent of an alloy for attachment of porcelain. Hydrogen gas evolved during porcelain firing is a frequent cause of porosity in the opaque porcelains. The physical properties of this palladium-free alloy appear very adequate for ceramic bonding.

* Degudent G. Degussa, West Germany.

Physical Characteristics of Degudent G

Vickers Hardness	195
Tensile Strength	530 N/mm^2
Yield Strength	470 N/mm^2
Elongation percent	Soft 15 %, Hard 9 %
Specific Gravity	18.4

For those clinicians who carry out extensive gold occlusal coverage of their porcelain restorations, the colour of this new alloy should be more appealing.

Gold-Palladium-Silver Alloys

The gold-palladium-silver alloys have only been on the market since 1972 (*Katz,* 1974; *Tuccillo,* 1976). The composition of these alloys has been given by Tuccillo as follows:

Gold	–	50 %
Palladium	–	30 %
Silver	–	12 %
Indium		
Tin	–	8 %

Since platinum is not present, there is little reason to add iron to this system. Hardening depends on solid solution hardening by the tin and/or indium of the gold-palladium binary. Indium is not so effective as tin but both atoms will randomly substitute for gold or palladium on the face-centred cube lattice. Since both are smaller in diameter and contribute more valence electrons, they force a lattice strain because of the negative attraction they have for each other and thus strengthen the alloy (*Tuccillo,* 1977). The high palladium content results in a melting range that is around 40 °C higher than that of the gold-platinum-palla-

Table 2-4   Physical and Mechanical Properties of Au-Pt-Pd and Au-Ag-Pd Alloys

Properties	Alloys			
	Gold-Platinum-Palladium		Gold-Silver-Palladium	
Tensile strength N/mm² (p.s.i.)	492−608	(71,300−88,200)	521−724	(75,600−105,000)
Yield Strength N/mm² (p.s.i.)	401−458	(58,100−66,400)	329−526	(47,700−76,300)
Modulus of Elasticity N/mm² (p.s.i.)	$86.2-93.8 \times 10^3$	$(12.5-13.6 \times 10^6)$	$102-117 \times 10^6$	$(14.8-16.9 \times 10^6)$
Per cent Elongation	5.0−12.9		13.9−30.6	
Vickers Hardness (DPN)	161−197		167−228	
Density	17.9−18.3		11.9−14.5	

After *Moffa, J. P.,* 1977, Physical and Mechanical Properties of Gold and Base Metal Alloys. NIH Conference Proceedings.

dium systems. The gold-palladium-silver alloys are therefore more resistant to metal creep during the firing of the porcelain. The increase in palladium and silver content, replacing gold and platinum, results in a 25 percent lower density and a cost saving. The fit of castings made from gold-palladium-silver alloys, when compared with Type III gold casting alloys, was similar (*Nitkin* and *Asgar,* 1976). Also *Huget* et al. (1976) found that of three "white gold alloys" tested, their strength and hardness was also comparable with a hardened Type III casting gold. However, as explained previously, high palladium content alloys can absorb hydrogen gases more readily and are not ideal for ceramic bonding. In addition, high silver contents can cause greening of the porcelain. Some patients also object to the lack of gold lustre in the castings but this is not a serious defect.

If a cheaper alternative is required to the gold-platinum alloys, then the gold-palladium-silver alloys appear to be the materials of choice.

Palladium-Silver Alloys

These alloys are relatively new to ceramic bonding and were first marketed in 1974. Palladium-silver alloys contain about 60 percent palladium with the balance being silver. Other elements that are added include indium and tin which harden the alloy by forming a solid solution. There is a geometrical increase in hardness with an increase in tin content (*Tuccillo,* 1977). Palladium-silver alloys have a low density (10.8 gm/cm³) and with their comparatively low metal cost can mean a substantial saving over the gold-platinum alloys. However, their handling properties are not good. The fit of castings is inferior to that of the Type III gold alloys (*Nitkin* and *Asgar,* 1976) and the technique for handling these alloys is more complicated and time-consuming because of the high silver content. Silver may impart a greenish hue to the porcelain by diffusion at the metal/porcelain interface (*Tuccillo,* 1977). The colour may be produced by silver atoms, with a zero charge, forming colloidal silver in the glassy porcelain. This can be accentuated in porcelains with a high soda content such as the metal-ceramic porcelains, since silver diffuses more rapidly in sodium containing glass.

In addition to the above defects, the high palladium content can increase the risk of hydrogen gas absorption.

Mechanical properties of the noble-metal alloys

The mechanical properties required in metal-ceramic type alloys for various types of crown and bridgework have yet to be fully established. However, it is generally agreed that for long span bridgework an alloy should possess both high yield strength and a high modulus of elasticity (stiffness) to avoid stress in the porcelain veneer. Ultimate tensile strength is a measure of the maximum stress which a structure such as a bridge can endure before rupturing but this is not a frequent occurrence in fixed bridgework. Fracture of the joints between crowns and pontics can occur if there is porosity in the casting or when the cross-sectional area of the joints is reduced below 2 mm in a vertical direction.

The mechanical properties of the various noble metal alloys are shown in Table 2-4 and *Moffa* (1977) has rightly drawn attention to the dangers of making generalisations when dealing with groups of alloys. However, as will be discussed later, the mechanical properties of the gold-platinum-palladium alloys are generally satisfactory for all types of crown and bridgework providing attention is paid to the design of the metal substructure.

Nature of the Porcelains used in Metal-Ceramic Systems

Dental porcelains developed for enamelling metals must fulfill certain definite requirements. The coefficient of thermal expansion must be slightly less than that of the metal (14.5×10^{-6} per degree Centigrade) in order to avoid undesirable tensile stresses developing in the enamel on cooling. The mineralogical structure of the porcelain must be maintained during successive bakings of the metal-ceramic crown to avoid problems of devitrification or hydrolytic instability.

The porcelains used in dental metal-ceramic work are similar in nature to the felspathic porcelains described in Monograph I, with the exception of their alkali content and minor additions of other oxides. The soda and potash content of these porcelains is higher than regular porcelain in order to raise the thermal expansion and be compatible with the metal substructure.

Some metal-ceramic porcelains contain leucite ($K_2O\ Al_2O_3\ 4\ SiO_2$) as a crystalline phase. Since leucite is a very high expansion phase (20×10^{-6} per degree Centigrade), its crystallisation in a porcelain made to match the high gold alloys is valuable. Increasing the K_2O (potash) content of the porcelain will move the composition into the leucite field and increase the tendency to crystallise, particularly in the presence of nucleating agents such as TiO_2 as shown below in the composition for the metal-ceramic porcelains. However, this crystallisation can be undesirable if it increases the opacity of the porcelain.

The opaque porcelain that is applied directly to the metal surface will generally approximate to a sodium/potassium felspar-glass flux mixture of the following composition:

				Weight per cent
Silica	SiO_2	Glass former		48.00 – 59.00
Alumina	Al_2O_3	Intermediate		16.30 – 20.00
Potash	K_2O	Alkali-fluxes		8.40 – 10.30
Soda	Na_2O			5.70 – 7.00
Calcium oxide	CaO	Fluxes		1.20 – 1.45
Boric oxide	B_2O_3			1.20 – 1.45
Titania	TiO_2			2.70 – 3.30
Tin oxide	SnO_2	Opacifiers		4.30 – 5.25
Zinc oxide	ZnO_2			1.20 – 1.50
Ferric oxide	Fe_2O_3			Trace
Fluorine	F_2			Trace

The opaque porcelains are heavily loaded with opacifiers in order to mask the metal sub-structure and reduce the thickness of opaque porcelain to the minimum.

Modern "paint-on" opaques can effectively mask the metal when applied in thicknesses as low as 100 μm. However, it should be noted that these materials tend to be highly light reflective and can introduce further problems with regard to their effect on the enamel porcelain's colour.

The dentine and enamel porcelains which cover the opaque layer will also consist of felspathic glasses and may correspond to the following analysis:

		Weight per cent	
Silica	SiO_2	59.2	– 66.2
Alumina	Al_2O_3	14.5	– 18.9
Potash	K_2O	9.5	– 12.3
Soda	Na_2O	4.7	– 9.7
Calcium oxide	CaO	0.4	– 2.10
Titania	TiO_2	0.25	– 0.29
Ferric oxide	Fe_2O_3	0.045	– 0.055
Fluorine	F_2	0.20	– 0.50

It will be noted that boric oxide or lithium oxide are not used as fluxes in the enamels in this case but they may constitute a small proportion of some dental enamels.

Although these enamel porcelains do not differ greatly from regular porcelains, it is important to recognise the influence of the alkali content on the final product. As described in Monograph I, Na^+ ions will disrupt the basic glass-forming network SiO_4, and when used in excess, devitrification of the glass may occur. The high expansion porcelains used in the metal-ceramic technique are therefore always more prone to problems of devitrification since it is essential to raise the alkali content in order to approximate to the alloy's thermal expansion. In addition, a high alkali content can increase the risk of hydrolytic instability.

The earlier porcelains used in metal-ceramic work were very prone to these problems but current products are considerably improved and the manufacturers have achieved a greater grasp of the problem of building stable dental glasses with high thermal expansions. Despite these improvements, none of the current porcelains used in the metal-ceramic technique can withstand repeated firings like regular or aluminous porcelains. The latter materials contain less alkali and in the case of the aluminous porcelain, the high combined alumina content produces a very stable glass, much less prone to devitrification. In addition, the regular or aluminous porcelains are more translucent since they are not formulated to cover metal. For this reason, the use of porcelains made for the metal-ceramic technique is to be strongly deprecated in the construction of the complete porcelain jacket crown. Each porcelain has been formulated for a specific situation and the regular or aluminous porcelains will give better results in the all ceramic restoration.

The Nature of the Metal-Ceramic Bond

The success of metal-ceramic crowns and fixed bridges depends upon the firmness of the bond between metal and ceramic. In order to appreciate the nature of this bond it is essential to consider all the stages of applying and baking porcelain to noble-metal alloys. The following description has been over-simplified but may assist in clarifying an area which has become somewhat confused.

Stage I. The metal coping or bridge sub-structure is cleaned by sand-blasting or steam cleaning the surface and then finally placed in an ultra-sonic cleaning bath. The roughened surface produced by sand-blasting provides an easily wettable surface and will assist in mechanical retention of the porcelain enamel.

Stage II. The metal is de-gassed by heating to 1000 °C in vacuo for around ten minutes and then slowly air-cooled in normal atmosphere. This procedure will not only de-gas the casting but also induce some age-hardening in the alloy (Fig. 2-6). At the same time, base metal atoms will diffuse to the surface of the metal and form an oxide film (e.g. Indium, tin or zinc oxide).

Stage III. An opaque porcelain slurry is applied to the surface of the casting so that an even and thin layer is formed. The metal and opaque porcelain are then slowly oven-dried and the o-paque porcelain will shrink onto the metal surface.

Stage IV. The opaque porcelain on the metal is introduced into the hot zone of the furnace and "lensing" and initial sintering of the grains of porcelain will occur. At this stage the porcelain will start to wet the face of the metal and, depending upon the efficiency of wetting, surface tension effects will come into play. The term *"van der Waals"* forces or wetting bonds have been used to describe these adhesive forces. However, whatever the nature of this wetting action, the main driving force is surface tension. It is known that the surface tension of a liquid is associated with the tendency to wet the surface on which it is in contact. The angle between the solid-liquid vector determines the wetting and the smaller this angle, the better will the molten porcelain wet the solid metal. If the wetting is efficient, the porcelain will enter all the minute irregularities on the metal surface and some mechanical interlocking must occur. In addition, base metal atoms will continue to diffuse to the surface of the metal by bulk diffusion and the oxide film will provide means for chemical bonding with the porcelain.

Stage V. The opaque porcelain is then raised to its final maturing temperature of around 930 °C to 960 °C. At this stage the porcelain will continue to shrink through sintering and pore elimination. During the firing cycle (sintering) of porcelain, at no time does the porcelain become molten or fluid, except for a 25 μm film of glaze that appears on the surface at the glaze temperature. Resultantly the porcelain exerts an increasingly restrictive effect on the expansion of the gold alloy that it surrounds (*Vickery* and *Badinelli,* 1968). On cooling, the gold will attempt to return to its original dimensions and because its expansion is greater than the porcelain it will contract faster than the porcelain. The gold, in trying to contract faster than the porcelain, will be placed under tension and the porcelain under compression.

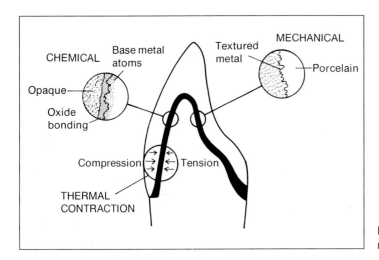

Fig. 2-7 Components of Cera-mo-Metallic Bond.

Stage VI. The enamel and dentine porcelain veneer is now applied and sintered to maximum density. This process will repeat all the stages of firing the opaque and similar compressive forces will be developed during shrinkage and cooling of the enamel porcelains. A gradation of thermal expansion coefficients from the enamel glaze to the opaque porcelain will further strengthen the entire ceramic body.

A study of all the stages of baking a metal-ceramic crown will reveal a fairly complicated system of bonding. The nature of this ceramo-metallic bond may be divided into the following components (Fig. 2-7).

Mechanical – Surface tension provides intimate contact of porcelain with all the micro-surface irregularities of the metal. Stage IV and V.

Chemical – Bulk diffusion of base metal atoms produces an oxide film on the metal surface which forms a chemical bond with the porcelain. Stage IV and V.

Compression – Sintering shrinkage and thermal contraction of the porcelain will be resisted by the metal and compressive stresses will be

set up in the porcelain. The porcelain will be firmly bonded to the metal. Stage V and VI.

Evidence to support the above components of the ceramo-metallic bond has become available through a number of investigations on the nature of the bond and these will now be discussed in detail.

Methods of Testing Bond Strength

The accurate measurement of the bond strength at the ceramo-metallic junction presents formidable problems, since the complexity of the bonding probably defies the development of a single test experiment.

Mechanical retention will be affected by the nature of the metal surface, i.e. surface contamination and degrees of roughness. Chemical bonding will be influenced by the trace elements incorporated in the alloy and the degree of wetting by the porcelain. Compression retention will depend upon the geometry of the metal substructure and the correct matching of the thermal expansions of both metal and porcelain.

Several tests have been used to assess the strength of the ceramo-metallic bond in dental

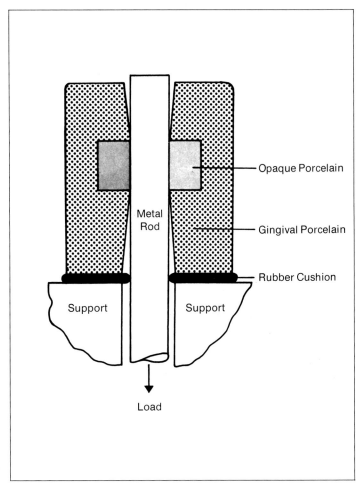

Fig. 2-8 Diagrammatic cross-section of the shear test specimen for determining the strength of the ceramo-metallic bond (after *Shell, J. S.,* and *Nielsen, J. P.* (1962) J. Dent. Res. 41, 32.

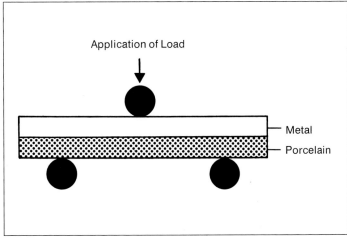

Fig. 2-9 Diagrammatic cross-section of the bend test specimen used for determining the strength of the ceramo-metallic bond (after *Lavine, M. H.,* and *Custer, F.* (1966) J. Dent. Res. 45, 32.

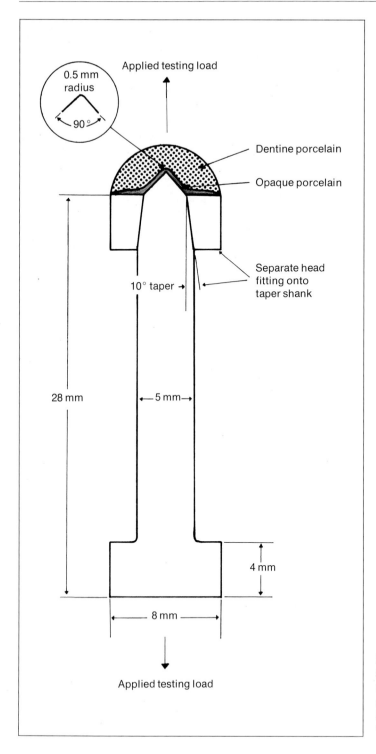

0.5 mm radius

90°

Applied testing load

Dentine porcelain

Opaque porcelain

Separate head fitting onto taper shank

10° taper →

28 mm

← 5 mm →

4 mm

← 8 mm →

Applied testing load

Fig. 2-10 Diagrammatic cross-section of the tensile test specimen for determining the strength of the ceramo-metallic bond (after *Sced, I. R.,* and *McLean, J. W.,* 1972, Brit. dent. J. 132, 232).

restorations. *Shell* and *Nielsen* (1962) devised a test in which a 14 G wire (1.63 mm dia.) was embedded in a block of porcelain to a depth of about 2.5 mm and the stress to pull it out was measured (Fig. 2-8). Exact matching of the gold and porcelain thermal expansion coefficients was claimed and a bond composed of 30 % *van der Waal's* wetting forces with the remaining chemical forces (a mixture of "ionic, covalent and metallic bonds") with no contribution from mechanical retention was proposed. Another test devised by *Lavine* and *Custer* (1966) used a flat strip of metal with the porcelain baked onto the tensile face which was then tested for transverse strength (Modulus of Rupture) (Fig. 2-9). *Knapp* and *Ryge* (1966) used a different approach and strained a porcelain-coated alloy rod and then measured the energy to initiate and propagate fracture. *Sced* and *McLean* (1972) designed a test piece based on a standard metallurgical tensile test piece, except for the modification of the metal face which was made conical in order to place the bond in the direction of maximum shear stress (Fig. 2-10).

However, none of these test methods can be regarded as ideal and the problem of residual stresses interfering with the results must be taken into account. The selection of the best test piece is therefore a question of deciding which one produces the least amount of residual stress at the bond.

Choice of Test Piece Design

A cylindrical pull-out test such as that due to *Shell* and *Nielsen* (1962) is open to criticism due to the possible retentive effect of thermal expansion mismatch stresses. This is due to the fact that the conditions laid down by *Shell* and *Nielsen* namely, that no thermal stresses develop due to differences in thermal expansion, cannot be generally achieved since:

a) Exact matching of the expansion coefficients of alloys and porcelain over a temperature range is unlikely.

b) Practical systems are generally designed with a small mismatch so as to leave the porcelain under slight compression.

In this case the thermally induced hoop stress in the *Shell-Nielsen* test would be similar to the state of affairs in a shrink fitted collar although of reverse sign, and an estimate of residual stress could be made on this basis. The hoop stress, however, has no component in the direction of the applied stress during testing so its calculation is of little value. There is, unfortunately, no simple calculation for determining the longitudinal stress in a collar which is the one which would contribute to the pull-out stress. Therefore, it is not possible to calculate accurately, the effect of thermal expansion mismatch in this case.

The transverse test used by *Lavine* and *Custer* (1966) is subject to criticism since the maximum tensile stress in the system is at the surface of the porcelain and it is likely that failure will initiate here. The bond itself is under a considerably lower tensile stress as it is near the neutral plane where the stress is zero, and by suitable dimensional adjustment of test-piece the bond could even be in compression.

The porcelain-coated rod test of *Knapp* and *Ryge* (1966) would also be subject to errors introduced by residual stresses, as in the *Shell-Nielsen* test. The modified metallurgical test-piece design of *Sced* and *McLean* (1972) is not entirely free from the problem of residual stresses. The contribution of residual stress to the test result should, however, be smaller than in the *Shell-Nielsen* test although it must be assumed that there will be some stress contribution arising from the algebraic sum in the testing direction of the residual stresses in the porcelain.

All the present tests can only give a measure of the strength of a metal-ceramic system under a defined state of loading. It is unlikely that any test can be devised which will give an absolute measure of the adhesion of porcelain to metal except in cases where the adhesion strength is lower than the tensile strength of the porcelain and the metal/porcelain couple is so exactly thermally matched as to be stress-free.

Results of Testing Bond Strengths

Vickery and *Badinelli* (1968) have discussed the gold porcelain bond in some detail and their conclusion that the strength of the bond is the sum of a number of components probably provides a realistic picture of the practical situation, although the magnitude and distribution of these components are questionable. Their conclusions regarding the contribution of *van der Waal's* forces do not agree with those of some earlier workers (*Ryge,* 1965; *O'Brien* and *Ryge,* 1965), who by contact angle measurement concluded that "wetting bonds" in one instance and *van der Waal's* forces in the other could adequately explain observed strengths. The concept of *van der Waal's* forces seems to be open to misinterpretation when applied to porcelain bonding and one would not expect their contribution to be large since such forces are inherently small (*McLean* and *Sced,* 1973).

There is, however, considerable evidence for some form of chemical bonding. *Nally, Monnier* and *Meyer* (1968), after electron microprobe examination, proposed that indium migrated to the alloy surface forming indium oxide which combined with the porcelain during firing. Similar work (*Szantho, von Radnoth* and *Leutenschlager,* 1969), elsewhere on a different alloy, showed the presence of a tin oxide layer which was thought to contribute to the bonding mechanism. *Knapp* and *Ryge* (1966) also concluded that the bond strength was improved in an oxidising atmosphere. By contrast, when the alloy surface was depleted of oxide, the bond strength was reduced by 30 percent (*Anthony* et al., 1970).

If a good bond has been achieved, the breaking stress should approximate to the tensile strength of opaque porcelain and *Nally* (1969)

has given a figure of 25 N/mm² for the tensile strength of one brand of European porcelain.

Experiments conducted by *McLean* and *Sced* (1973) support the above evidence and indicate that a base metal oxide, when formed at the gold alloy interface, has an important function in producing a good bond. High fusing gold-platinum-palladium alloy test specimens in Group A (Table 2-5) illustrate the ideal state of affairs where fracture has occurred through the porcelain. By contrast, those specimens in Group B which had been cleaned in 5% hydrofluoric acid, were considerably weaker due to the removal of the surface oxide by the acid. Resultantly, failure of the bond occurred predominantly at the metal/porcelain interface. The difference in fracture characteristics between Groups A and B are illustrated in Figs. 2-11 and 2-12. Further support to the chemical bonding theory is lent by a study of Fig. 2-13 showing a microsection of a gold alloy/porcelain bond. Evidence of internal oxidation near to the metal surface is clear. It should also be noted that removal of the oxidisable elements from the surface by acid etching will hinder the further formation of oxide. When such specimens were re-machined to expose fresh metal and allow formation of the oxide film, the test results (Group C) once again compared favourably with those in Group A.

The effectiveness of the wetting of a sand-blasted metal surface by the porcelain is also illustrated in Fig. 2-13 and the increase in surface area provided by a slightly rough surface may also improve the bonding. However, it should be noted that very rough surfaces, producing sharp re-entrant angles, might increase the stress concentration at the bond (*Kelly* et al., 1969) so the use of coarse stones is to be deprecated. The ideal surface is one that has been finally textured with Aluminium oxide grit (30 μm).

Although there is still some confusion and controversy over the nature of the ceramo-metallic bond, a number of points can be made.

Table 2-5 Bond Strength of High-fusing Gold-Platinum-Palladium Alloy/Porcelain Specimens

Specimen Group	Specimen type and treatment	No. of tests	Mean breaking stress N/mm²	p.s.i.	Standard deviation	Remarks
A	Conical-ended outgassed for 2 hrs. at 900 °C and better than 10^{-3} torr.	6	29.4	2,027	2.16	Failure through porcelain near to interface. No porosity in porcelain.
B	Group C outgassed as Group A and again cleaned with 5 % HF.	6	18.5	1,272	0.98	Failure predominantly at metal/porcelain interface. Slight porosity.
C	Conical-ended specimens remachined to expose fresh metal. Outgassed as Group A.	12	28.0	1,930	7.05	Failure through porcelain near to interface. Standard deviation increased by two exceptionally low test results. Standard deviation of high group only = 2.14 (mean 30.4)

1. Base metal additions to the gold alloys contribute to the bonding process by forming a surface oxide film which reacts with the porcelain and brings it into atomic contact with the metal. Reaction here does not necessarily mean formation of an identifiable compound but rather a disappearance of the interface by interdiffusion between oxide and porcelain. Chemical etching of the surface of the alloy immediately prior to porcelain application is therefore highly undesirable.

2. Good wetting of the metal or metal oxide by the porcelain is essential. In the case of the gold alloys, wetting by the porcelain is excellent. It is likely, therefore, that surface roughness will contribute to the bond strength by increasing the surface area of the bond and possibly by providing a "keying" effect, thus resisting shear stresses. Current practice of texturing the metal with 30 μm Al_2O_3 appears to provide a good surface for retention of the porcelain. Excessive roughening of the surface could prove detrimental by providing undesirable stress concentration at the bond.

3. In practical systems the contribution of residual stresses due to slight thermal expansion mismatch of the alloy and porcelain could be significant in providing residual compressive stresses in the porcelain, thus requiring the application of higher stresses in service before tensile failure at the bond could be initiated. These residual stresses must not be too high, otherwise they could contribute to failure of the bond.

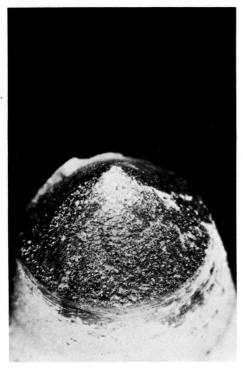

Fig. 2-11   Fracture surface of a gold alloy specimen showing considerable retention of porcelain. Conical-ended testpiece after the design of *Sced* and *McLean* Fig. 2-10. (Mag × 20 approx.)

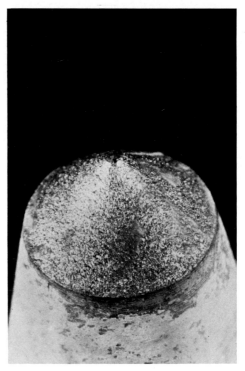

Fig. 2-12   Fracture surface of conical-ended gold alloy test-piece previously cleaned in HF for re-use. Considerable exposure of metal surface is evident with little retention of porcelain. (Mag × 25 approx.)

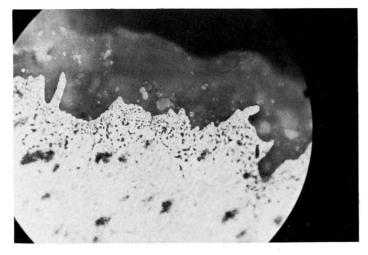

Fig. 2-13   Oblique microsection through a gold alloy/porcelain bond showing good wetting of the metal by the porcelain, and internal oxidation in the alloy adjacent to the bond. Mag × 700 (from *McLean, J. W.,* and *Sced, I. R.* (1973). The gold-alloy/porcelain bond. Trans. Brit. Ceram. Soc., 5:229.

The current evidence on metal-ceramic bonding confirms that the bond can be divided into the three categories of compression, chemical, and mechanical bonding. The assignment of definite figures or percentages to each one of these components will be a matter of controversy for some time.

From a clinical standpoint, it is probably more important to examine the type of fracture in a metal/porcelain system, e.g. interfacial or through the porcelain. In the absence of tensile failure through the porcelain, the clinical safety of any metal/ceramic system must be suspect since the maximum possible strength is not being achieved and is likely to be variable, depending on the precise conditions of preparation of the restoration.

furnace vacuum is reasonably effective if held at temperature (1000 °C) for at least ten minutes.

3. Sandblasting the casting with 30 μm Aluminium oxide aids in mechanical retention of the porcelain without producing high stress concentration at the bond.
4. Do not use strong acid etching to clean the casting after preparatory treatment. Acid etching will reduce the amount of surface oxide available for chemical bonding.
5. Do not contaminate the casting with the fingers or any other contaminant prior to applying the porcelain.

Technical Considerations

Noble-Metal Alloy Systems

If a good bond has been achieved between porcelain and metal, the breaking stress should approximate to the tensile strength of the opaque porcelain and any fracture should occur through the porcelain. The technical requirements for achieving a strong bond are as follows:

1. Do not use large quantities of old metal in which depletion of the base metals has taken place. Use at least 50 percent new metal for every casting.
2. Outgassing of the metal in vacuo is essential. Failure to outgas the alloy may result in a high degree of porosity at the porcelain bond which reduces the effective load bearing cross-section. High vacuum (better than 10^{-3} torr) is ideal but the standard dental

Base Metal Alloy/Porcelain Systems

The satisfactory nature of the gold alloy/porcelain bond has been confirmed by experimental and clinical experience. However, with the rising cost of precious metal and the demand for stronger alloys with greater creep resistance when the porcelain is applied, the interest in base metal alloys is increasing. These alloys are all based on either nickel chromium or cobalt-chromium and typical analyses and mechanical properties are given in Table 2-6 a and b.

Poggioli et al. (1968) have studied the following alloys:

a) austenitic Fe-Cr alloy
b) austenitic Fe-Cr alloy + Ta + Nb
c) a Ni-Cr-Mo alloy
d) a Co-Cr stellite + 10 percent Ni.

They found that the nickel-base alloy was best, forming a strong bond with several opaque porcelains, whereas the stellite formed a weak bond and failed by detachment along the metal/

Table 2-6 a

Typical Analyses of Base-Metal Alloys

Cobalt-Chromium		Nickel-Chromium	
Co	65.8	Ni	67.1
Cr	26.7	Cr	17.1
Mo	5.2	Co	0.39
W	0.65	Mo	4.85
Mn	0.98	Mn	3.86
Ni	0.54	Mg	0.19
Fe	0.1−0.5	Al	4.75
Si	0.90	Si	0.75
Cu	up to 0.10	Be*	1.00
C	0.49	C	0.014
		Fe	0.002−0.05
		Ti	0.01−0.05
		Cu	0.01−0.10

* Beryllium omitted in some alloys.

Table 2-6 b

Physical and Mechanical Properties of Base-Metal Alloys

Properties	Beryllium Containing		Non-Beryllium	
Tensile strength, N/mm² (p.s.i.)	778−1350	(112,800−196,000)	539−919	(78,200−133,300)
Yield strength N/mm² (p.s.i.)	466−838	(67,600−121,500)	260−858	(37,700−124,400)
Modulus of Elasticity N/mm² (p.s.i.)	$165-210 \times 10^3$	$(24.000-30.4 \times 10^6)$	$141-248 \times 10^3$	$(20.5-36 \times 10^6)$
Per cent Elongation	3.0−23.9		2.3−32.6	
Vickers Hardness	307−357		175−436	
Density g/cm²	7.9−8.7		7.9−8.7	

After *Moffa, J. P.*, 1977, Physical and Mechanical Properties of Gold and Base-Metal Alloys. NIH Conference Proceedings.

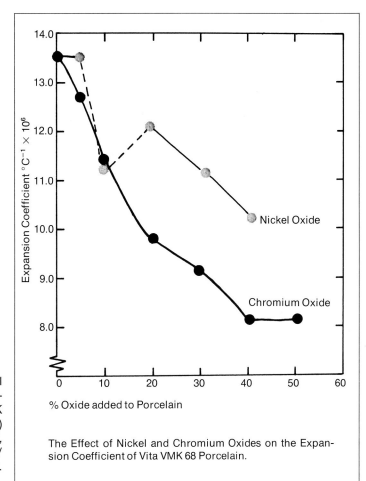

Fig. 2-14 The effect of Nickel and Chromium oxides on the expansion coefficient of Vita VMK 68 porcelain (20 °C – 600 °C) (from *McLean, J. W.,* and *Sced, I. R.* (1973). The base-metal alloy/porcelain bond. Trans. Brit. Ceram. Soc. 5:235.

The Effect of Nickel and Chromium Oxides on the Expansion Coefficient of Vita VMK 68 Porcelain.

metal oxide interface. They concluded that, in practical prostheses, design played a considerable part in preventing fracture and agreed with *Vickery* and *Badinelli* (1968) that much of the strength of the bond was due to compressive stresses set up by the small thermal mismatch between porcelain and metal.

The evaluation of the shear bond strength of noble metal and base metal alloys by *Moffa* et al. (1973) showed that there was no difference between the two base metal alloys and that both values were significantly higher than that for the control gold-based alloy.

A later study by *Lubovich* and *Goodkind* (1977) on three base metal alloys, produced bond strengths smaller than or in excess of those of traditional gold-based alloys. These studies indicate that great variations can occur in recorded bond strengths of the base metal alloys and could be related to either the method of test, differences in metal casting and preparation, or differences in the dental porcelains used.

Some light has been shed on this problem in a study by *McLean* and *Sced* (1973) showing that the strength of the bond between dental porcelain and base metal alloys containing chromium or nickel is adversely influenced by the formation of chromium or nickel oxide. When these oxides are combined in the dental porcelain, they reduce the thermal expansion coefficient of the porcelain (Fig. 2-14) thus incurring the danger of a high degree of residual stress at the bond. In addition, it was found that if oxidation of the base metal alloy was suppressed by atmosphere control, direct chemical reduction of some constituents of the porcelain by chromium is still likely, with chromium oxide as one of the products. If hydrogen atmosphere was used it would probably reduce K_2O at 1000°C, whilst chromium metal is likely to reduce K_2O Na_2O and SnO_2. This reduction process is also likely to occur in dental practice since, once the porcelain matures, the bond interface is effectively shielded from the furnace atmosphere. Any reaction would therefore be independent of the oxidising potential of this atmosphere. This probably explains a frequent complaint that in base-metal porcelain systems the metal "shows through". It is not, in fact, the metal that is seen, but a region of the porcelain containing the products of reduction which appear grey in colour (Fig. 2-15).

Bond Strength of Base Metal Alloy/Porcelain Systems

Because of the high degree of residual stress at the bond, the bond strength of both cobalt and nickel-chromium alloys may appear to be higher than the gold alloys when fired in oxidising atmosphere and the mean breaking stress can be above that at which tensile failure of the porcelain occurs with gold alloys (McLean and Sced, 1973). However, such results can be misleading since the high degree of residual stress created at the bond by the lowering of the thermal expansion by chromium oxide must be accounted for. If this residual stress was acting in opposition to the applied stress it would be necessary to overcome it before a positive

stress was applied and the indicated load at failure could be misleadingly high.

Although the bond strength of the base metal alloy/porcelain systems can be as high as 36 N/mm^2 when tested as in Fig. 2-10, the type of fracture, for example, through the porcelain or interfacial, may be as important as the actual strength. Base metal alloy systems generally break at the interface (Fig. 2-16) whereas the gold alloys usually exhibit a cohesive fracture in the porcelain (Fig. 2-11). In the absence of tensile failure through the porcelain as in the gold alloy systems, the clinical safety of any metal-ceramic system must be suspect since the maximum possible strength is not being achieved and is likely to be variable depending on the precise conditions of preparation of the restoration.

Types of Metal/Porcelain Failure

Classification of ceramo/metal failures has been made by O'Brien (1977) and is related to the interfaces formed at fracture (Fig. 2-17).

1. Metal-Porcelain

The interfacial fracture occurs leaving a clean surface of metal. This type of fracture is generally seen when the metal surface is totally depleted of oxide prior to baking the porcelain or when no oxides are available. It may also be due to contaminated or porous metal surfaces.

2. Metal Oxide-Porcelain

The porcelain fractures at the metal oxide surface, leaving the oxide firmly attached to the metal. This is a common type of failure in the base metal alloy system.

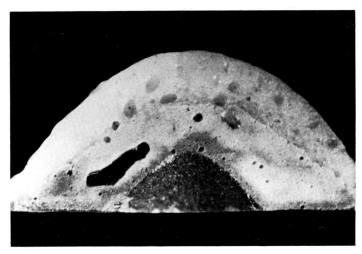

Fig. 2-15 Section through porcelain removed from conical-ended test-piece cast in nickel-chromium alloy after firing in vacuo. Darkening of the opaque porcelain adjacent to the original metal/porcelain interface shows the extent of interaction between metal and porcelain caused by diffusion of chromium ions. Mag × 8 approx. (from *Sced, I. R.,* and *McLean, J. W.,* 1972). The Strength of Metal/Ceramic Bonds with Base Metals Containing Chromium. Brit. dent. J. 132, 232.

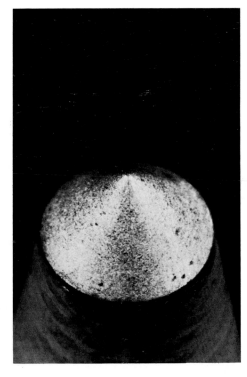

Fig. 2-16 Fracture surface of a conical-ended test-piece cast in nickel-chromium alloy showing no retention of the porcelain and a classical interfacial fracture. (Mag × 20 approx.)

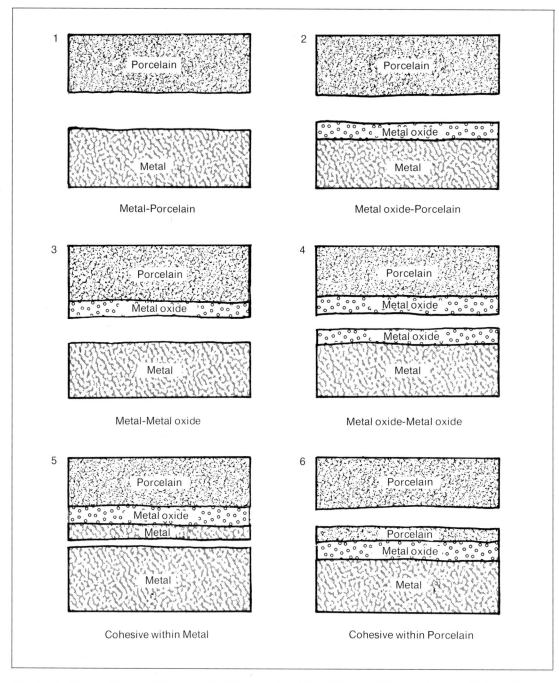

Fig. 2-17 Type of Bond Failure in Metal-Ceramic. After *O'Brien, W. J.* Cohesive Plateau Theory of Porcelain-Alloy Bonding. Conference Proceeding. University of Southern California. 1977. Dental Porcelain. State of the Art.

3. Metal-Metal Oxide

This is an interfacial fracture in which the metal oxide breaks away from the metal substrate and is left attached to the porcelain. This is a common cause of failure in the base metal alloy systems when there is over-production of chromium and nickel oxide at the interface.

4. Metal Oxide-Metal Oxide

This fracture occurs through the metal oxide at the interface and results from an over-production of oxide causing a sandwich effect between metal and porcelain.

5. Cohesive within Metal

This type of fracture would only occur in cases, for example, where the joint area in bridges breaks. It is a most unlikely type of fracture for the individual metal-ceramic crown.

6. Cohesive within Porcelain

This is the optimum type of fracture in which tensile failure occurs within the porcelain. In this case the bond strength exceeds the strength of the porcelain. An ideal situation is created when the oxide film is only a few molecules thick and forms a solid solution with the porcelain. This is the most common type of fracture in the high gold content alloys, confirming their consistent clinical results.

Prolonged or repeated firing of a metal-ceramic crown can cause excessive dissolution of the oxide layer in the glassy porcelain. In this instance, tensile failure could still occur in the porcelain and not reveal the residual stresses at the bond interface caused by differential thermal expansion. Fractures of this type may occur with the base metal alloys.

In view of the effect of the oxide formation at the metal interface on the porcelain's expansion, it is clear that any future metal systems must incorporate base metals which produce oxides that will conform to the following requirements:

1. The oxide should form only a very thin layer on the alloy but still be sufficient to bring the porcelain into atomic contact with the metal.

2. The oxide should have good adhesion to the alloy surface.

3. The oxide should react with the porcelain but in doing so must not appreciably alter those characteristics of the porcelain which are important to the success of the final product, e.g. thermal expansion, strength, colour, and opacity.

In the case of indium or tin oxides which are formed on gold based alloys, their properties conform to the above requirements. Chromium oxide, which is the main constituent of the oxidation product in chromium bearing base-metal alloy, does not, and this must place the use of base metal alloys for porcelain bonding in question. It must also be recognised that in order to produce a corrosion-resistant alloy, a high level of chromium is almost essential to any base-metal alloy.

Although many thousands of base metal alloy/ceramic crowns have been placed, it is possible that at any time the high degree of residual stress at the bond may be the cause of sudden and catastrophic failure.

Effect of the Degree of Oxidation and Cooling Rate on the Strength of the Bond

It has been established that there is no definite correlation between the degree of pre-oxidation and bond strength of the base metal alloys other than the more highly pre-oxidised specimens tend to be stronger (*McLean* and *Sced*, 1973). However, despite this higher strength, interfacial fracture of the porcelain always oc-

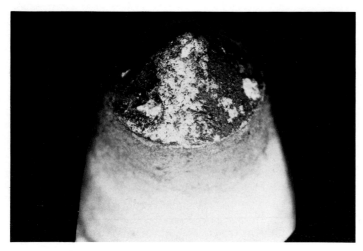

Fig. 2-18 Fracture surface of a conical-ended test-piece cast in cobalt-chromium alloy which was given a prolonged pre-oxidation period. Considerable reaction of the porcelain with the metal oxides has occurred and detachment of the porcelain has revealed a strong greenish oxide layer. Mag × 20 approx. (from *Sced, I. R., Hopkins, B. E.,* and *McLean, J. W.,* 1970. Report on the Strength of Metal to Porcelain Fused Bonds as used in Dental Restorations, National Physical Laboratory, England.)

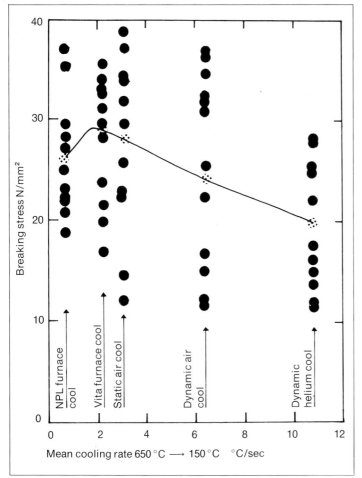

Breaking stress N/mm^2

NPL furnace cool

Vita furnace cool

Static air cool

Dynamic air cool

Dynamic helium cool

Mean cooling rate 650 °C ⟶ 150 °C   °C/sec

Fig. 2-19 The effect of cooling rate on the strength of the bond between a cobalt-chromium alloy and Vita VMK 68 Porcelain. (From *McLean, J. W.,* and *Sced, I. R.* (1973). The Base-Metal Alloy/Porcelain Bond. Trans. Brit. Ceram. Soc. 5:235.

curred, leaving considerable amounts of greenish oxide on the surface of the metal (Fig. 2-18).

The effect of cooling rates on the bond strength does have an effect. A steady fall in strength has been observed with higher cooling rates (Fig. 2-19). This may be the direct consequence of higher residual stresses relaxing by crack formation during, or soon after cooling. At the fastest cooling rate (dynamic helium cool) cracking extended right through the porcelain and was easily visible. These results do not give strong support to the theory of strengthening by deliberate induction of internal stress. The increase in mean breaking stress for a cooling rate of 2.1 °C/sec had a significance of 85 % when compared with that for the lowest cooling rate. One must conclude, therefore, that to deliberately try and introduce high residual stresses either by increasing the expansion mismatch or the cooling rate would be a dangerous practice, since the margin between any slight benefit and the introduction of permanent damage is narrow.

An ideal cooling rate should be one in which the crown is allowed to cool slowly at the muffle entrance of a dental furnace. Dynamic air-cooling in which the crown is removed too soon from the furnace aperture is highly detrimental (Fig. 2-19).

Technical Considerations –
Base-Metal Alloy Systems

It is apparent that the base-metal alloy systems are technique sensitive and the question is "How do we control oxide production so that consistent bonding of porcelain may be obtained?" Successful bonding of porcelain to base-metal alloys is very dependent upon both casting and firing techniques. A clean and homogeneous casting is the basic requirement for successful work. Spruing of the pattern should satisfy the following criteria:

1. Sprues should be within the thermal centre of the mould with the pattern close to the orbital plane.
2. No sharp angles – glass smooth surfaces.
3. All facial margins of single units facing the same direction and trailing the direction of the thrust of the casting machine.
4. Sprues must be attached to the thickest section of the pattern.
5. For adequate feed of metal, sprues should be 3.5 mm in diameter and taper slightly as they enter the mould. The restricted throat will prevent back pressure or premature cooling in the sprueway.
6. Sprues should fan out from a central reservoir and allow uninterrupted flow of metal directly into the pattern. Runner bars are contraindicated since they alter the path of metal flow and cause turbulence.

After casting and finishing, the base-metal copings should be thoroughly cleaned by sandblasting with 30 μm aluminium oxide grit and then by steam cleaning. Porcelain should be applied immediately on the metal surface before the casting can become contaminated. After the opaque porcelain is applied, the cardinal point to bear in mind is that vitrification must be rapid and complete before a thick oxide layer can form and interfere with bonding. The use of metal firing trays to improve thermal conduction, and furnace muffles with even heat distribution will assist the technician. Short firing cycles of one or two minutes are also recommended and opaque porcelains which can vitrify in this time are now available. Enamel and dentine porcelains should be applied with the minimum number of bakes.

Work is now in progress to try and eliminate excessive oxide formation, or reduction of the porcelain by base-metal constituents, by using various coating agents. One such material* utilizes aluminium powder blended with a ceramic frit as the coating agent. Presumably it is intended that the aluminium competes with the nickel and chromium for oxygen, thus preventing rapid oxidation of the base-metal alloy. This is an interesting approach and merits further investigation. However, the exact role of aluminium oxide has yet to be established since during oxidation it could weaken the glass interface or form a porous weak interlayer.

Other methods which may also be of some interest rely on the electro-deposition of a precious metal, such as gold or rhodium on the surface of the base-metal casting. In this case it is hoped that the precious metal surface will act as a barrier to any oxide formation. Bonding to the porcelain would then be achieved by electro-deposition of a thin coating of tin on the surface of the precious metal which is subsequently oxidised during porcelain application (*McLean* and *Sced,* 1976).

Despite all these improvements in technique and surface bonding, a further criticism must be levelled at the base-metal alloy systems. The casting fit of the current materials still remains in doubt and *Nitkin* and *Asgar* (1976) concluded that in terms of fit, base-metal castings were inferior to castings made from high or low gold content alloys. However, they rightly concluded that base-metal alloys show potential despite the poor results obtained and they considered that two areas of technology needed improving. Firstly, improved casting techniques such as induction casting and, secondly, the development of a different type of investment with higher expansion.

In addition to the above requirements, it may also be desirable to develop opaque porcelains that cannot be reduced by nickel or chromium ions.

* Ceramalloy. Ceramco Inc., New Jersey.

From the clinician's point of view he must recognise that when using base-metal alloys, he will probably sacrifice some fit and that aesthetically the metal is not ideal in colour. In addition, the technique sensitivity of these materials demands greater skill from the ceramist and any failure to follow precisely the correct procedures or submitting the metal-ceramic restoration to too many bakes could result in bond failure. On the other hand, the base-metal alloys can be used in thinner section and show almost negligible metal creep on firing the porcelain (*Moffa* et al., 1973).

Further clinical requirements need to be taken into account, for example when removing a crown or bridge. In the case of the base-metal alloys, this presents a formidable problem.

Evaluation of Metal-Ceramic Systems

The development of metal-ceramic systems in dentistry imposes severe disciplines, and good aesthetics are obviously a high priority. If a strong bond between metal and porcelain is to be achieved which also satisfies aesthetic demands, then a metal-ceramic system should meet the following requirements:

Oxide Formation

1. Good wetting of the metal or metal oxide by the porcelain is essential.
2. The oxide should be soluble in the porcelain.
3. The oxides formed on the surface of the metal should not discolour the porcelain or interfere with glass formation.
4. The metal or metal oxides should not react in any way so as to reduce the strength of the

porcelain or introduce high internal stresses, e.g. by raising or lowering the thermal expansion of the interfacial porcelain.

5. The metal or metal oxide should not corrode or produce toxic effects in surrounding tissue.

Strength and Castability

The metal should be clinically acceptable both in regard to castability, accuracy of fit and appearance. It should also exhibit minimal creep during firing of the porcelain and possess adequate mechanical strength for multiple splinting and bridgework. The relationship between the mechanical and physical properties of the metals used in porcelain bonding and clinical requirements are as follows:

1. Yield Strength

The stresses placed on the porcelain will be reduced if the metal resists plastic deformation during function. A high yield strength will also allow the use of thinner sections of metal but the strength must be at least 50 percent above that of the gold-platinum alloys before any significant clinical advantages are obtained.

2. Modulus of Elasticity

Alloys with a high modulus of elasticity will also reduce stress on the porcelain. However, if the modulus is very high the stresses developing in the porcelain during cooling cannot be easily relieved by metal deformation so that cracking problems can become more serious. Deformation of the metal if too high can, of course, affect the fit of the casting.

3. Creep or "sag-resistance"

The metal framework in a metal-ceramic combination must not melt during firing of the porcelain. In addition it must also resist thermally induced stresses which can cause the metal to creep or "sag". Resistance to metal creep is obviously related to the melting temperature of the alloy and generally those alloys with higher melting temperatures will resist distortion better during firing of the porcelain. Precipitation hardening is also another way of improving resistance to creep at high temperatures.

4. Hardness

A material with a high hardness is usually more difficult to grind, polish and adjust in the dental laboratory. The high gold content alloys are therefore the easiest materials to finish.

5. Burnishability

Accuracy of fit not only depends upon castability but also the ease with which the metal can be burnished. A metal margin may only be burnished if the operator can overcome the inherent yield strength in the metal and the metal also has a reasonably high elongation percent. Burnishability is thought to depend on yield strength, elongation percent, rate of strain hardening and the modulus of elasticity.

An assessment of the various metal-ceramic systems and how they meet the above requirements may now be made.

Gold-platinum-palladium alloys

Advantages

Excellent bonding to porcelain. The permanency of the bond has been well established experimentally and clinically.

Good castability and will reproduce fine margins.

Easily finished and polished.

Corrosion resistant and non-toxic.

Yield strength and modulus of elasticity adequate for most types of crown and bridgework.

Excellent for reproducing occlusal surfaces.

Disadvantages

Low sag or "creep" resistance, can distort at fine margins or warp on long span bridges during porcelain firing.
Yield strength and modulus of elasticity can be inadequate on long span bridges unless used in fairly thick section.
High cost.

Gold-palladium-silver alloys

Advantages

Higher melting range (ca. 1200 °C – 1260 °C) produces better sag or creep resistance than the gold-platinum alloys (*Moffa*, 1977).
Yield strength can be higher in some brands than gold-platinum alloys.
Modulus of elasticity higher than the gold-platinum alloys. Useful in long span bridgework.
Good castability and will reproduce fine edges.
Easily finished and polished.
Will reproduce occlusal surfaces accurately.
Non-Toxic.
Lower cost.

Disadvantages

Higher palladium content can increase the risk of gases being entrapped in the casting and spoil the porcelain bonding. High silver content may cause greening of porcelain.
Bonding to porcelain not yet well established clinically or experimentally.
Some patients object to white colour and metal collars tend to show through grey in the mouth.

Palladium-silver alloys

Advantages

High yield strength and modulus of elasticity, suitable for long span bridges.
Non-toxic.
Low cost.

Disadvantages

Difficult to cast accurately. Does not reproduce fine margins like the high gold alloys (*Nitkin* and *Asgar,* 1976).
High silver content can interfere with bonding of porcelain and may cause discolouration.
High palladium content can increase problems of gassing at interface.
Patients may object to colour and metal collars show through grey in the mouth.

Base-metals
Nickel-chromium alloys

Advantages

Modulus of elasticity 2 to 2.5 times higher than the gold alloys.
Yield strength can be higher than the gold alloys but non-beryllium alloys can be significantly lower in strength than the gold alloys.
Low cost.

Disadvantages

Very difficult to cast accurately.
Margins may be short and the surface rougher.
Bonding of porcelain and its colour can be affected by oxide production. Permanence of bond not yet established experimentally or clinically.
Can be toxic in nickel-sensitive patients.
Patients may object to colour and metal collars can look black in the mouth.
Alloys with very high yield strengths cannot be burnished easily and are difficult to finish. (N.B. These are usually beryllium-containing alloys).
More difficult to remove from teeth than the gold alloys.

An examination of the advantages and disadvantages of the alloys used for ceramic bonding still shows that the gold-platinum-palladium alloys offer the most advantages. The permanency of the porcelain bond is well established clinically and the alloys meet most of the requirements for casting fit and mechanical strength. It is for this reason that the beginner in ceramics is strongly advised to use only gold-platinum alloys. With more experience he may then experiment with other systems.

The only reason for wishing to replace gold-platinum alloys is one of cost and mechanical strength. However, the cost of a gold restoration in the laboratory involves less than one-quarter of the total fee, so that if labour costs are increased the saving in metal cost is marginal (*Smith,* 1977). A more sensible approach to the problem of selection of alloys should be one of improved clinical performance since the overall cost to the patient, even assuming gold doubled in price, would still be very low ($<8\%$).

It is essential to establish in what areas other metal systems can improve the clinical performance of metal-ceramic restorations. There is little doubt that improvements in creep resistance, yield strength and modulus of elasticity are desirable in the gold-platinum alloy systems. The gold-palladium-silver or nickel-chromium alloys cannot achieve this goal without sacrificing other desirable properties. In the case of the base-metal alloys, more work has yet to be done on casting accuracy and development of new investments. The low density nickel-chromium alloys need more force during casting to adapt them to fine margins. They also require investments that are easily wetted and retain smooth surfaces at high temperatures.

Induction casting machines may be effective in standardising casting procedures but they are no guarantee that the alloy will be properly melted. Base-metal alloys differ in emissivity, and induction casting machines equipped with optical pyrometers are prone to make serious errors. Setting the controls of the machine to the alloy manufacturer's suggested casting temperatures does not always result in satisfactory results. *Moffa* (1977) has found that even with these sophisticated devices, an empirical approach is necessary to achieve sound castings.

Even assuming the casting problem is overcome, no solution has yet been found to controlling oxide production at the interface of a nickel-chromium/porcelain interface. Use of these materials should therefore be confined to the specialist and research laboratory.

A more promising alternative to the gold-platinum systems may be found in the gold-palladium-silver alloys. These materials have several desirable properties such as higher creep resistance, and modulus of elasticity. However, due to their high palladium content, they must present greater problems with regard to gas absorption since, as previously explained, palladium is a known hydrogen acceptor. In addition, both dentist and patient must accept the white colour of these alloys. As the gold content is lowered and palladium and silver are added, the yellow colour is lost. Tarnish resistance in vivo can also be another problem, together with possible greening of the porcelain due to silver contamination.

To summarize all the above properties must lead to certain generalisations and *Moffa* (1977) has drawn attention to the impossibility of classifying all the base metals under one group of properties. However, certain basic features do emerge from a study of both gold and base-metal alloys:

1. The higher the gold content the greater the casting accuracy and ease of fabrication.
2. Lower palladium content lessens the risk of gas absorption.
3. Replacement of palladium by tantalum can produce more yellow gold coloured ceramic bonding alloys.
4. The greater the base-metal content, particularly of nickel and chromium, the greater the problem of controlling oxide production to molecular layers.
5. The higher the melting temperature of the alloy the greater resistance to metal creep on firing porcelain.
6. High modulus of elasticity and yield strength allows the use of thinner metal sections on longer spans of bridgework.

Other aspects that are sometimes overlooked concern the application of porcelain. For example, the use of alloys with very high modulus of elasticity require porcelains with very close matching thermal expansions since the metal has little give in it during cooling. High yield strengths and modulus of elasticity therefore exert a discipline on the ceramic manufacturer. Burnishability of alloys is frequently referred to and often related to percent elongation. However, alloys with a high percent elongation may also have a high yield strength and to overcome the strength of these alloys, very heavy pressure is required to burnish them. In the author's experience, burnishing of ceramic bonding alloys is not a practical proposition. Even the gold-platinum alloys are difficult to burnish on a metal die and to suggest that they can be burnished in the mouth is stretching the realms of practicability. During cementation the viscosity of the cement is rising rapidly and the dentist only has a very limited time for burnishing if he is to seal a margin. Burnishing after the cement has set is highly dangerous since, even assuming the metal deforms, the cement will crumble and a potential site for dissolution is created.

In view of the many problems involved in using alternative alloys, the gold-platinum-palladium alloys described in Table 2-3 must still be considered the best alloys to use for all-purpose bridgework. In the case of individual crowns where aesthetics are of prime importance, the newer gold-platinum tantalum alloys (Degudent-G) may be used to provide a yellower gold colour at the margins.

Bonding of Porcelain to Precious Metals Using Tin Oxide Coatings

Improvements in the aesthetics of metal-ceramic crowns are dependent upon:

1. Reduction in the thickness of the metal coping.
2. Reduction in the light reflectivity from the metal opaque porcelain.

A new method of bonding porcelain to metal using tin oxide coatings offers possibilities for achieving the above objectives (McLean and Sced, 1976). The method consists of bonding aluminous porcelains to platinum foil copings. Attachment of the porcelain is secured by electroplating the platinum foil with a thin layer of tin and then oxidising it in a furnace to provide a continuous film of tin oxide for porcelain bonding. It was considered that combining a high strength aluminous porcelain with a crack-free metal surface might result in a composite which possessed the optimum properties of both materials. The bonded platinum foil acts as an inner skin on the fit surface, reducing subsurface porosity and micro-cracks in the porcelain and increasing the strength of the unit. Experimental work by Sced et al. (1977) conducted on discs of aluminous porcelain (Vitadur S) fired onto plated and non-plated platinum foil showed that for specimens prepared in pure platinum foil the mean breaking stress for ten tests was 70.48 N/mm^2. For specimens with tin oxide coated foils (the bonded foil) the mean value was 128.96 N/mm^2, representing an increase in strength of approximately 83 percent. In addition, it was shown that the bond strength for aluminous porcelain fired against pure platinum (sand-blasted with 30 μm Al_2O_3) was approximately 15 N/mm^2 as compared with 53 N/mm^2 for a similar tin-plated specimen (McLean and Sced, 1976). A detailed study of the effect of coating thickness for tin on platinum showed that there is a practical working

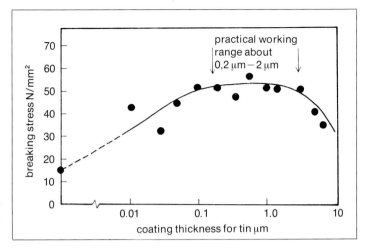

Fig. 2-20 Optimum thickness of tin-plating to obtain the best porcelain bond strengths.

range of 0.2 – 2.0 μm for the optimum strength of around 50 N/mm^2 (Fig. 2-20). In this range failure is always cohesive in the core porcelain. Below 0.2 μm the strength falls and the incidence of interfacial failure increases until failure is almost totally interfacial at zero coating thickness. There is a minimum tin coating thickness below which either the coating is inadequate due to discontinuity or possibly because oxidation of these very thin tin layers occurs without adequate diffusion bonding to the platinum. Above 2.0 μm thickness another fall-off in strength occurs. Failure in this region is still cohesive but the porcelain is weakened. Excessive formation of tin oxide when dissolved in the porcelain could be the cause.

The Platinum Bonded Alumina Crown

This new system of bonding porcelain to metal by electroplating techniques has been developed commercially with the introduction of the platinum bonded aluminous porcelain crown. New core powders (Vita-Pt)* with sufficient covering power to mask the platinum foil also pro-

* Vita Zahnfabrik, Bad Saeckingen, West Germany.

vide a neutral colour for the overlying dentine and enamel porcelains (Vitadur-N)*. In addition, an electroplating machine, the "Ceramiplater"* has been designed to deliver the correct coating thickness of tin for porcelain bonding.

Principles of the technique

The bonded alumina crown consists of an aluminous porcelain crown bonded to a 0.025 mm thick platinum coping. In order to provide a porcelain butt fit and eliminate the dark shadow produced by a metal collar, the crown is baked onto an inner platinum foil matrix (unplated) which is removed after baking and provides space for the cement (Fig. 2-21).

Twin Foil technique

The twin foil technique involves the laying down of two platinum foils in close apposition to each other. The inner foil of 0.025 mm platinum provides a matrix for the baking of the porcelain and the outer foil which forms the inner skin to the crown is tin-plated and oxidised to achieve strong chemical bonding with the aluminous core porcelain (*McLean* et al., 1976). The outer or "bonded foil" remains in position on the internal fit surface of the crown and will eliminate

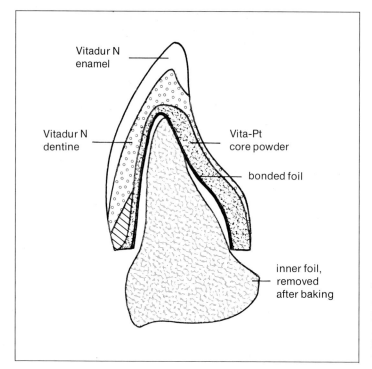

Fig. 2-21 Diagram of the twin foil technique for making a platinum bonded crown. The inner foil is removed after baking the crown, leaving the tin oxide coated foil bonded to the inner surface of the aluminous core porcelain.

Fig. 2-22 Diagram showing the bonding of tin oxide coated platinum foil to aluminous porcelain and glass-ionomer cement. Bonding is achieved via the oxide surfaces of all materials. Atoms are drawn to scale according to their atomic radii.

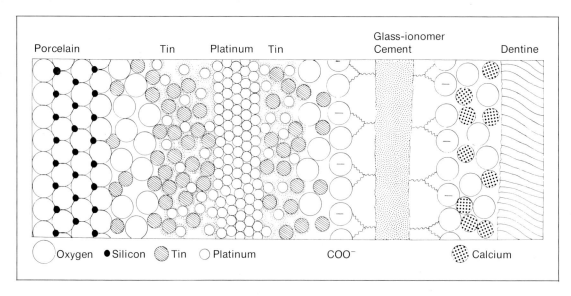

surface microcracks in the porcelain (Fig. 2-21). The bonded alumina crown was developed with the following objectives:

1. Reduction of metal and labour costs in construction.
2. Provision of a porcelain butt fit on the labial or buccal surface of the crown, eliminating the dark shadow of a metal collar.
3. Reduction of stresses at the porcelain metal interface during cementation procedures.
4. Improvement in strength of the aluminous porcelain crown by reducing internal microcracks and sub-surface porosity which are the sites for crack propagation.

Cementation

After tin-plating and oxidising the platinum foil, a tin oxide layer will also be present on the fit surface of the crown. Due to the presence of this layer and also to the availability of stannic or stannous ions in the tin oxide, hydrogen and metal ion bridges can be formed between the polar oxide layer and the polyanions in carboxylate or glass-ionomer cement. In simple terms, the platinum can be linked with the cement by a metal bond forming between the carboxyl groups of the cement and the tin oxide in the platinum. It may be represented as follows:

$$Platinum\ foil + tin\ oxide$$
$$Pt-Sn-O$$

$$M^{n+}-OOC-CH_2$$
$$Carboxyl\ group-cement$$

M^{n+} are metal ions available either as stannous or stannic ions from the tin oxide layer or as aluminium, zinc or calcium ions from the carboxylate or glass-ionomer cements (Fig. 2-22).

Tin-plating of inlays made from cast gold alloys will also facilitate bonding to polyacrylic acid-based cements (*McLean, 1977*). For the best results, it is advisable to clean the surface of the inlay and teeth with a proprietary cleaner such as Cavilax (Espe, W. Germany) before cementation. The bonded foil in the crown may also be cleaned with Cavilax.

On cementation of the crown or inlay it is possible to obtain strong physico-chemical bonding between the platinum, the cement and the tooth, thereby reducing future risks of microleakage. When cementing the bonded alumina crown, it is important to use the correct powder/liquid ratio as recommended by the manufacturer. Indications for the use of the bonded alumina crown are given in Monograph IV.

Dispersion Strengthening of Glasses

Glassy materials such as dental porcelain may be strengthened by dispersing ceramic crystals of high strength and elasticity in the glass matrix. If the glass has a similar thermal expansion to the crystals, the strength and elasticity of crystal-glass composites may increase progressively with the proportion of the crystalline phase (*Binns, 1962*). The rate of increase in modulus of elasticity is independent of the grain size of the included crystalline phase and suggests that these composite solids are behaving partly as a constant strain system. The resulting uneven stress distribution may be responsible for the increase in strength and it is probable that the high strength crystals bear a greater proportion of any load applied to the composite ceramic body and act as a reinforcing phase.

The choice of reinforcing crystals that can be used in dental porcelains is fairly limited since consideration must be given to factors such as fusion temperature, coefficient of thermal expansion, bonding properties with dental porcelain, colour, mechanical strength and resistance to thermal shock during rapid firing cycles.

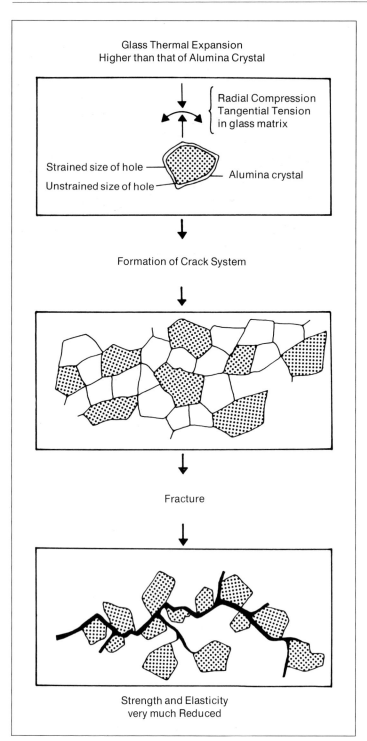

Glass Thermal Expansion
Higher than that of Alumina Crystal

Radial Compression
Tangential Tension
in glass matrix

Strained size of hole

Alumina crystal

Unstrained size of hole

Formation of Crack System

Fracture

Strength and Elasticity
very much Reduced

Fig. 2-23 Diagram illustrating the fracture path in an alumina-glass composite where the thermal expansion of the glass is higher than the alumina. (After *Binns, D. B.,* 1962. The Science of Ceramics, vol. 1. Academic Press, London.)

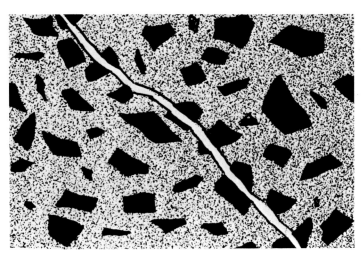

Fig. 2-24 Diagram of the fracture path occurring in an alumina-glass composite where the coefficients of expansion match. The crack will then pass indiscriminately through both glass and crystal phases. (From *McLean, J. W.,* and *Hughes, T. H.,* 1965. Brit. dent. J. 119, 151.)

Types of Reinforcing Crystals

Quartz

As explained in Monograph I, quartz crystals have been used as a filler in regular dental porcelain for many years. In the case of the high-fusing porcelains, quartz may constitute up to 15 percent of the ceramic body. However, there has been considerable disagreement as to the effectiveness of quartz as a reinforcing phase in ceramic bodies, due to the inversion of the quartz crystals during heating causing stressing of the glass matrix upon cooling. *Marzahl* (1955) and *Mattyasovszky-Zsolnay* (1957) regard the stressing of the glass matrix as a source of strength, whereas *Genin* (1958) and *Weyl* (1959) consider that a weakening effect occurs. More recently, *Jones* (1970) determined the strength of dental porcelain bodies containing 10 percent by weight of quartz and found a marked reduction in the flexural strength of the fired bodies. He suggested that the high coefficient of thermal expansion and inversion of the quartz crystals were the determining factors in the lowered strengths observed. It is apparent that a more efficient reinforcing agent is desirable in dental porcelain if any significant degree of reinforcement is to be obtained.

Alumina

When alumina crystals are dispersed in a glass matrix, the stress pattern set up on cooling is determined by differences in thermal expansion between the glass and the alumina. Any such stress may be added to the applied load and result in a lower measured strength. For example, if the thermal expansion of the glass matrix is higher than the alumina crystals then the strength and elasticity of the composite is very much reduced (*Binns,* 1962). On cooling, the glass will be placed in radial compression and tangential tension (Fig. 2-23). However, providing the thermal expansion of the glass matrix matches that of the alumina, sudden volume changes of crystal structure such as occurs with quartz do not occur with alumina-glass composites. The alumina crystals bear a greater proportion of any load applied (Fig. 2-24) and the strength of the alumina-glass composite is increased roughly in proportion to the alumina concentration.

Types of Alumina

The physical properties and characteristics of alumina (Al_2O_3) have been described in Mono-

Table 2-7 Characteristics and Properties of Fused Alumina Crystals

		Sample – 400 mesh	
		Fused Alumina	Oversize
		Diameter microns	Cum. Wt. %
Specific Gravity	3.911		
Hardness (Knoop K 100)	2,100		
Thermal Conductivity	0.06	38.30	0,00
	(Room Temp.)	36.82	0.00
		35.22	0.00
(C.G.S. Units)	0.012	33.45	0.32
	(1,000 °C)	31.48	1.72
		29.22	5.52
Coefficient of Expansion	6×10^{-6}	26.55	13.05
	(20 °C – 100 °C)	23.20	37.55
	8.5×10^{-6}	21.07	55.78
	(20 °C – 1,000 °C)	18.41	83.07
		14.62	97.34
		11.62	99.37
Chemical Analysis		9.24	99.89
		7.37	99.98
SiO_2	0.10 %	5.90	100.00
Fe_2O_3	0.15 %	4.76	100.00
CaO	0.02 %	3.90	100.00
Na_2O	0.026 – 0.3 %	3.29	100.00
Al_2O_3	99.53 – 99.57 %		
		Interpolated Points (%)	
		25	24.91
		50	21.75
		75	18.96
		Specific surface	1153 sq. cm/g.

graph I. In order to obtain suitable crystals of alumina for reinforcing dental porcelain, it is necessary to select aluminas of very high purity and certain characteristics.

Calcined Alumina

Calcined alumina of the alpha-type may be obtained with purities in excess of 99 percent. The fine powdered alumina consists of agglomerates of tiny crystals and when incorporated in dental porcelain tends to cause excessive opac-ity due to differences in refractive indices between the glassy porcelain and the alumina crystals. Single crystals of alumina are therefore preferred for dental purposes.

Fused Alumina

In order to obtain single crystals of alumina, it is necessary to fire alumina at much higher temperatures than employed during calcination. Single crystals of alumina may be prepared by fusing "pigs" of high purity alumina (99.6 percent) in an electric arc furnace at 2,150 °C. The crystals formed on cooling are generally very large and may be subsequently ground and sized according to standard mineralogical techniques. Typical properties for these fused alumina crystals are given in Table 2-7.

The viscosity and transition temperature of the glasses used in making an alumina-glass composite should not be too high, otherwise very high temperatures are required in order to obtain easy flow of the glass grains around the alumina crystals. The firing temperatures of these glasses is therefore restricted to temperatures within the ranges of 850 °C to 950 °C by the use of appropriate fluxes such as boric oxide, soda, and potash.

Types of Glass used with Alumina

The coefficient of thermal expansion of fused alumina crystals is in the range of 6.4 to 7.8 $\times$ 10^{-6} °C depending on temperature (Table 2-7). When these crystals are dispersed and fused in a glass matrix, the glass must not only match the crystals in thermal expansion, but also form a strong chemical bond with the alumina. In addition, the glass must be sufficiently pyroplastic to wet the surface of the crystals and flow easily around each grain.

Types of glasses used in making alumina-glass composites are generally based on a special borosilicate glass, containing a high dissolved alumina content or alternatively, a completely dissolved (fritted) felspar-glass flux containing additional quantities of alumina both in the free state and dissolved in the glass. The free alumina crystal content of these glasses is restricted to about 5 to 10 percent. Glasses used for the incorporation of alumina crystals will generally correspond to the following formulation:

Aluminous Porcelain

Alumina-glass composites used in dental ceramic work have been termed "Aluminous Porcelains" (McLean and Hughes, 1965).

There are three main types of aluminous porcelain. A high-strength core material containing as much as 50 percent fused alumina crystals and dentine and enamel veneer powders made from high alumina content glasses which overlay the high-strength core and give colour and translucency to the jacket crown.

Aluminous Porcelain Core Powders

The aluminous porcelain core powders provide the main reinforcement in a porcelain jacket

			Weight per cent
Silica	SiO_2	Glass former	62.0 − 65.0
Alumina	Al_2O_3	Intermediate	17.0 − 20.0
Potash	K_2O		6.5 − 7.7
Soda	Na_2O	Fluxes	4.2 − 4.7
Lime	CaO		1.6 − 1.8
Boric oxide	B_2O_3		6.7 − 7.3

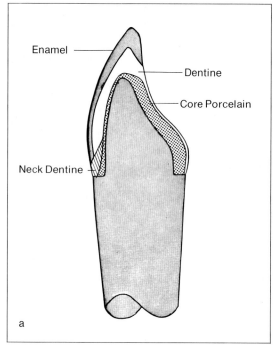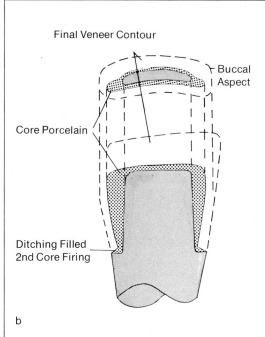

Enamel

Dentine

Core Porcelain

Neck Dentine

a

Final Veneer Contour

Buccal Aspect

Core Porcelain

Ditching Filled 2nd Core Firing

b

Fig. 2-25   Diagram of the correct placement of alumina core and veneer porcelains in an aluminous porcelain jacket crown. The core porcelain must be used to the maximum advantage on the lingual surface.

crown (Fig. 2-25), and their free alumina content will vary between 40 to 50 percent by weight.

The grain size of the fused alumina crystals is selected to provide optimum strength without producing undesirable opacity.

Influence of Grain Size on Opacity and Strength

The strength and opacity of aluminous porcelain is related to the grain size of the alumina crystals used. The finer the grain size the greater the strength, but this is accompanied by increased opacity of the fired body due to differences in refractive indices between the crystals and the glass matrix (*McLean* and *Hughes,* 1965). Very high opacity in opaque or core por-

celains is not desirable since it increases the amount of light reflection from the surface when translucent enamel veneers are applied. Undesirable colour influences are then inevitable from the opaque porcelain and increase the incidence of metameric colour effects which are discussed in Monograph III. An aluminous core porcelain is therefore formulated so that it will transmit some light and not produce a "mirror" effect when the enamel porcelains are applied.

The influence of grain size on light transmission may be seen in Figure 2-26. Alumina crystal concentrations of 40 percent by weight produce considerable differences in light transmission according to their fineness or specific surface area. It will be seen that very fine crystals in the range of 4,000 to 7,000 cm²/gram (600 to 850 mesh) will produce almost total opacity

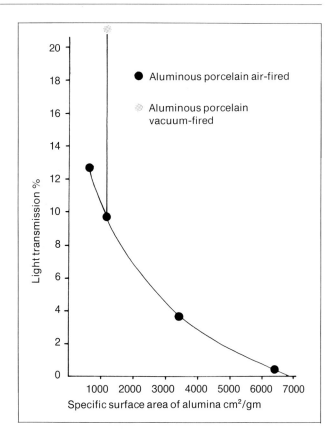

Fig. 2-26 Effect of alumina particle size on the light transmission through 1 mm thick discs of aluminous core porcelain.

with light transmissions of less than 0.5 percent on 1 millimetre thick discs. By contrast, fused alumina crystals of around 1,200 cm²/gm (400 mesh) will transmit up to 12 percent light and this can be increased to over 20 percent when low pressure atmosphere or vacuum firing is used.

Very fine alumina will increase the strength of the fired body (Table 2-8) and at a specific surface area of 3528 cm²/gram (Aluminous Porcelain C), the strength of an aluminous porcelain containing 40 percent by weight of fused alumina crystals will be in the region of 134 N/mm² (19,500 p.s.i.). Coarser grades of alumina (specific surface area 737 cm²/gram) markedly reduce strength (Aluminous Porcelain A) probably due to the increased "notch effect" created at the grain boundaries of the crystals as explained by *Weyl* (1959).

It is clear that a compromise must be reached between strength and opacity and for this reason fused alumina crystals are selected of a size range that will provide at least 10 to 15 percent light transmission on 1 millimetre thick discs but at the same time are sufficiently fine in grain size to impart substantial strength improvements. Aluminous porcelain B in Table 2-8 represents a typical example of the size range of alumina crystals used and this will correspond to a mean diameter of 25 microns (400 mesh) with a top size of approximately 37 microns. It should also be noted that the size range of the glass powder also plays a significant part in obtaining maximum sintered densities (*McLean*, 1966). Fine powders (<40 μm) suitable for vacuum sintering will soften and flow more easily around the alumina grains and high sintered densities can then be obtained.

101

Table 2-8 Effect of Grain Size of Alumina on the Strength of Aluminous Porcelain

	Specific surface of alumina cm²/g	Modulus of Rupture N/mm²	p.s.i.
Aluminous Porcelain A	737	92.5	13,407
Aluminous Porcelain B	1,153	127.6	18,509
Aluminous Porcelain C	3,528	134.8	19,547

Alumina crystal content 40 percent by weight.
Glass matrix – single phase low fusing felspathic.

Influence of Alumina Crystal Concentration on Strength

The concentration of free alumina crystals in aluminous porcelain is limited by the ability of the glass phase to flow round and wet every crystal. It has been found that concentrations of alumina above 50 percent by weight cannot be sintered to high densities (*McLean,* 1966). This is due to the angular nature of the fused alumina crystals causing interference to the flow of the glass phase. In general, it may be said that, if the grains are not well separated by the glass phase, it is impossible to produce a reasonably pore-free body. Rounded grains of alumina are therefore preferred to sharp-angled crystals.

Binns (1962) has shown that when alumina crystals are sintered in a glass matrix of matching thermal expansion, the strength and elasticity of the mixture will increase with volume proportions of up to 40 percent of alumina. Similar strength increases were found in the dental aluminous porcelains (*McLean,* 1966) and typical strengths are given in Fig. 2-27. The strength of sintered or high alumina and regular dental porcelain has been included for comparative purposes. In the case of the aluminous porcelain containing 50 percent by weight of free alumina crystals the sintered densities can be improved by pre-fritting the alumina crystals and glass powder at 1200 °C and then re-grinding the crystal-glass composite. When this powder

is refused during construction of the jacket crown, the crystals are thoroughly wetted by the glass and strong chemical bonds are formed. Unfortunately the high strength 50 percent alumina bodies are more opaque and these powders are generally used for constructing lingual reinforcements or all-ceramic bridge sub-structures combined with high-alumina rods.

Crack-propagation in Aluminous Porcelain

The strengthening effect of alumina crystals dispersed in a glass matrix may be explained by two theories. The constant-strain theory discussed on page 97 and the limitation of flaw size theory which has been proposed by *Hasselman* and *Fulrath* (1966). They performed experiments on spheroidal alumina incorporated in a matched expansion glass matrix and reported considerable improvements in strength for their composites. It was hypothesised that hard crystalline dispersions within the glass matrix limit the size of Griffith flaws and strengthen the composite. At high volumes of dispersed alumina, the flaw size was governed by the average distance between particles dispersed in the matrix.

The reduction in the flaw size on the surface of aluminous porcelains may account for the improved impact strength found with these materials (*Southan,* 1968) but it should be noted that the constant-strain theory also finds support in

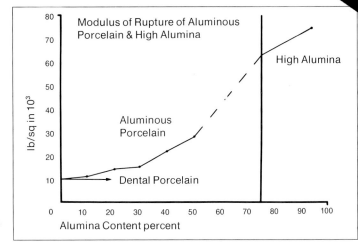

Fig. 2-27 Graph of the strength of dental porcelain compared with the aluminous porcelains and high alumina.

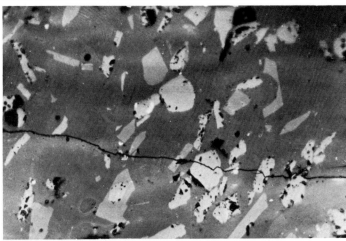

Fig. 2-28a Photomicrograph of the fracture path in a two-phase system of dental porcelain reinforced with fused alumina crystals. (From *McLean, J. W.,* and *Hughes, T. H.,* (1965) Brit. dent. J. 119, 151.)

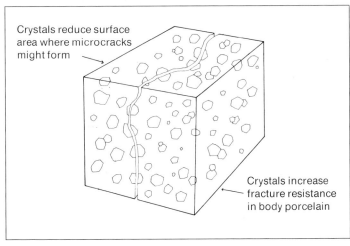

Fig. 2-28b Diagram of the two methods by which the strength of alumina/glass composites is increased.

polished sections of fractur-
~~~elains~~~ which have been cor-
~~~always~~~ show fracture paths
~~~iminately~~~ through both glass
and c₁, ~~~ig.~~~ 2-28a and b). It seems likely
that in this ~~~case~~~ the alumina crystals have modified the flaw system throughout the entire
ceramic body.

Glazed dental porcelain is subject to a marked
reduction in flexural strength when the glaze is
removed by grinding (Table 2-1), but the aluminous porcelains do not appear to be so affected by mild surface abrasion. Rods of aluminous
porcelain which were tested in the glazed and
abraded condition revealed very little difference
in strength as illustrated in Table 2-1. This effect
could again be accounted for by the theory that
the alumina crystals modified the flaw system in
both the surface and body of the fired ceramic.

Sintering Aluminous Porcelain

The strength of aluminous porcelain, unlike
dental porcelain, is very much affected by the
density of the fired ceramic. Porosity, particularly when present at the grain boundaries of
the alumina crystals, can cause considerable
weakening of aluminous porcelain (*McLean,*
and *Hughes,* 1965).

Aluminous porcelain must be very carefully condensed and the sintering or firing schedule will
also play an important part in obtaining high
densities. Aluminous porcelain is preferably
fired in low pressure atmosphere and a vacuum
furnace is really essential.

The firing schedule should be slow in order to
allow porosity to escape at the grain boundaries
and the porcelain should not be allowed to
reach its maximum recommended maturing
temperature much under five minutes. For example, an aluminous core porcelain maturing
at 1050 °C should be introduced into the hot
zone of the furnace muffle at 800 °C and a firing
schedule of 50 °C per minute would then ensure
a slow maturation period. Prolonged firing

under vacuum at the maximum maturing
temperature is strongly deprecated,
since at these elevated temperatures the glass
may "bloat" or swell. Vacuum must therefore be broken immediately any aluminous
porcelain reaches the manufacturer's recommended maturing temperature, otherwise the
porcelain can become honeycombed by porosity. It is important to bear in mind that the
glass matrix powders will soften and become
very viscous at temperatures at least 100 °C
below that of the aluminous porcelains' firing
temperature.

Once vacuum has been broken, an aluminous
porcelain may be safely fired in normal atmosphere for prolonged periods.

Effect of Sintering Time on the Strength of Aluminous Porcelain

In order to obtain the maximum mechanical
strength from aluminous porcelain, it is essential that the chemical bonding of the glass to
the alumina crystals is strong enough to form a
constant strain system (Fig. 2-28). In this way,
cracks will pass indiscriminately through both
glass and alumina crystal phases and maximum
strengths will be obtained. If the wetting of the
alumina crystals by the glass phase is inadequate, then a weak bond is formed at the interfaces and a crack will tend to deviate at a crystal
boundary. The alumina crystals will interrupt
the crack by forcing the fracture path to pass
round a crystal but the alumina crystals will not
be bearing a greater proportion of the stress
applied as in a constant strain system. In this
case the high modulus of elasticity of the alumina is not used to its full advantage.

As previously explained, the high fusing aluminous core porcelains (1100 °C) are usually pre-

pared by pre-fritting the alumina-glass composite and then regrinding to a fine powder. This results in a pre-coating of the alumina crystals with the glass phase prior to supplying the core powder to the technician. In this way effective chemical bonding has already been achieved in the factory.

In the case of the low-fusing aluminous core porcelains (1050 °C), these powders generally consist of a simple mixture of 45 percent by weight of alumina crystals and glass powder. Efficient wetting of the alumina crystals can only take place at the time of firing the core powder on the platinum matrix. If short sintering periods are used, the glass may not be sufficiently viscous to flow round and chemically bond to the alumina crystals. The ceramist is therefore advised to prolong the sintering period of the aluminous core porcelains beyond the time recommended by the manufacturers. This additional sintering time must be done in normal atmosphere in order to prevent "bloating" of the ceramic and a period of fifteen minutes will generally be sufficient to provide high densities and maximum chemical bonding of the crystal-glass composite. Longer firing or sintering schedules for aluminous porcelain will not harm these materials since, unlike the glassy dental porcelains, alumina reinforced ceramics are more resistant to pyroplastic flow and are not subject to devitrification (McLean, 1970).

The higher strengths obtained with alumina core porcelains using longer firing schedules have been confirmed by Jones et al. (1972). They observed significant increases in strength of the alumina-core porcelains which had been fired at 1150 °C for fifteen minutes. In this case, both the time and temperature had been increased beyond that recommended by the manufacturer.

Dispersion Strengthening of Glass with Alumina Whiskers

Alumina whiskers are filamentary single crystals having both high surface and crystalline perfection. Their strength at room temperature can be as high as 1.38×10^4 N/mm^2 (2×10^6 p.s.i.) with a modulus of elasticity of 4.83×10^5 N/mm^2 (70×10^6 p.s.i.).

Dispersion of these whiskers in a glass matrix may be done in several ways (McLean, 1969). Two methods that were tried in jacket crown work were as follows:

The whiskers were intimately mixed with a finely ground glass powder used for making aluminous porcelain and applied to a platinum matrix by standard technique. It was found that whisker concentrations above 15 percent created difficulties with regard to sintering behaviour, and high densities could not be obtained. It became clear that if sufficient whiskers were to be incorporated in the glass powder and make a significant contribution to strength, then alternative methods would have to be used. Vacuum hot-pressing techniques allow high whisker concentrations to be used but such methods are not commercially viable in dentistry.

An alternative method was tried in which preformed "green" whisker tapes were incorporated in the jacket crown. These tapes were produced by using the finely ground glass powder and highly oriented whiskers held in an organic binder (Wakelin, 1967). The tapes were incorporated in aluminous core porcelain on the lingual surface of the crown by a laminated technique. Once again problems of sintering the alumina whisker-glass composite arose, since the layers of porcelain in between the tapes tended to be very porous despite firing in vacuo. It was considered that future research might make it possible to produce lingual alumina whisker reinforced glass shells which could be lightly ground to fit the jacket preparation. In this case the shells could be produced by vacuum hot pressing. However, it is doubtful

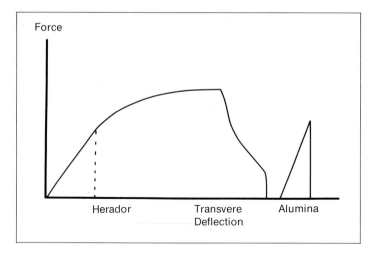

Force

Herador   Transvere   Alumina

Deflection

Fig. 2-29 Graph depicting the strength of a typical gold alloy used in the metal-ceramic technique against high alumina. Testing was done on 3 mm diameter rods of each material. Note that the yield strength of the metal was slightly below the modulus of rupture of the high alumina rod.

whether this method could rival the comparative simplicity of the fused porcelain to gold technique.

Enamelling of High Strength Crystalline Ceramics

The improved strengths obtainable with the aluminous porcelains are still not sufficient to warrant using them in very thin sections of 0.5 mm, and it is doubtful whether ceramics of this type will ever seriously rival the metal-ceramic systems in resistance to tensile failure. However, metal sub-structures are by nature unaesthetic and costly to produce, with the result that considerable interest is always shown by the clinician in all-ceramic systems.

If metals could be replaced by ceramics of high flexural strength which compare favourably with the level of permanent deformation obtainable on current high-fusing gold alloys, then real possibilities exist for the development of fracture-proof ceramic crowns and bridges.

Very high strengths in ceramics are generally to be found amongst materials that undergo

some form of recrystallisation during firing. The resultant interlocking crystalline system is better able to withstand high stresses than the felspathic dental glasses. In addition, the crystalline materials must be selected for their inherent high strength and this will depend upon the nature of the bonding of the atoms as outlined in Monograph I. Sintered or high alumina is one such material possessing high flexural strength (Fig. 2-27).

High-alumina is classified as having a minimum content of 75 percent alumina; anything below this level is termed aluminous porcelain.

At the present time, high alumina may only be used as a pre-fabricated reinforcement in the construction of crowns and bridges and techniques for using these materials will be described in future monographs. Basically the high-alumina is used to reinforce the anchorage areas of crowns and bridge pontics and thus prevent tensile failure of the enamel porcelains applied to the surface. This type of reinforcement is similar to the mode of action of the metals used in the metal-ceramic techniques.

Experiments have been conducted on sintering high-alumina powders directly onto platinum matrices similar to the standard porcelain jacket techniques (*McLean,* 1966). Few problems were encountered in firing these powders at 1500 °C

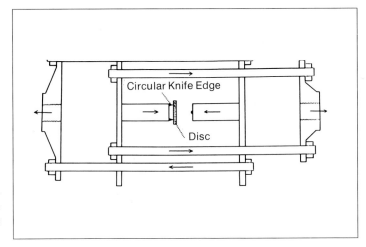

Fig. 2-30 Diagram of the apparatus used for determining the *Timoshenko* discs breaking stress test.

to 1650°C and suitable furnaces are already available for these purposes. However, due to the negligible glass phase in high-alumina, these materials are very resistant to pyroplastic flow. As a result they will not flow and adapt themselves to a platinum matrix in the same way as dental porcelain. High-alumina will either fissure or contract and distort the platinum matrix so that an accurate fit is very difficult to obtain. With our present powder technology and sintering techniques, it is doubtful whether high-alumina jacket copings could be made a commercially viable system without debasing (fluxing) the alumina to provide greater pyroplasticity. In this event strength will be reduced.

The development of techniques for using preformed high-alumina reinforcements with enamel veneers has been described by *McLean* and *Hughes* (1965) and the strength of these laminates is similar in some aspects to the metal-ceramic systems.

Strength of Alumina-Enamel Laminates

The strength of high-alumina compares quite favourably with the high fusing gold alloys, and this is illustrated in Fig. 2-29 which shows the

failure of a rod of high-alumina and a heat treated high-fusing gold alloy under transverse loading. The yield strength of the metal is slightly less than the modulus of rupture of the high-alumina; however, it should be noted that high alumina is more brittle than metal and could not be used to restore thin edges.

When aluminous porcelain veneers are applied to high-alumina, it is possible to measure the strength of the composite. Discs of high-alumina 1 millimetre thick can be veneered with aluminous porcelain and a laminated disc of exactly 2 millimetres thick is then made by grinding the veneer porcelain to a thickness of 1 millimetre.

Timoshenko (1959) in his Theory of Plates and Shells proposed a method whereby the maximum breaking stress of a specimen disc may be determined by supporting the disc on a circular knife edge and applying a concentrated load at the centre of the opposite face (Fig. 2-30). The load is increased steadily until the disc fractures and, given this load and the dimensions of the specimen, the maximum disc breaking stress on the tension side of the disc may be calculated. The disc breaking stress of the aluminous porcelain enamel face may then be determined.

Table 2-9 illustrates the strength of discs of

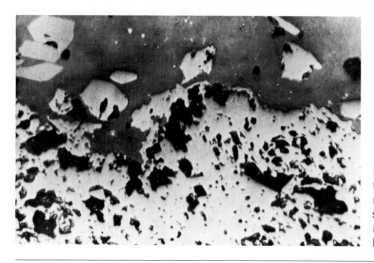

Fig. 2-31 Photomicrograph of the interface between high alumina and aluminous porcelain showing good wetting of the alumina interface by the porcelain. Mag × 170.

Table 2-9 Strength of Porcelain and Alumina – Glass Composites

Composition of disc	Maximum breaking stress	
	N/mm²	p.s.i.
Medium fusion air-fired porcelain	60.5	8,780
Low fusion air-fired porcelain	66.4	9,640
Medium fusion vacuum-fired porcelain	66.4	9,639
High Alumina veneered with Aluminous Porcelain	364.9	52,968
High Alumina	575.1	83,260

high-alumina veneered with an aluminous porcelain enamel and for comparison purposes equivalent discs of regular porcelain are included. The alumina-enamel porcelain laminates will be seen to be approximately five times stronger than the regular porcelain discs. Pure discs of high-alumina are over eight times stronger and illustrate the excellent mechanical properties of this material.

It was concluded from these experiments that the use of high-alumina as a preformed reinforcement in ceramic crowns might provide similar strengths to those obtained with the metal-ceramic systems and this would appear to be borne out by subsequent clinical evidence (*McLean,* 1966).

Bonding of Aluminous Porcelain to High Alumina

The bonding at the interface between aluminous porcelain enamels, having the required thermal expansion, and high-alumina, is of a chemical nature and an ionic bond between the oxide constituents of both materials is probably achieved (*McLean,* and *Hughes,* 1965). This was shown by observation of the fluorescent effect at the interface when examined under ultraviolet light, porcelain ions having diffused into the surface of the alumina.

The wetting of porcelain enamels on high-alumina is excellent and very small contact angles are obtainable. In addition, the interface will reveal no porosity (Fig. 2-31) as can occur at some metal-ceramic interfaces.

Controlled Crystallisation of Glasses

Controlled crystallisation of glass was developed by Stookey at the Corning Glass Works in the United States and new and unique properties were observed in these glass ceramics. Not only was the strength of these materials markedly improved but very high thermal shock resistance was imparted.

Controlled crystallisation of glass depends upon the fact that glass, at ordinary temperatures, is a super-cooled liquid which does not crystallise on cooling from a melt. It can be made to crystallise by heating to a suitable temperature with crystal seed or nuclei present. The glass is then converted to a dense mass of very tiny interlocking crystals. Titanium dioxide is an effective nucleating agent and the starting glass must be homogeneous with qualities like optical glass. Spodumene is a suitable glass, compounded from the oxides of lithium, aluminium and silicon and has been used extensively to make "Pyroceram" cooking ware. Normally the ware is heated to a temperature where the glass shows the first signs of softening. After myriads of nuclei have been formed in this way, the glass is slowly heated to higher temperatures where tiny spodumene crystals grow on the nuclei, converting the transparent glass to an opaque white mass composed chiefly of spodumene crystals.

The opacity of these glass ceramics makes them unsuitable for dental application but more recently *McCulloch* (1968) has reported on experiments with a glass-ceramic based on lithia, zinc oxide, silica in which metal phosphates were used as nucleating agents. The glass was transparent and amber in colour in the glassy state but became translucent and toothlike after crystallisation or ceraming for 1 hour at 600 °C. At this stage, modulus of rupture figures in excess of 124 N/mm² (18,000 p.s.i.) were obtained.

This glass ceramic was used to produce posterior teeth by moulding in a die and counterdie. These production teeth were only made in a single shade but further experiments were performed in which bars of the vitreous glass were made photo-sensitive by using silver as a nucleating agent. On cooling, the bars responded to ultra-violet light so that by differentially irradiating the surface, the glass, on heating to the ceraming temperature, could be made to crystallise at different rates, thus creating a polychromatic effect. It was shown that further characterisation might be accomplished by applying printed transfers, containing tooth pigments, to the surface.

These experiments have not yet reached the stage of commercialisation and considerable problems in fabrication and colour control must still present themselves to the tooth manufacturer. The current high standard of aesthetics in a vacuum-fired anterior porcelain tooth has been created by building in concentrated colours and multiblended veneers of dental porcelain by manual application. The fact that this process has not yet lent itself to automation is indicative of the tremendous problems encountered in duplicating both the depth of translucency and colour of human enamel and dentine. Dentistry still demands a high degree of artistic skill even in a mass-produced porcelain tooth.

Production of Pre-stressed Surface Layers in Dental Porcelain via Ion-exchange

The term diffusion in a solid applies to the internal process by which an atom is handed on or changed from one lattice position to another. The movement of atoms or ions from a saturated surface layer through the interior, as atoms or ions, constitutes diffusion proper. The driving force for diffusion is the concentration gradient.

When sodium ions lying in the surface of dental alumino-silicate glasses are exposed to surface contact with liquids containing metallic cations,

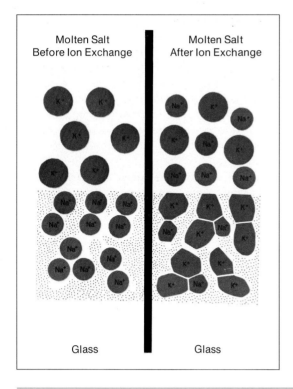

Molten Salt
Before Ion Exchange

Molten Salt
After Ion Exchange

Glass

Glass

Fig. 2-32 Diagram of ion-exchange in the surface of dental porcelain showing exchange of potassium ions with sodium ions producing a crowding of atoms at the surface. A pre-stressed surface layer results from this effect. (After *Southan, D. E.,* 1968, Ph. D. Thesis, University of Sydney).

the sodium ions may be exchanged with certain types of metallic cations. *Southan* (1968) has shown that dental porcelains with sufficient soda content (Na_2O) may be chemically treated in a potassium nitrate salt bath and the potassium ions will diffuse into the surface of the porcelain and be exchanged for some of the sodium ions. The larger potassium ions result in crowding of atoms at the surface of the porcelain (Fig. 2-32) and a pre-stressed surface layer is produced. This surface compression resulted in an increase in strength of the glazed or abraded condition of the porcelain. The flexural strength of the porcelains tested was improved by 47 to 122 percent depending on the shape of the test piece. Southan showed that thin sections of ion-exchanged porcelains were stronger than comparable test pieces of aluminous porcelain and that in thicker sections both materials were similar in flexural strength. However, the impact resistance of aluminous porce-

lain was found to be considerably greater than the chemically treated porcelains.

The strengthening of dental porcelain via ion-exchange is also very dependent upon the time/temperature cycling. It appears that the limiting factor in the diffusion rate of ions at temperatures below the annealing range of the porcelain is the rate of diffusion within the glass itself. The limiting factor at temperatures above the annealing range of the porcelain depend upon the rate of ionic exchange at the glass-salt boundary. *Southan* (1968) performed experiments on the regular Vita vacuum porcelain 1130 °C and determined the strength of ion-exchanged samples of abraded and glazed specimens. These specimens were treated for 17 hours at 475 °C in molten potassium nitrate. On thick specimens of the porcelain, the modulus of rupture was increased by 68 percent but in the case of thin wafer-like specimens the average measured strength rose by 122 percent.

Glazing of the specimens prior to ion-exchange treatment produced slightly higher strengths but these were not of great significance.

Southan (1968) considered that the treatment of aluminous porcelain crowns would produce significant increases in strength even when the outer surfaces were ground, since the internal or fit surface would still be stronger. The clinical significance of strengthening crowns by ion-exchange has yet to be established but this area of research merits further study.

Technical Considerations

Aluminous Porcelains

1. The alumina core porcelains must be well condensed to avoid porosity on firing. Low pressure (vacuum) firing will not eliminate large pores in a crystalline ceramic. Condensation is very dependent upon the effects of surface tension. Always work the porcelain when it is wet and never allow it to dry out.

2. The strength of the alumina core porcelains is very dependent upon good wetting and chemical bonding of the crystals to the glass phase. Core porcelains containing 45 to 50 percent alumina crystals are better fired for at least 15 minutes at their maturing temperatures. Never fire core porcelains for prolonged periods in vacuo. This will cause bloating or swelling.

Recommended Firing Schedule

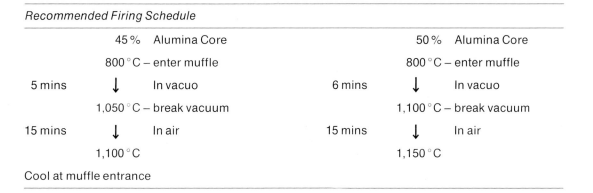

	45% Alumina Core			50% Alumina Core	
	800°C – enter muffle			800°C – enter muffle	
5 mins	↓	In vacuo	6 mins	↓	In vacuo
	1,050°C – break vacuum			1,100°C – break vacuum	
15 mins	↓	In air	15 mins	↓	In air
	1,100°C			1,150°C	

Cool at muffle entrance

Monograph II

References

Anthony, D. H., Burnett, A. P., Smith, D. L., and Brooks, M. S. (1970). Shear test for measuring bonding in cast gold alloy-porcelain composites. J. dent. Res. 49, 27.

Binns, D. B. (1962). Some physical properties of two-phase crystal-glass solids. I. The Science of Ceramics, vol. 1. London, England. Academic Press pp. 315 – 334.

Binns, D. B. (1964). British Ceramic Research Association, Personal Communication.

Cook, J., and Gordon, J. E. (1964). A mechanism for the control of crack propagation in all-brittle systems. Proc. Roy. Soc. A. 282:508.

Craig, R. G., and Farah, J. W. (1977). Finite Element Stress Analysis of Porcelain and Porcelain-Fused-to-Metal Crowns. In: Dental Porcelain: The State of the Art. University of S. California. Ed. Yamada, H. N., and Grenoble, P. B.

El-Ebrashi, M. K., Craig, R. G., and Peyton, F. G. (1969). Experimental stress analysis of dental restorations. Part III. The concept of the geometry of proximal margins. J. Pros. Dent. 22:333.

El-Ebrashi, M. K., Craig, R. G., and Peyton, F. A. (1970). Experimental stress analysis of dental restorations. Part VII. Structural design and stress analysis of fixed partial dentures. J. Pros. Dent. 23:177.

Genin, L. G. (1958). Effect of quartz on the strength of porcelain. Glass and Ceram. (Moscow) 15:35.

Gurney, C. (1964). Source of weakness in glass. Proc. Roy. Soc. A. 192, 537.

Hasselman, D. P. H., and Fulrath, R. M. (1966). Proposed fracture theory of a dispersion-strengthened glass matrix. J. Amer. Ceram. Soc. 49:68.

Hodson, Jean T. (1959). Some physical properties of three dental porcelains. J. Pros. Dent. 9:235.

Huget. E. F., Dvivedi, N., and Cosner, H. E. (1976). Characterisation of gold-palladium-silver and palladium-silver for ceramic-metal restorations. J. Pros. Dent. 36:52.

Jones, D. W. (1970). Ph. D. Thesis, University of Birmingham.

Jones, D. W., Jones, P. A., and Wilson, H. J. (1972). The relationship between transverse strength and testing methods for dental ceramics. J. of Dent. 1:85.

Katz, M. (1974). U.S. Patent 3,819,366.

Kelly, M., Asgar, K., and O'Brien, W. J. (1969). Tensile strength determination of the interface between porcelain fused to gold. J. Biomed. Mat. Res. 3:403.

Knapp, F. J., and Ryge, G. (1966). Study of bond strength of dental porcelain fused to metal. J. Dent. Res. 45:1047.

Kulp, P. R., Lee, P. W., and Fox, J. E. (1961). An impact test for dental porcelain. J. Dent. Res. 40: 1136.

Lavine, M. H., and Custer, F. (1969). Variables Affecting the Strength of Bond between Porcelain and Gold. J. Dent. Res. 45:32.

Leinfelder, K. F., Servais, W. J., and O'Brien, W. J. (1969). Mechanical properties of high-fusing gold alloys. J. Pros. Dent. 21:523.

Lubovich, P. R., and Goodkind, R. J. (1977). Bond strength of ceramic-metal alloys. J. Pros. Dent. 37:288.

Marzahl, H. (1955). Effect of quartz on the strength of porcelain. Ber. Dtsch. Keram. Ges. 32:203.

Mattyasovsky-Zsolnay, L. (1957). Mechanical strength of porcelain. J. Amer. Ceram. Soc. 40:299.

McCulloch, W. J. (1968). Advances in dental ceramics. Brit. Dent. J. 125:361.

McLean, J. W. (1966). The development of ceramic oxide reinforced dental porcelains with an appraisal of their physical and clinical properties. M. D. S. Thesis, University of London.

McLean, J. W. (1969). N. B. S. Special Publication, Dental Materials Research. Proc. 50th Ann. Symposium, pp 77 – 83.

McLean, J. W. (1970). Alumina Reinforced Ceramics.

In Tylman, S. D. Theory and Practice of Crown and Fixed Partial Prosthodontics (Bridge). C. V. Mosby Co., St. Louis.

McLean, J. W. (1977). A New Method of Bonding Dental Cements and Porcelain to Metal Surfaces. Operative Dent. 2:130.

McLean, J. W., and Hughes, T. H. (1965). The reinforcement of dental porcelain with ceramic oxides. Brit. dent. J. 119:151.

McLean, J. W., Kedge, M. I., and Hubbard, J. R. (1976). The Bonded Alumina Crown. 2. Construction using the Twin Foil Technique. Austral. Dent. J. 21:262.

McLean, J. W., and Sced, I. R. (1973). The gold-alloy/porcelain bond. Trans. Brit. Ceram. Soc., 5:229.

McLean, J. W., and Sced, I. R. (1973). The base-metal alloy/porcelain bond. Trans. Brit. Ceram. Soc. 5:235.

McLean, J. W., and Sced, I. R. (1976). The Bonded Alumina Crown. 1. The Bonding of Platinum to Aluminous Dental Porcelain using Tin-Oxide Coatings. Austral. Dent. J. 21:119.

Moffa, J. P., Lugassy, A. A., Gucker, A. D., and Gettleman, L. (1973). An evaluation of non-precious alloys for use with porcelain veneers. J. Pros. Dent. 30:424.

Moffa, J. P. (1977). Physical and mechanical properties of gold and base-metal alloys. In: Alternatives to Gold Alloys in Dentistry pp 81 – 93. Conference proceedings N.I.H.

Nally, J. N., Farah, J. R., and Craig, R. G. (1971). Experimental stress analysis of dental restorations. Part IX. Two-dimensional photo-elastic stress analysis of porcelain-bonded-to-gold crowns. J. Pros. Dent. 25:307.

Nally, J. N., Monnier, D., and Meyer, J. M.: Distribution topographique de certains elements de l'alliage et de la porcelaine au niveau de la liaison ceramo-metallique. Schweiz. Mschr. Zahnheilk. 78:868-78, Sep 68 (Fre) Ref. cited in Index to Dental Literature, 1969.

Nally, J. N. (1969). Chemico-physical analysis and mechanical tests of the ceramo-metallic complex. Int. Dent. J. 18:309.

Nitkin, D. A., and Asgar, K. (1976). Evaluation of alternative alloys to Type III gold for use in fixed prosthodontics. J. A. D. A. 93:622.

O'Brien, W. J., King, J. E., and Ryge, G. (1964). Heat treatment of alloys to be used for the fused porcelain technique. J. Pros. Dent. 14:955.

O'Brien, W. J., and Ryge, G. (1965). Contact angles of drops of enamels on metals. J. Pros. Dent. 15:1094.

O'Brien, W. J. (1977). Cohesive plateau theory of porcelain-alloy bonding. In: Dental Porcelain – The State of the Art, pp. 137 – 141. University of Southern California. Ed. Yamada, H. N., and Grenoble, P. B.

Peyton, F. A. (1968). Restorative Dental Materials p. 294. C. V. Mosby Co., St. Louis.

Poggioli, J., Montagnon, J., and Lambart, J. (1968). Emaillage d'un alliage non precieux avec la porcelaine dentaire. Rev. Franc. Odontostomat. 15:1215 – 20, Nov. 68 (Fre). Ref. cited in Index to Dental Literature, 1969.

Ryge, G. (1965). Current American research on porcelain fused to metal restorations. Int. Dent. J. 15:385.

Saachi, H., and Paffenbarger, G. C. (1957). A simple technique for making Dental Porcelain Jacket Crowns. J. A. D. A. 54:366.

Sced, I. R., and McLean, J. W. (1972). The strength of metal/ceramic bonds with base metals containing chromium. Brit. dent. J. 132:232.

Sced, I. R., McLean, J. W., and Hotz, P. (1977). The strengthening of aluminous porcelain with bonded platinum foils. J. Dent. Res. 36:1067.

Shell, J. S., and Nielsen, J. P. (1962). Study of the bond between gold alloys and porcelain. J. Dent. Res. 41:1424.

Shevlin, T. S., and Lindenthal, J. W. (1959). Mechanical Testing of Porcelain. Ceram. Bull. 38:491.

Shillingburg, H. T., Hobo, S., and Fisher, D. W. (1973). Preparation design and margin distortion in porcelain-fused-to-metal restorations. J. Pros. Dent. 29:276.

Smith, D. L. (1977). Economics of Gold Alloys in Dentristry. In: Alternatives to Gold Alloys in Dentistry, pp. 19 – 27. Conference Proceedings N.I.H.

Smith, D. L., Burnett, A. P., Brooks, M. S., and Anthony, D. H. (1968). Iron-Platinum Hardening in Casting Golds for Use with Porcelain. J. Dent. Res. 49:283.

Southan, D. E. (1968). The Physical properties of modern dental porcelain. Ph. D. Thesis, University of Sydney.

Szantho von Radnoth, M., and Leutenschlager, E. P. (1969). Metal surface changes during porcelain firing. J. dent. Res. 48:321.

Timoshenko, S. (1959). Theory of Plates and Shells, p. 76. McGraw-Hill, New York.

Tucillo, J. J. (1976). U.S. Patent 3,961,420. Dental restoration combining dental porcelain and improved white gold alloy and U.S. Patent 3,981,723. White gold alloy.

Tuccillo, J. J. (1977). Composition and functional characteristics of precious metal alloys for dental restorations. In: Alternatives to Gold Alloys in Dentistry pp. 40–67. Conference proceedings N.I.H.

Vickery, R. C., and *Badinelli, L. A.* (1968). Nature of attachment forces in porcelain-gold systems. J. Dent. Res. 47:683.

Wang, F., and *Tooley, F. V.* (1958). Influence of reaction products on reaction between water and soda-lime-silica glass. J. Am. Ceram. Soc. 41: 521-4. Ref. cited in Chemical Abstracts 53: 3625e, 1959.

Wakelin, R. J. (1967). Personal Communication.

Warpeha, W. S., and *Goodkind, G. J.* (1976). Design and technique variables affecting fracture resistance of metal-ceramic restorations. J. Pros. Dent. 35:291.

Weyl, von D. (1959). The effect of internal stresses on the structure and mechanical strength of porcelain. Dtsch. Keram. Ges. 36:319.

Wilson, H. J., and *Whitehead, F. I. H.* (1967). Comparison of some physical properties of dental porcelain. Dent. Practit. 17:350.

Monograph III

Aesthetics of Dental Porcelain

Aesthetics of Dental Porcelain

The replication of the form and colour of natural teeth in dental porcelain remains an art rather than a science. Thus correct colour matching of natural teeth by the clinician is dependent upon his subjective assessment and, even with the use of the most modern types of shade guide and colour corrected lighting, he will experience difficulty in producing consistent shade matchings. This point has been well illustrated by *Culpepper* (1970). Thirty-seven practising dentists were invited to match the shades of six natural teeth using four shade guides and four different light sources, including daylight. *Culpepper* concluded:

1. There was a lack of consistency between the individual dentists participating in the experiments in matching natural tooth shades.
2. The shade guides employed in the study did not always correspond to the gradations of predominant colours observed in the natural teeth.
3. None of the four prosthetic shade guides tested produced consistent results in matching six natural teeth under four different light sources.
4. None of the four light sources tested contributed to consistency in clinically matching the shades of six natural teeth. Lights included daylight, fluorescent light, and two prototype shade-matching lights (*Comparator* and *MacBeth*).

5. Critical colour perception varied from one individual to another.

6. Some individuals were unable to duplicate with any reliability their shade selections from one time to another.

This study is of particular value in demonstrating what occurs in normal clinical practice. Colour matching of natural teeth, being of necessity subjective in nature, limits the use of scientific instruments. Modern colour measuring instruments used for determining a single colour will give a precision only of about ±0.005 in chromaticity, which is worse than that achieved by visual colorimeters. If we accept the limitations of subjective assessment of colour, then the understanding of the variables involved in duplicating human enamel with dental porcelain is more important to the clinician than the acquisition of a detailed knowledge of the nature of light and its effect on colour perception. However, there are certain aspects of the behaviour of light that are of use to the practising clinician and which can assist him in making his shade selections.

The Nature of Light

Light is a form of radiant energy which is in the wavelength region detectable by the human eye. Without light, colour does not exist. As *Newton* explained in his "Optiks": "The rays (of light) to speak properly are not coloured. In them there is nothing else than a certain power to stir up a sensation of this or that colour." The sensation is a subjective experience, whereas the beam of light, which is the physical stimulus that produces the sensation, is entirely objective.

Light is emitted when solids, such as metals or metal oxides, are heated to incandescence, when electric currents are passed through gases or as the result of nuclear reactions as, for example, in the sun. Whatever the nature of the light source, colour response results from either a reflected or a transmitted beam of white light or a portion of that beam. There must be enough light before colour is seen and no object appears coloured in low levels of illumination because the sensitive rods in the eye cannot detect colour, unlike the less sensitive cones.

The colour that is seen by an observer in matching a tooth shade will depend upon:

1. The spectral energy distribution of the light source, e.g. daylight or artificial light.
2. The spectral characteristics of the tooth, in respect to absorption, reflection, transmission.
3. The sensitivity of the eye.
4. The conditions under which the colour of the tooth is being viewed, e.g. oral background, wet or dry conditions, angle and intensity of illumination.

In order for the clinician to obtain correct colour rendering, he must try and use a source of light that contains a full spectrum, without any excessive dominance of energy at any wavelength. In order to understand this phenomenon a short description of the spectrum is necessary.

When a beam of light is passed through a glass prism, the light beam is dispersed and emerges as bands of colour, including violet, blue, green yellow, orange, and red. The colours result from a difference in wavelength from the violet to the red end of the spectrum. These series of coloured bands are often termed "the spectrum of the light source." The wavelengths and colour bands in visible light are illustrated in Fig. 3-1. The eye is sensitive to light radiations from about 380 mμ to 780 mμ and will be capable of registering all the colours from violet to red. The spectra of light sources are not identical (e.g. sunlight to artificial light) and this explains why tooth colours may change according to the light source.

If any of these colours are viewed under a light source that has greater energy in one or more specific wavelengths (colour bands) then this colour will be dominant to the observer. For example, a clinical situation can arise when a tooth or porcelain crown appears quite different in colour when viewed under daylight or tungsten light. The relative energy distribution of average daylight and tungsten filament light is graphically depicted in Figs. 3-2 and 3-3. The light from tungsten filament light has a very low energy at the blue end of the spectrum (400 mμ) and relatively high energy at the red end (700 mμ). A tungsten light would therefore have a dominantly orange red energy and its colour rendering of porcelain or tooth structure would be to emphasise the orange-redness of the tooth crown and minimise the blue-greenness. By contrast average daylight has a slight dominance in the blue end of the spectrum (450 − 500 mμ) and teeth would not appear so orange in colour but take on the more natural hue of the blue-grey enamel.

In the case of fluorescent tubes, as these are gas discharge lamps, the bulk of their radiant energy is in very narrow spectral bandwidths. Although the lamp can be made to emit energy

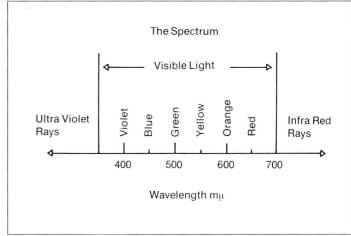

Fig. 3-1 Diagram of the colour bands and wavelengths of visible light.

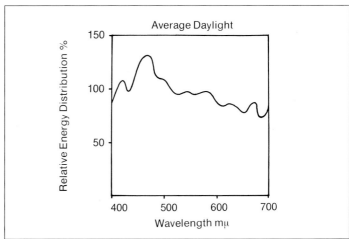

Fig. 3-2 Diagram of the relative energy distribution in daylight.

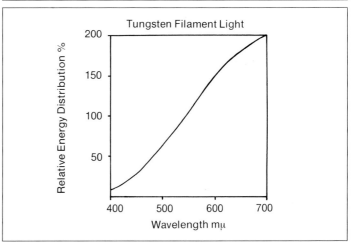

Fig. 3-3 Diagram of the relative energy distribution in tungsten filament light.

throughout the spectrum by the use of fluorescent phosphors, much of the energy is always in narrow bandwidths related to the particular gases being used. It is for the above reasons that natural daylight is still the best source for matching shades.

Primary Colours

It is possible to make nearly all colours by mixtures of three primary colours – red, green, and blue. Equal amounts of a red, a green, and a blue light will give the appearance of white and this enables a mathematical system to be devised for the specification of colour. The white produced with the mixture of red, green, and blue light is not physically a true white light, for it does not contain all the components of normal white light. In the case of pigments that are used in dental porcelain, these have the quality of absorbing some part of the white light and the colour which the ceramist sees results from the remainder of the light which is left. The colour is therefore produced subtractively.

The Three Dimensions of Colour

Colour has a three-dimensional quality and when describing it the following three variables will influence the observer's colour rendering.

1. Hue. The type of colour, e.g. red, orange, blue, etc.
2. Chroma. The strength or purity of a colour at any given value level.
3. Value. The total reflectance or luminance. This property is related to brightness or lightness.

Hue

The colour sensation experienced by the observer when viewing a tooth is the result of the amount of absorption of the various colour rays of the tooth dentine and enamel. The observer will then become aware that the tooth has a definite hue, for example pinky-yellow, grey-yellow, or bluish-yellow. If the clinician can become accustomed to grouping teeth in specific ranges of hue then shade selection will already be made easier. Porcelain tooth manufactures have, in recent years, made considerable strides in grouping their teeth into various ranges of hue, as will be described later. However, it should be remembered that, under good conditions, the eye can distinguish about two-hundred different hues.

Chroma

When two teeth have the same hue, it may be observed that one of them appears more intense or pure in colour. This intensity depends upon the saturation of colour or the strength of hue and may be easily seen when comparing two similar specimens of dental porcelain. Although both specimens may be of the same hue, it will be noticed that when the thickness of either specimen is reduced, the intensity or pureness of colour of one specimen may deteriorate more rapidly than the other. Ceramists loosely call this a "washed-out effect" and it is due to loss of colour saturation. The hue is de-saturated with white because of the increase in translucency (i.e. increase in white light). Marked changes in the colour of dental porcelain occuring in enamel veneers of different thickness present the greatest problem to the ceramist and porcelain manufacturer. This is particularly noticeable in the porcelains used in the metal-ceramic technique. The degree of colour saturation of the teeth is therefore of great importance since this will often depend upon the thickness and translucency of the enamel and the degree of calcification of the underlying dentine. Unless the clinician makes a careful note of the thickness of the overlying layer of human enamel and its effect on the tooth colour, then the technician will be placed in great difficulty when duplicating this enamel.

The consistency of colour saturation in dental porcelain when varied in thickness from 0.5 to 1 mm is also an excellent guide to the ceramist of the porcelain's quality. Materials that are subject to devitrification or separation of the colour pigments can often be detected when the porcelain is baked in different thicknesses. Ideally a dental porcelain should retain its colour saturation over a range of thicknesses between 0.5 to 1 mm. This saturation of colour should not be obtained at the expense of translucency since porcelain crowns must have depth of translucency if they are to match natural teeth.

Value

Value is a photometric quality. When all the colours of the spectrum from a white light source are reflected from an object with the same intensity as received, then the object appears white. Conversely, when all the spectrum colours are absorbed equally, the object appears black. This colour contrast between black and white is well-known and accounts for the difference in brightness between objects. In the case of a human tooth, the younger patient has generally made little secondary dentine and resultantly his tooth is "whiter and brighter". Dental porcelains which can match these younger tooth dentines and enamels will therefore have to contain more whitening agents such as zirconium oxide. The porcelain enamels should be made from very high purity glasses in order to avoid a grey-green affect influencing the final colour or hue.

Chroma and Hue together define the quality aspect of the colour. Value can be defined as the quantitative aspect of colour.

When opaque or core porcelains are placed near to the surface of porcelain crowns, they generally increase the value or brightness. In-creasing the enamel thickness will reduce value.

Colour Measurement

The three dimensions of colour – hue, chroma and value – can be used in various ways to define and measure colour.

The *Munsell* Colour System described on page 143 arranges all the colours through the interior of a cylinder. Value varies vertically, hue varies with position about the centre in a horizontal plane, and chroma varies with the distance outward, normal to the centre vertical.

Other methods use the C.I.E. System (Commission Internationale d'Eclairage). In this system the colour of a material is specified by the intensity of the three primary colours (red, green and blue) reflected under standard conditions. The reflected tristimuli (red, green and blue) intensities are then compared with those from a white reference standard and the tristimulus values of the specimen are calculated. Further calculations lead to a complete specification of the colour of a material in terms of its dominant wavelength, percentage luminance or brightness, and its excitation or spectral purity.

The use of a colour measuring instrument is of some value as a research tool in dentistry and can definitely assist the manufacturer in determining and grouping his shade selection. However, from a clinical standpoint, there is little evidence up to date that shade selections in the mouth could be determined by instrumentation.

The eye can detect differences in colour often better than the most sensitive instruments available.

Complementary Colours

Certain hues when places alongside each other appear to have a higher chroma. These colours are called complementary. For example an orange colour will appear brighter when placed in a blue field. However, when complementary colours are mixed together they have a neutralising effect on each other and appear greyer. When blended in unequal amounts, the hue which is present in greatest chroma will be reduced in value (less bright and greyer) and will appear to have been reduced in colour saturation (chroma).

A knowledge of complementary colours may assist the ceramist when altering shades by intermixing colours but as will be shown in volume II, "Laboratory Procedures in Dental Ceramics", the use of surface stains to alter a shade has severe limitations.

Optical Properties

Translucent objects will both reflect and transmit some light. The human tooth may therefore be regarded as a translucent material, and as the enamel approaches the tip of the incisal edge, the amount of light transmitted will increase to a degree where it almost becomes transparent. Translucency in human enamel is influenced by the reflection and refraction of light in the enamel rods. In order to understand this important area relating to dental aesthetics, the clinician should be familiar with the effects of refractive index on light dispersion and the effects of light scattering.

Reflection

Regular or Specular Reflection

Definition:

Reflection without diffusion in accordance with the law of optical reflection as in a mirror.

Diffuse Reflection

Definition:

Diffusion by reflection in which, on the macroscopic side, there is no regular reflection.
(Definition in International Lighting Vocabulary. C.I.E. No. 17. 1970.)
High spots on a metal-ceramic crown are produced by high reflection from opaque porcelains on the metal. In this case the opaque porcelain is acting like a mirror surface and is increasing the value of the crown.

High reflection is undesirable in porcelain crowns since natural teeth seldom produce areas of high reflectivity. Translucent enamel reduces reflection but increases light transmission. Methods of decreasing specular and diffuse reflection will be described.

Refractive index and dispersion

When light passes from a vacuum into a denser material, its velocity is decreased. The ratio between these velocities determines many optical phenomena and is called the index of refraction.

The refractive index is a function of the frequency of light, normally decreasing as the wavelength increases. This change with wavelength is known as dispersion of the refractive index (*Kingery,* 1960).

Reflection and Refraction

The relative index of refraction between phases (ratio of refractive indices) determines the reflectance and refractive properties of a phase boundary. For example, the change in velocity of light when passing through an alumina crystal and its surrounding glass matrix will cause the light to bend as it passes through the glass/crystal interface (phase boundary). However, some is reflected from the surface of the crystals, and it is this light that increases reflection and makes a crown look brighter.

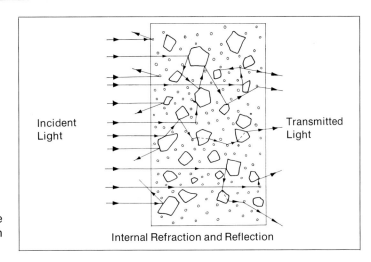

Incident
Light

Transmitted
Light

Internal Refraction and Reflection

Fig. 3-4 Diagram showing the internal refraction and reflection of light in dental porcelain.

Light Scattering

The effects of light scattering are probably the most important aspects to understand in formulating dental porcelain.

Dental porcelain can be regarded as optically heterogeneous, i.e. it is a transparent medium containing small particles such as metallic oxides (opacifiers), crystals or glassy grains of dissimilar refractive indices to the porcelain. When a beam of light enters such a system, a portion of the beam is scattered and the intensity of the beam is reduced (Fig. 3-4). In any ceramic system the greatest light scattering effect is obtained with an increasing difference in refractive index between the particles (opacifiers) and the main bulk of the porcelain phase. In addition, the scattering is strongly dependent on particle size, so that the maximum scattering occurs at a particle size of the same magnitude as the radiation wavelength. For particle sizes much smaller than the wavelength of incident radiation, the scattering constant (referred to as K) increases with particle size and is inversely proportional to the fourth power of wavelength. The scattering coefficient reaches a maximum when the particle size is about equal to the wavelength of incident radiation and decreases at larger particle size values (*Kingery,* 1960). The scattering constant K, reaches a constant value for particle sizes substantially larger than the wavelength of incident radiation, so that for a fixed concentration of second phase the measured scattering coefficient is inversely proportional to particle size.

The refractive index of dental porcelain is similar to that of a typical soda-lime-silica glass which is in the range of 1.51 to 1.52. Potash felspar generally has a higher refractive index than soda felspar.

In order to increase the light scattering in dental porcelain and simulate the prismatic effect of human enamels, it is necessary to introduce opacifiers, crystals or a second phase of porcelain powder to the basic frit. The various materials used in these techniques have been described in Monograph I, "The Nature of Dental Ceramics".

Opacity

When a beam of light consisting of a large number of light rays strikes a smooth surface, the rays will be reflected in a regular manner. However, in all dental porcelains the way the light is scattered is much more complex and will

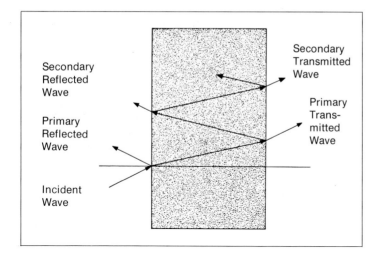

Secondary Reflected Wave

Primary Reflected Wave

Incident Wave

Secondary Transmitted Wave

Primary Transmitted Wave

Fig. 3-5 Diagram of the scattering effect of an incident beam of light in dental porcelain. The primary reflected wave tends to increase with a higher glaze whereas the secondary reflected wave is much more dependent on the reflectivity of the opaque background used. Transmitted waves of light would only occur in the absence of metal backgrounds and would be at their maximum in the incisal area of a crown.

have a varied effect on the aesthetics of the porcelain crown, depending on its method of construction.

The important optical characteristics seen when a beam of light enters a typical dental porcelain is illustrated in Fig. 3-5. A fraction of the light is reflected (specular reflection) and this determines the degree of glaze or gloss on the surface. Of the remaining light, a fraction is diffusely reflected, (Fig. 3-4) and the remainder directly and diffusely transmitted (Fig. 3-5).

Depending upon the difference in refractive indices between the dispersed particles (opacifiers etc.) in dental porcelain, the light transmission, diffusion and reflectance can be varied to produce highly translucent enamels, less translucent dentines, and opaque backgrounds to cover metal or cement surfaces.

The importance of understanding the role of opaque porcelains in dental ceramic work will be discussed later. However, at this stage it is essential to consider the main factors determining the production of opaque porcelains in dentistry.

As explained previously, for maximum scattering power the particles (opacifiers etc.) should have an index of refraction far different from that of the matrix material, they should have a particle size nearly the same as the wavelength of the incident radiation, and the volume fraction of particles present should be high. Since the opacifiers must have an index of refraction substantially different from dental porcelain, this limits the number of materials available. In addition, opacifiers must be able to be formed as small particles in a silicate liquid matrix and this further limits the materials that can be used.

Opacifiers used in dental porcelain can be materials that are completely inert with the glass phase, they can be inert products formed during melting, or they can be crystallised from the melt during cooling or reheating, as discussed in Monograph I.

Materials used in dental porcelain as opacifiers are listed as follows with their refractive indices:

Opacifier		Refractive Index
Tin dioxide	SnO_2	2.0
Zirconium dioxide	ZrO_2	2.2
Titanium dioxide	TiO_2 (anatase)	2.52
Aluminum trioxide	Al_2O_3	1.8
Dental Porcelain		1.5

The fractions of incident light that are reflected, absorbed, and transmitted in an opaque dental porcelain depend on the thickness of the specimen as well as the scattering and absorption characteristics. For practical applications the use of opaque porcelains in dentistry is concerned with the reflectance of an opaque layer in contact with a backing of some reflectance. The backing could be either metal or the cement under a complete porcelain crown.

Kubelka and *Munk* (1931) have indicated that the reflectance from ceramics increases as the backing reflectance increases. In the case of dental ceramics the backing reflectance would be dependent upon the texture of the metal surface or the reflectance and absorption powers of the dental cement. The reflectance from the surface of ceramics will also increase as the scattering coefficient increases, as the thickness of the opaque coating increases, and as the reflectivity increases. The reflectivity is determined by the ratio of the absorption coefficient and the scattering coefficient.

Paint-on-Opaques

Good opacification is obtained with high values of reflectivity, thick coatings, and high values of the scattering coefficient or some combination of these (*Kingery,* 1960). Unfortunately, all of the above criteria are probably the least desirable from a dental standpoint. Although the metal surface of a crown can be easily masked with an opaque porcelain with the above properties, the high reflectance from these paint-on-opaques must cause high reflectivity from the crown's surfaces and introduce metameric problems. The significance of these problems in dental porcelain will be discussed later.

In the case of metal-ceramic crowns, a thin coating applied by spraying or brushing is currently used by the technician. These opaques have high covering power, generally obtained by using high light scattering power metallic oxides such as tin or zirconium oxide. The gold alloys can be masked with opaques using coatings often as thin as 100 microns. The light transmission through the opaque porcelains used in the metal-ceramic technique is very low and is within a range of 0.2–0.5 percent light transmission on one millimetre thick specimens. (*McLean* and *Hughes,* 1965).

It is now possible to see the great difference between the two materials. Aluminous porcelain crowns will allow both diffuse and regular transmission of light (Fig. 3-6). By contrast, the metal-ceramic opaque will only permit diffuse reflection and specular reflection of light (Fig. 3-7). These differences are by far the most significant causes for poor aesthetics on the front teeth when metal-ceramic restorations are fitted, since a natural tooth always permits diffuse transmission and regular transmission of light (Fig. 3-8).

In order to simulate natural teeth an artificial crown must have depth of translucency. Only in this way can an anterior crown become submerged in the mouth. Surface colourants can never provide the answer to the ultimate aesthetic result since colour must be seen in depth. Surface colourants behave like opaque porcelains and produce highly reflective surfaces. The role of opaques in dentistry has been determined by our necessity to mask undesirable metal or cement backgrounds. The aesthetic problems arising from their use will be discussed later.

Translucency

Diffuse reflection of light produced by internal scattering must not be too great in dental porcelain, otherwise anterior crowns look very artificial. By contrast the fraction of incident light which emerges as diffuse transmission is vital in a ceramic crown. It is this diffused light that

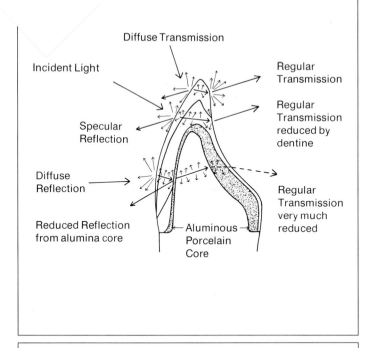

Diffuse Transmission

Incident Light

Regular
Transmission

Regular
Transmission
reduced by
dentine

Specular
Reflection

Diffuse
Reflection

Regular
Transmission
very much
reduced

Reduced Reflection
from alumina core

Aluminous
Porcelain
Core

Fig. 3-6 Diagram of the reflection and transmission of incident light in an aluminous porcelain crown. Note the transmission of light through the entire body of the crown.

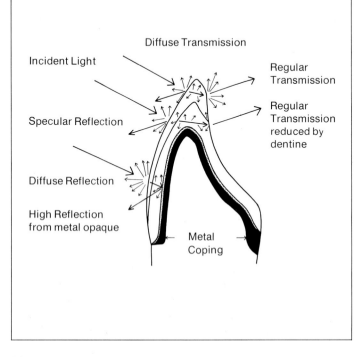

Diffuse Transmission

Incident Light

Regular
Transmission

Specular Reflection

Regular
Transmission
reduced by
dentine

Diffuse Reflection

High Reflection
from metal opaque

Metal
Coping

Fig. 3-7 Reflection and transmission of incident light in a metal-ceramic crown. Note the increased reflectance from the metal opaque.

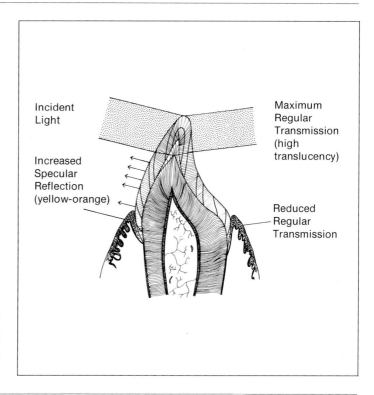

Incident Light

Increased Specular Reflection (yellow-orange)

Maximum Regular Transmission (high translucency)

Reduced Regular Transmission

Fig. 3-8   Diagram of a cross-section of a human tooth showing areas of maximum light reflection and transmission. Gingival colour would also be influenced by the gum and root dentine.

produces translucency in dental porcelain (Fig. 3-6).

In order to produce translucent enamels which also give a prismatic effect, similar techniques are used in dental porcelain to those for producing an opal glass. For example, we require minimal light absorption but maximum light scattering to give an effect similar to enamel prisms. In this case the dispersed phase (opacifiers, crystals etc.) in the enamel porcelain should have a refractive index not much different from that of the porcelain matrix. The use of two-phase materials, nucleation, and dispersion of particles has been described in Monograph I together with techniques used to enhance the blue-grey effect of dental enamel porcelains.

In addition, high translucency in modern dental felspathic porcelains has been achieved by increasing the amount of glass at the expense of mullite formation. Although this reduces strength, the translucency of the porcelain is greatly improved. The aluminous porcelains compensate for the reduction in strength of the veneer porcelains by the high strength core porcelains.

Surface Gloss

The glaze or gloss on the surface of a ceramic crown is intimately related to the relative amount of specular and diffuse reflection. *Dinsdale* and *Malkin* (1955) consider that surface gloss is closely related to the sharpness and perfection of the reflected image, that is, to the narrowness of the specular reflection band and its intensity. These factors are primarily determined by the index of refraction and by the surface smoothness.

Kingery (1960) considers that because ceramic systems are not perfectly smooth, there is considerable diffuse reflection from the surface. If

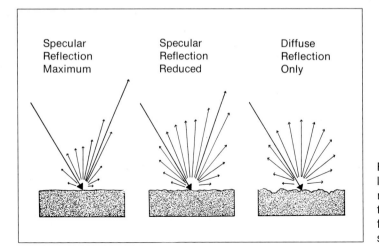

Specular Reflection Maximum

Specular Reflection Reduced

Diffuse Reflection Only

Fig. 3-9 Diagram illustrating the light scattering from increasingly rough surfaces. Specular reflection is reduced and diffuse reflection increased with increasing surface roughness.

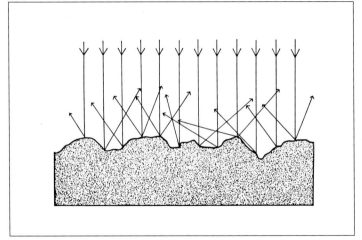

Fig. 3-10 Diagram illustrating how the diffuse reflection of light occurs from opaque porcelains or cements.

the amount of energy reflected at different angles from a single incident beam is measured for an opaque material of increasing roughness, results such as those shown in Fig. 3-9 are obtained. In opaque materials, such as silicate cements and dental opaque porcelains, the degree of diffuse reflection is related to surface roughness, as illustrated in Fig. 3-10.

It is therefore undesirable to apply dentine and enamel porcelains onto highly glazed opaques since a mirror surface is created and bright spots may appear particularly at the incisal third of the preparation. A rougher surface can be produced by lightly blasting the surface of the opaque with 30 μm aluminium oxide grit. This type of surface will increase diffuse reflection (Figs. 3-9 and 3-10).

In the case of the translucent enamel and dentine porcelains, subsurface reflections are most important. This is why the building-in of colour in depth is so important if a three-dimensional quality to the crown is to be obtained. (See Fig. 3-6 and frontispiece.)

Effect of Metal Surface Treatment on the Masking Power of Opaque Porcelain

The surface treatment of the metals used in the metal-ceramic technique can have an effect on the masking power of the opaque porcelain. One investigation showed that sandblasted and fineground surfaces required comparable thicknesses of porcelain to achieve the same degree of opacity at selected wavelengths, whereas specimens conditioned with a gold flashing agent required 40 to 60 percent less opaque porcelain to achieve the same result (*Herzberg* et al., 1972). A change in reflectivity was noted for all surfaces as porcelain of increasing thickness was applied. It is interesting to note that in this research work, porcelain samples equal to, or more than, 0.65 mm thick were assumed to be completely opaque, because no changes in spectral curves were noted at greater thicknesses.

Any optical differences that can be detected clinically between a sand-blasted or finely ground metal surface are probably marginal and it is for this reason that a change in colour of the metal surface or its spectral reflectivity is the most likely way of improving the aesthetics of the metal-ceramic crown.

The current high fusing gold alloys are dark grey in colour and it is for this reason that "gold flashing" agents have been introduced. These surface conditioners have been given various names such as "bonding agents", "bright coat", "gold glaze" or "metal conditioners". In general they have not become very popular with the dental ceramist and most technicians find that they can mask the metal surface very effectively without their use. These surface coating agents are all colloidal dispersions of gold in an organic base and it must be recognised that pure gold cannot form a chemical bond with dental porcelain. The use of these coating agents may, therefore, reduce the potential oxide surface area for bonding to porcelain.

The ultimate solution to the problem of producing a good colour to the metal surface probably lies in "gold flashing" but such a surface must be left chemically reactive in order to provide a strong bond between gold and porcelain. In addition, great care must be exercised in the use of very thin coats of opaque porcelain since these can be highly reflective and therefore increase the risk of metameric and other undesirable colour effects.

Ultra-Violet Radiation and Fluorescence

Natural teeth will fluoresce under ultra-violet radiation and this is particularly noticeable in dancehalls and discotheques where lamps are used which emit the blue end of the spectrum in addition to some ultra-violet radiation. By this means, an "effect" is created in which white shirts and teeth are "luminous" but some dental restorations are black.

It is thought that the "fluors" (i.e. the compounds causing fluorescence) in natural teeth are organic in nature (*Horsley,* 1967), are possibly protein, and that the fluorescence may be due to the energy transfer from phenylalanine and tyrosin to tryptophane (*Hefferen* et al., 1967; *McDevitt* and *Armstrong,* 1969). In addition, part of the inorganic matrix of teeth has also shown to be fluorescent since inactivation of the protein by heat does not cause complete failure of response of teeth to ultra-violet radiation.

Since natural teeth fluoresce vividly in both sunlight and in the lighting of discotheques, it is desirable that dental porcelain should contain substances that can make the ceramic crown simulate the natural fluorescence of the human tooth.

In order to understand the phenomenon known as fluorescence, clinicians should be aware of certain fundamentals. An excellent account of fluorescence has been given by *Wilson* (1969). Fluorescence is the absorption of radiation of a particular wavelength and its re-emission as a radiation of longer wavelength. For example, when ultra-violet light strikes natural teeth or certain restorative materials, visible radiation is emitted. As previously stated, light is radiation which is in the wavelength region detectable by the human eye. The radiation from the sun, or white light, includes all the wavelengths from the visible spectrum; violet has the shortest wavelength, approximately 400 mμ, and red the longest, approximately 700 mμ. Ultra-violet radiation has a shorter wavelength between 300 – 390 mμ (Fig. 3-1). Radiation can be considered as discrete units called photons; the energy associated with each is inversely proportional to its wavelength.

Ultra-violet radiation has greater energy than visible light because it has a shorter wavelength. If ultra-violet radiation falls on a body, then some energy transformation can occur, energy being imparted to the atoms or molecules in the body, producing excited states. When the atoms or molecules return to a less excited state, but not the original state, radiations of less energy can be emitted, sometimes in the visible range. This fact has been known for over a hundred years as *Stokes'* Law. It can be stated simply as "The wavelength of the light emitted by a fluorescent substance is greater than that of the exciting radiation". In a solid fuorescent material known as phosphor, fluorescence is bound up with the molecular structure of the material. It is exhibited by many materials such as sulphurs, oxides, tungstates and silicates. With these materials the phenomenon of fluorescence is often associated with the presence of small amounts of impurities, such as manganese, bismuth, copper, antimony and chromium. The intensity of the fluorescence depends upon the concentration of the impurity; an optimum value exists for each material which is usually between 0.001 percent and 0.1 percent. The importance of such impurities is well illustrated by the ruby which consists of aluminium oxide containing a very small amount of chromium oxide. In a ruby, artificially prepared in the laboratory, the small amount of chromium oxide is absolutely essential if the artificial stone is to exhibit the fluorescent characteristic of the real stone. Without the chromium oxide there is no fluorescence, but with it the fluorescence is identical with that of natural ruby.

The fluorescence of natural teeth is greatest when the wavelength of the exciting radiation is about 300 mμ, whilst the emission of light is most pronounced at a wavelength of about 400 mμ. Carious dentine does not fluoresce, and it is believed that this is due to the presence of a material in the carious dentine which masks the effect of the fluorescent coumpound. This masking agent in carious dentine absorbs strongly in the ultra-violet region 230 to 330 mμ with maximum absorption at 265 mμ. It is therefore probable that the masking agent protects the fluorescent component from excitation by the ultra-violet radiation.

Radio-active compounds in dental porcelain

The yellow-white fluorescence of natural teeth may be reasonably simulated by incorporating a small percentage of sodium diuranate into the porcelain frit. The uranium content does not usually exceed 0.15 percent and will produce a brilliant canary-yellow colour. The yellow can then be dampened down by the incorporation of cerium salts which are blue. In this way the yellow becomes desaturated to a blue-white fluorescence. All modern aluminous and metal-ceramic porcelains will fluoresce a blue-white and although the manufacturers have not yet succeeded in exactly simulating the yellow-white fluorescence of natural teeth, the current methods are a great improvement over earlier products.

Radiation hazards

Moore and *MacCulloch* (1974) have determined the radio-activity of porcelain powders by comparing them with the "normal background radiation" in the atmosphere. They concluded that crown and bridge porcelains were the most active of the groups studied, emitting on average 3.01 times that of the background level of radiation. Porcelain artificial teeth have an average increase of 1.74 times the background level. Although they concluded that the danger to patients from these emissions may be assumed to be negligible, they did warn the ceramist against sucking brushes and instruments used to apply the powders. This would reduce any skin dosage and the amount of powder ingested. Adequate ventilation of the laboratory or air conditioning would also minimise the inhalation of powder.

The danger to full-time dental ceramists should be appreciated. Carcinoma of the bladder is stated to be one of the effects of uranium intoxication and any long-term ingestion of radioactive substances known to predispose to malignant disease should be avoided.

Medical and dental procedures involving the therapeutic or diagnostic use of radiation are exempt from specific dose limitations, and reliance is placed on the clinician's appreciation of the balance between risk and benefit in any given circumstance. It cannot be claimed that the use of radioactive fluorescers in dental porcelain is a diagnostic or therapeutic procedure (*O'Riordan* and *Hunt,* 1974): consequently, the dose limit appropriate to these circumstances is that recommended in the medical and dental code of practice (HMSO 1972) for single organs of members of the public, namely 1.5 rem in a year averaged over the organ. This figure is adopted from the recommendations of the International Commission on Radiological Protection (ICRP Publication 9) for unspecified organs or tissues.

The above statements in the report by *O'Riordan* and *Hunt* (1974) resulted in the following recommendations being published by the National Radiological Protection Board (NRPB Report 25, 1974):

"An examination of the use of uranium compounds in dental porcelain to simulate the fluorescence of natural teeth shows that the irradiation of the tissue of the mouth may well exceed the limit recommended by the International Commission on Radiological Protection for the average dose to the general organs or tissues of members of the public. The performance of fluorescing agents is unsatisfactory in ultraviolet light, and they may be unnecessary in normal light. It is recommended that the practice be discontinued and that non-radioactive fluorescers be considered.

This requirement is now being incorporated in future standards.

Colour Blending

As explained previously, of all the visible colours and shades, there are only three primary colours consisting of red, green, and blue. All other colours may be produced by the correct combination of these colours. Although knowledge of colour blending can be useful to the dental ceramist, it is doubtful whether he will be able to blend shades as accurately as the tooth manufacturer. Even the most experienced ceramists are tending to use pre-blended shades of porcelain which can be modified by the addition of concentrated colours or "effect masses". Pre-blended shades of porcelain can be used separately or mixed together to produce a custom-built shade guide. This probably represents the ideal and will give intermediate shades between the manufacturer's selected colours. It has been the author's experience that attempts to vary the colour of porcelain jacket crowns by minor additions of concentrated colour pigments to the dentine powders is more likely to confuse the beginner rather than assist him. If the ceramist is to produce his own shades then

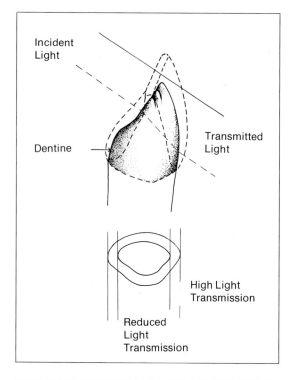

Incident Light

Dentine

Transmitted Light

High Light Transmission

Reduced Light Transmission

Fig. 3-11 Diagram showing the effect of the underlying dentine on colour production in a young tooth.

he must have an extensive knowledge of blending primary colours and preferably acquire this knowledge in a porcelain factory. The beginner is better advised to work with pre-blended shades and use shade buttons or preferably a custom-built shade guide.

Colour Production in Natural Teeth

Human enamel contains approximately 97 percent by weight mineral matter, mostly in the form of hydroxyapatite, $Ca_{10}(PO_4)_6(OH)_2$ though carbonapatite, fluorapatite, calcium fluorides,

calcium carbonate may be present in varying small amounts in different individuals. The hydroxyapatite crystals in enamel are extremely small (3000—5000 Å in length by 50—1200 Å in width) with a consequent high surface area/volume ratio. The enamel rods or prisms are bound together with organic material (the collagen matrix) which represents approximately 1 percent of the total mass. Enamel is therefore very translucent and may transmit up to 70 percent light through a 1 mm thick section.

By contrast the dentine only contains about 70 percent by weight of hydroxyapatite and the apatite crystals are much smaller than in enamel (200—300 Å long by 40—70 Å wide). Consequently they have an even greater surface area/volume ratio. The organic matrix of dentine constitutes about 20 percent by weight of the total tissue, or about 30 percent on a volume percent basis. It is mostly collagen with a small quantity of mucopolysaccharide ground substance. The dentine is still translucent but will generally not transmit much more than 30 percent light on a 1 mm thick section.

It is possible that the smaller apatite crystals in dentine may also be responsible for an increase in the opacity values. The small crystals would correspond with the very fine powders (high specific surface area) used as opacifying or re-inforcing agents in porcelain. Dispersion of fine powders in matrices of different refractive indices results in an increase in opacity. The colour in dentine is probably produced from a combination of the refraction of light in the prisms combined with an increase in emission of rays of light in the yellow to orange range, compared with the tooth enamel. The collagen matrix in the dentine would play a significant role in causing this light refraction.

The total colour effect in a natural tooth is there-fore derived from a combination of light directly reflected from the tooth surface combined with light that has been reflected from the dentine and which has already undergone some internal reflection. The dentine is the prime source of colour and the reflected rays of light which are emitted via the enamel are modified by the thickness and degree of translucency of the enamel and the dark oral background.

The effect of enamel thickness and translucency on colour is illustrated in Fig. 3-11. The dentine in the younger tooth will often form two or three lobes over the pulp which will appear as finger-like extensions under the enamel.

Incisal Third

The highly translucent enamel covering the dentine produces what one might term "a wrap-around effect". This results in increased trans-lucency not only at the incisal one-third but also in the approximal areas. The enamel will, at the same time, delineate the finger-like extensions of the dentine. The grey translucency at the incisal tip is accentuated by the dark oral background.

Middle Third

The middle-third of the tooth contains a major quantity of dentine. The overlaying enamel will therefore take on some of the dentine hue but this will be modified by the translucent blue-grey enamel so that the final colour is often a mixture of yellow-orange, blue, and grey.

Cervical Third

As the enamel approaches the cervical line of the tooth crown, it thins down to a chisel or chamfer edge. The influence of the underlying dentine on the colour of the tooth is therefore quite marked. The neck of the tooth will take on a deeper hue which will vary in colour from orange-yellow to often a distinct brown, depend-ing upon the degree of calcification of the den-tine (Fig. 3-8).

Reproducing Natural Teeth in Dental Porcelain

The main features in a natural tooth that must be reproduced in dental porcelain are colour, texture, and translucency. The aesthetic re-placement of human tooth enamel with dental porcelain is limited more by our methods of fixation rather than by the inherent aesthetic properties of dental glasses. Unfortunately there are no biologically inert cements that are transparent and which match the refractive indices of tooth structure. Resultantly it is im-possible for the basic colour of the tooth den-tine to influence markedly, the colour of the por-celain enamel veneer. We are therefore forced to provide an underlying artificial dentine col-our which may or may not resemble the human

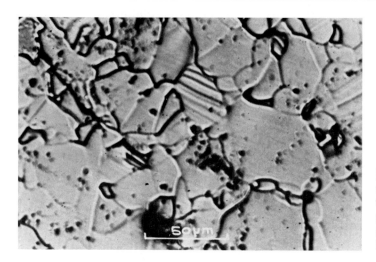

Fig. 3-12 Photomicrograph of an etched surface of aluminous veneer porcelain showing the grain boundaries which produce a "prismatic effect". Courtesy of Dr. *D. Jones,* Univ. Birmingham.

dentine. Here, then, is the first variable factor encountered in simulating natural teeth. The second factor is the duplication of the enamel colour and translucency. Natural enamel, being prismatic in nature, may only be duplicated if one could produce a material which was also made up of minute and closely-packed prisms. Dental porcelain will not fulfil this requirement but, on the other hand, it is probably the closest material to human enamel that is available. Fine dental glass powder can be made to give an opalescent or "prismatic effect" (see page 37, Monograph I) when the glass grains are only partially sintered at their grain boundaries, producing some refraction of light. (Fig. 3-12). Over firing of dental porcelain will obliterate the grain boundaries and produce a glassy porcelain which lacks the life-like qualities of correctly fired enamels.

Types of Porcelain Crowns

In order for the student to appreciate the variables involved in duplicating human tooth crowns in dental porcelain, it is useful to consider the evolution of the various types of porcelain crown.

These may be grouped as follows:

1. Regular felspathic air-fired porcelain crowns.
2. Regular felspathic vacuum-fired porcelain crowns.
3. Metal-ceramic crowns.
4. Aluminous porcelain crowns.

Felspathic crown – air-fired

The early porcelains used for jacket crown construction were of the high temperature maturing variety.

At that time, vacuum-firing techniques had not been introduced and the aesthetics of the finished porcelain jacket crown was influenced by the air-firing techniques used in platinum wound furnaces. Porcelain powders used in air-firing methods of construction must, of necessi-

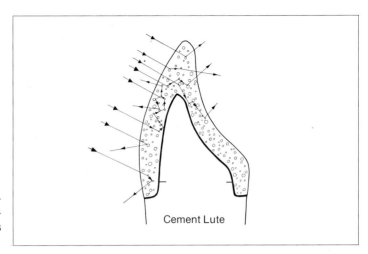

Cement Lute

Fig. 3-13 Diagram of the cloudiness produced in air-fired porcelain by the entrapped air-bubbles causing high light refraction.

ty, be fairly coarse in nature if excessive opacity in the fired ceramic is to be avoided (see page 47, Monograph I). However, if the dentine porcelains are too translucent, then the risk of the cement lute reflecting through the porcelain veneer is increased. The manufacturers utilized the slight cloudiness produced by the entrapped air-bubles in the fired ceramic to decrease this light reflection from the cement lute (Fig. 3-13). Small additions of opacifying agents would also be made to the coloured porcelain. The air-fired dentine porcelains were therefore capable of reproducing the background colour of the dentine very accurately. The major faults in the aesthetics of the air-fired crowns were to be found in the enamel veneers where translucency could be difficult to obtain. The natural "wrap-around" translucency of the approximal enamel could only be produced if very coarse glass powders were used since these materials, when fired, contained fewer but larger entrapped air bubbles (see page 47, Monograph I). These rather coarse powders were difficult to handle and the refinement of the surface could be most difficult. In addition, the characterisation of the incisal one-third of the enamel was also difficult since the building-in of concentrated colours or check lines lacked the control given by the finer vacuum-fired powders. Final-

ly, an air-fired surface could not be ground and re-polished but required further glazing if porous areas were not to be left on the surface.

Despite these defects, porcelain jacket crowns which were made in these materials reached extremely high aesthetic standards. Various coloured luting cements of the zinc phosphate type were produced to "back-up" the dentine colours. There are still many clinicians today who advocate altering the colour of the porcelain crown with these cements, if the shade is not quite accurate.

Felspathic crown – vacuum-fired

Vacuum-firing of porcelain jacket crowns was introduced to improve the aesthetics of the enamel veneers and also to produce dense surfaces. Additional benefits were derived from this research since finer powders could be used which gave lower firing shrinkages and better handling properties. In addition, colour control of the crowns was improved by the increase in density of the powders both in the unfired or "green" state and in the fired or sintered state.

Because a vacuum-fired porcelain is more translucent than the regular air-fired porcelains, the manufacturers were given much more scope in developing natural enamel effects. It is easier to develop exact colours from a transparent or nearly-transparent glass than it is from a cloudy material. Control of hue, degree of saturation and brightness all being more easily obtained from a clear glass.

With the introduction of the vacuum-fired porcelains, the use of opaque porcelains to mask the cement lute was first attempted. These o-paque porcelains generally transmitted very little light (ca. 0.2 percent through 1 mm thick discs) and could be used in very thin sections, often of less than 0.3 mm. Various colours of dentine porcelains could then be made with im-proved translucency when compared with the air-fired porcelains. However, although this was of some benefit, the most significant improve-ment was to be found in the depth of trans-lucency achieved with the enamel veneers. For the first time concentrated colours (effect mas-ses) or stains could be utilized to provide a "wrap-around" enamel effect and to highlight any finger-like extentions of dentine in the youn-ger tooth (Fig. 3-11).

There is little doubt that the vacuum-fired porce-lains offered the ceramic technician almost un-limited scope in simulating natural enamel effects and these materials continue to set the standard for all our cosmetic dentistry.

The Metal-Ceramic Crown

The use of metal copings to reinforce the veneer porcelains is very widely used. However, it must be clearly understood that the introduction of the metal-ceramic crown was brought about by the demand from clinicians for greater strength in their veneer crowns. Inevitably this has been accompanied by a loss of aesthetics due to the increased light reflectivity from the opaque por-celains used to mask the metal coping (Fig. 3-7).

The masking of metal surfaces with opaque por-celains presents considerable problems to the ceramic manufacturer. In order to reduce the thickness of the opaque layer to the minimum, it is necessary to formulate porcelains with minimal light transmission. This in turn means that these materials, when covered with a trans-lucent enamel, become highly light reflective. The opaque porcelain acts like a mirror sur-face and this is very noticeable where light rays can penetrate the crown surface and are directly reflected back again. The upper incisors are particularly susceptible to this type of direct light reflection. Two critical paths of reflectance will be observed, at the incisal one-third of the preparation and at the cervical one-third where the porcelain becomes thinner (Fig. 3-14). In order to avoid this reflection of the opaque por-celain, the ceramic technician tends to over-contour the labial face of his crown, as indicat-ed by the dotted line in Fig. 3-14. This over-con-touring creates a cervical stagnation area and increases the risk of gingival inflammation. In order to mask the opaque porcelain and create a sense of depth of translucency, an enamel veneer of at least 0.8 to 1 mm thickness is requir-ed. Unfortunately the manufacturers are placed in a dilemma in this situation since they could very easily produce dentine colours with high translucencies similar to regular porcelains, if these porcelains were used in con-sistent thickness. Unfortunately the variable thicknesses encountered in crowns made for clinical use will often necessitate the use of den-tine porcelains of less than 0.5 mm thickness. In this situation a commercially-produced porce-lain powder must have a built-in safety factor, and light transmission through the porcelain must be reduced to a level where the opaque porcelain does not have a dominating influence on colour. The porcelains used in producing the dentine colours for the metal-ceramic technique are generally more opaque than regular porcelain where light reflectivity from the opaque layers is less severe. Un-fortunately, an increase in the opacity of dentine porcelains will also cause an increase in surface reflectance, and this

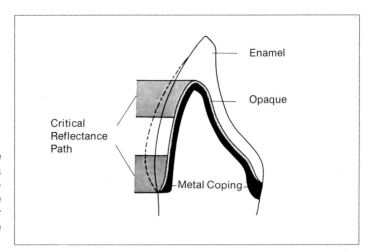

Enamel

Opaque

Critical
Reflectance
Path

Metal Coping

Fig. 3-14 Diagram illustrating the areas of high light reflection in a metal-ceramic crown. In order to overcome this colour problem the technician tends to over-contour the crown as illustrated by the dotted line.

is why the metal-ceramic crown tends to look less vital and has little depth of translucency when compared with a human tooth (Fig. 3-8). It is for this reason that the author tries to avoid their use on the upper incisors where the "mirror-effect" of the opaque porcelain is at its greatest. By contrast the posterior teeth receive more indirect illumination. If the opaque porcelain has a dominating influence on colour, then the clinician will face serious problems once the patient experiences varying artificial lighting conditions. This apparent change in colour of the crown is due to "metamerism" and to understand the problem, a brief description of this phenomenon is essential.

Metamerism

A pair of samples of any material are said to be "metameric" when their spectral characteristics are different but they appear similar in colour under certain conditions of illumination. For example, a manufacturer may produce a pink-coloured enamel bath and then make a set of ceramic wall tiles to match. He may be forced to use different pigments in the enamel bath glaze to those in the tiles, i.e. the spectral characteristics of the two materials are different. In natu-

ral daylight the tiles may match the colour of the bath perfectly. However, when the bathroom light is switched on, the tiles no longer match the colour of the bath. This is a classical example of "metamerism" which has plagued the ceramic industry for so long. The metameric pairs (in this case the bath and the tiles) do not continue to be colour matches under different sources of illumination. By changing the spectral distribution of the illuminant, the differences in the spectral characteristics of two materials become apparent. Pairs of ceramic materials containing similar metallic oxide pigments will be only slightly metameric whereas a ceramic made to match the colour of a tooth can be highly metameric since the spectral characteristics of the two materials are very different. It is now possible to see why the opaque layers of porcelain in metal-ceramic crowns can have such marked influences on the colour. Opaque porcelains will generally contain pigments which are at the red end of the spectrum, e.g. orange (see Fig. 3-1). These colours will appear fairly normal in average daylight but when the patient moves under tungsten filament light, an immediate colour change is apparent. The dominant orange-red energy of the lamp will emphasize the orange-redness of the opaque porcelain and, at the

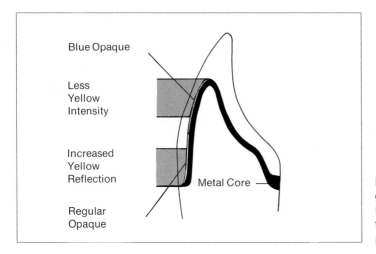

Blue Opaque

Less
Yellow
Intensity

Increased
Yellow
Reflection

Metal Core —

Regular
Opaque

Fig. 3-15 Use of blue or blue-grey opaques in the metal-ceramic technique to reduce yellow reflection at the incisal end of the preparation.

same time, the change in the spectral distribution of the illuminant (daylight to tungsten light) will increase any metameric effects. This phenomenon can often account for the apparent colour change seen in metal-ceramic crowns, when viewed under subdued tungsten filament light. The clinician may meet one of his patients at a party and suddenly be confronted with a central crown which appears quite out of character with the patient's other teeth. This mismatch in colour may not have been evident at the time of cementation of the crown and often the clinician finds it hard to believe that he could have made such a restoration. The reflection of the rays of tungsten filament light from the opaque porcelain have highlighted an inherent deficiency in the metal-ceramic system. Crowns which possess sufficient labial enamel and dentine porcelain to provide a proper depth of translucency will not be highly metameric. Translucent porcelains do not generally appear so metameric as opaque porcelain. Once the opaque layer becomes dominant, then metameric problems must arise and we see the typical "metal-ceramic smile".

The clinician can assist the ceramist in avoiding metameric effects by providing a preparation with adequate depth for the metal coping and enamel veneer. Generally it is recognised that a total depth of 1.5 mm is required in which the metal occupies 0.5 mm and the porcelain 1 mm. The ceramist must then ensure that the opaque porcelain does not have a dominating influence on colour. In cases where the labio-incisal third of the preparation has insufficient depth it is often a good plan to use an opaque colour in the blue end of the spectrum. By using a blue or grey-blue opaque in place of the more yellow-orange colours, artificial light, particularly of the tungsten filament type, will not highlight the orange colours (Fig. 3-15). At the same time, a grey colour can enhance the effect of translucency. The judicious use of multi-blended opaque porcelains in the metal-ceramic technique can alleviate some metameric problems.

The Aluminous Porcelain Crown

The aluminous porcelain crown was developed in an attempt to obtain similar aesthetics to the regular vacuum-fired felspathic crowns, combined with improved strength (*McLean* and *Hughes,* 1965). The aluminous core porcelains were formulated with the object of obtaining maximum translucency without sacrificing too much strength (*McLean,* 1966). Although these materials may appear to be very opaque to a

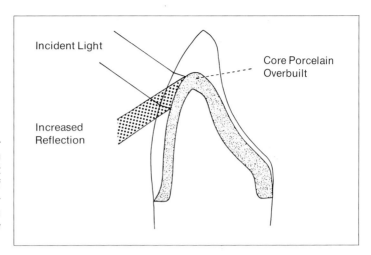

Fig. 3-16 Diagram showing increased light reflection from an aluminous porcelain core built too thickly in the incisal third of the preparation. The core porcelain will increase in opacity with thickness and become highly light reflective.

casual observer, they do in fact transmit some light, the paler shades of aluminous core porcelain transmitting up to 20 percent light through a 1 mm thick disc.

Providing these materials are used in their correct thickness, it is possible to make crowns as aesthetically pleasing as any regular vacuum-firing felspathic porcelain. Incorrect placement of the aluminous core porcelains can produce metameric effects similar to those of the metal-ceramic crowns, the commonest fault being found in the labio-incisal third of the preparation. If the core porcelain is built up too thickly in this area, there will be insufficient space for the dentine and enamel porcelain to provide depth of translucency. The core porcelain may then influence the colour of the enamel veneers (Fig. 3-16). Generally a minimum thickness of 0.8 mm of dentine and enamel porcelain is required to obtain the best effects. The ceramist may also fail to provide maximum thickness of aluminous core porcelain for reinforcing the lingual and approximal surfaces (Fig. 3-17). Correct core placement should not only provide good aesthetics but also provide maximum cervical and lingual reinforcement for the crown. A strong lingual strut of core porcelain may be extended approximally without marring the aesthetics of the finished crown (Fig. 3-18 a

and b). The thinner core porcelain overlaying the incisal one-third of the preparation will allow some light transmission, but it will also prevent the cement lute from having a marked influence on colour. Providing the labial aluminous core porcelain has not been built too thickly, it will be less light reflective than the regular opaque porcelains. This, in turn, will ensure that any metameric effects are reduced to the minimum. In order to reduce the influence of the aluminous core porcelains on the final colour of the enamel veneers, manufacturers are now providing a wide range of neutral core colours. Each dentine colour is provided with an aluminous porcelain core colour that does not cause a change in hue from the original dentine colour. In this way, dentine colour may be selected and should remain reasonably close to its original shade after it has been baked onto the neutral coloured core porcelain. In essence the core and dentine porcelains are in the same range of hue, but differ in their total reflectance or luminance.

A natural tooth may be reproduced in aluminous porcelain very accurately. Enamel translucency is provided by using single-phase glasses of high clarity (see page 99, Monograph II). The dentine and reinforcing core porcelain are

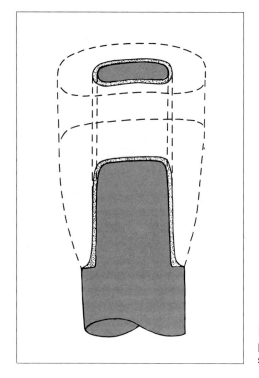

Fig. 3-17   Incorrect build-up of aluminous core where porcelain is built too thinly. The crown will not be sufficiently reinforced by such a thin layer.

matched in hue so that any light reflection from the core porcelain will give a close colour rendering to the dentine hue. Since the labial core porcelain will also transmit some light, the apparent depth of translucency in the crown is increased. However, the refraction of light at the alumina crystal boundaries is still sufficient to prevent the cement lute from altering the basic hue of the crown. By using highly translucent dentines and enamels combined with neutral tone aluminous core porcelains, the manufacturers have provided the ceramist with a versatile system for simulating natural teeth. The labial aluminous core porcelain is used as a light diffusion zone which provides a natural background for the enamel and dentine porcelains, but at the same time masks the cement lute (Fig. 3-18). Building the labial aluminous core porcelain too thickly will completely defeat the action of this colour filtration, turning the core porce-

lain into a classical opaque layer which is highly reflective (Fig. 3-16):

The Role of Opaque Porcelains in Obtaining Aesthetics

It has been argued that opaque porcelains are not required in dental ceramics and that the original air-fired crown could provide the best system. By using various coloured cements the clinician could alter the colour of the crown and eliminate the use of opaque layers of porcelain. This argument is perfectly valid for materials when the translucency of the enamel and den-

Fig. 3-18a and b   Correct build-up of aluminous core porcelain so as to provide optimum aesthetics and strength. Note that labial surface is kept as thin as possible and the lingual surface as thick as possible.

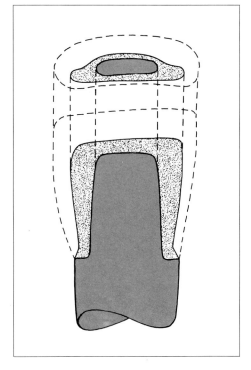

Figure 3-18a

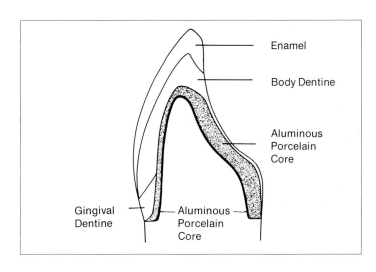

Figure 3-18b

tine porcelains is restricted to a level where the cement lute does not become clearly outlined against the tooth stump. However, if a porcelain crown is to simulate many natural teeth, greater degrees of light transmission in the enamel porcelains may be necessary. When these highly translucent enamels overlay the dentine, the latter porcelains should also be made more translucent, if sharp demarcation lines are to be avoided. Once this greater degree of translucency has been achieved, then light transmission through the crown is increased. At this level, the cement lute will become clearly outlined against the dentine stump. The ceramist has only to bake a regular vacuum-fired porcelain crown without the opaque base to see the validity of this statement. If a wide range of coloured cements was used, it might be possible to approximate the cement hue to that of the porcelain. However, in this case, a much closer degree of colour matching would be required than when an air-fired porcelain is used. For this reason, the manufacturers provide a range of coloured opaque porcelains which more closely simulate the hue of the dentine porcelains. It will be seen that the evolution of the opaque porcelains was necessary if a greater depth of translucency was to be achieved with the vacuum-fired crowns.

The use of opaque porcelain in the metal-ceramic crown was dictated by the metal background and, unfortunately, the aesthetic benefits of vacuum-firing have been partially lost. As explained previously, the dentine porcelains are generally more opaque in the metal-ceramic technique and the crowns lack depth of translucency. The benefits accruing to the regular vacuum-fired porcelains have been dissipated in metal-ceramics by the total opacity of the metal background. This is not serious in posterior crowns but becomes more and more acute as the central incisors are approached.

The term "opaque porcelain" has, perhaps, been a little misleading since, in the clinician's mind it signifies total opacity. From the previous discussion on the various types of porcelain, it will be seen that the opaque porcelain or opaque luting cement can have a dominating influence on aesthetics. The degree of opacity or, conversely, the amount of light transmission in opaque porcelains has a vital part to play in the development of good aesthetics.

Total opacity creates a "mirror-effect" and enhances any metameric effects. This type of opacity is inherent in the metal-ceramic system. Light transmissions of 15 to 30 percent in 0.5 mm thick layers of aluminous core porcelains will reduce this "mirror-effect" and consequently any metameric changes. At the same time, this lesser degree of opacity will still allow a more translucent dentine veneer porcelain to be used without causing any highlighting of the tooth dentine stump. Such a system can only be employed where the crown is constructed entirely in dental porcelain. For this reason the complete porcelain crown will continue to challenge the efforts of the ceramic manufacturer to replace it with metal-ceramics of comparable aesthetics.

In the case of metal-ceramics the surface texture or the gloss of the opaque porcelain can have a distinct effect on the aesthetic result. A highly-glazed opaque must increase reflection of light as illustrated in Fig. 3-9.

This will result in an increase in "Value" or brightness and is generally most undesirable since the tooth stump may be highlighted by a bright spot. If the opaque surface is rough, then the increased diffuse reflection will tend to lower "Value" and make the tooth appear darker or less bright. In addition to the aesthetic value of low glaze opaques it should be noted that the application of dentine porcelains should never be made to highly-glazed surfaces (see Monograph I) due to possible separation of the component porcelains.

As explained previously, the manufactures have attempted to reduce the dominant colour effect of opaque porcelains by the use of neutral opaque colours. In essence this means that the dentine and opaque colours should be matched for Hue, Value and Chroma. This is, of course, a counsel of perfection and cannot be achieved in practice since the opaque porcelains can never be exactly matched to translucent dentine porcelains. However, by formulating opaque porcelains that do not cause a visibly-marked change in colour of the dentine porcelain, a practical result can be achieved as described unter the section dealing with aluminous porcelain crowns.

High light transmission and reduction of specular reflection is well illustrated in the two "Vitadur" crowns shown on the frontispiece of this book. The purity of colour and depth of translucency would be difficult to achieve with a metal background.

Requirements for a Tooth Shade Guide

The prime requirements for a tooth colour guide have been considered by *Sproull* (1973) and should include

1. a logical arrangement in colour space and
2. an adequate distribution in colour space.

Sproull recommended that shade guides should be based on the *Munsell* Colour Order System (*Munsell*, 1961) and he thought that if the proper limit for the colour space of the natural teeth has been determined, and small enough intervals in Hue, Brightness (Value) and Saturation (Chroma) have been established, a match can be rapidly chosen. (An "ideal" colour space is one in which each colour is the centre of a sphere of colour, and the next closest matches in colour surround it). Sproull considered that a guide which did not fulfill the prime require-

ments of an adequate and logical arrangement in colour space would pose certain problems:

1. It takes too long to decide where to begin;
2. it is impossible, rapidly or logically to check the chosen match for accuracy;
3. the volume of colour space occupied by the materials to be matched may be impossible to reach within the guide.

The *Munsell* Colour Order System

The *Munsell* Colour System can be likened to a sphere or to a cylinder, [*Judd* and *Wyszecki* (1963); *Nickerson,* (1964)] as it is an irregular, three-dimensional figure that has characteristics of both. The relationship of one colour to another becomes apparent when the organisation of the colours within the three-dimensional solid is understood. When considered as a cylinder, a colourless or achromatic axis entends through the centre of the cylinder, pure white at the top, pure black at the bottom. A series of greys, progressing from black to white in equal visual steps, connects these extremities. Colours (Hues) are arranged around this axis, and within each Hue, the colours are arranged in scales according to their brightness (Value) and their saturation (Chroma). Light colours are placed towards the top of the cylinder and dark colours towards the bottom. The colours are purest on the outer skin of the cylinder, and they become progressively greyer as they approach the grey Value axis. Within each of these scales of Hue, Value and Chroma, the intervals were chosen to represent equal visual spacing under a standard light source.

The *Munsell* Colour Order System, when treated as a cylinder, may be considered, as a series of wheels stacked one upon the other, each wheel of ascending lightness as they progress to the top of the cylinder (Fig. 3-19). The three dimensions in colour are represented as follows:

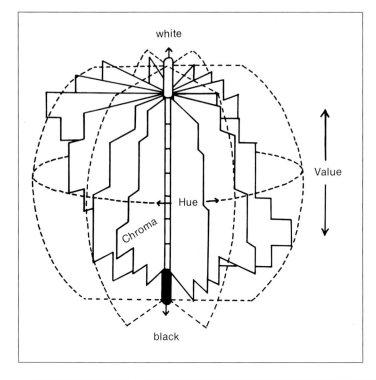

white

Value

Hue

Chroma

black

Fig. 3-19 The *Munsell* colour cylinder.

1. The brightness or "Value" axis is represented by the hub of the wheel.
2. The Hues are arranged sequentially around the rim.
3. The gradations of Saturation or "Chroma" are represented by the spokes of the wheel and run from the colourless axis at the hub to the purest hues or colours at the rim.

The *Adams* Co-ordinate System

This system which is popularly known as the "Lab" system is illustrated in Fig. 3-20. The Lab system is now being used increasingly in the ceramic industry and is made up of three co-ordinates. L signifies the vertical colour space or neutral axis; a, the horizontal axis and b the rectangular axis. A study of the diagram will reveal that the *Adams* System is a natural follow-up to the C.I.E. system, and similar to the *Munsell* Co-ordinate System.

Colour of Natural Teeth related to Modern Shade Guides

A limited spectrophotometric study on natural teeth by *Sproull* (1973) using the *Munsell* Colour Order System,* established a Hue range of 7.5 YR to 2.7 Y, a Value (Brightness) range of 5.8/ to 8.5/, and a Chroma (Saturation) range of /1.5 to /5.6.

Previous studies by *Clark* (1933) on 6,000 teeth established a Hue range of 6 YR to 9.3 Y, a Value range of 4/ to 8/ and a Chroma range of /0 to /7. *Clark* stated that the extreme ranges of Hue were seldom seen; only 1.1 percent of the

---

* The notation used places Hue at the left; Value (expressed by a number) above and to the right of the Hue symbol; and Chroma, also expressed by a number, below and to the right of the slanting line. Format in common usage is HV/C. H is preceded by a number to indicate the precise subdivision of the line.

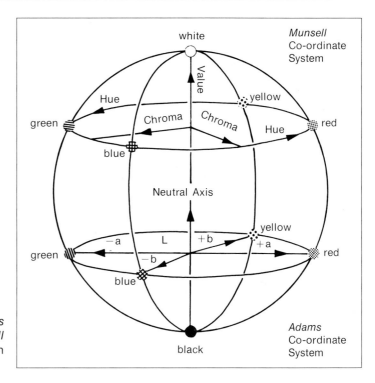

Fig. 3-20 Diagram of the *Adams* co-ordinate system and *Munsell* system. Courtesy of the British Ceramic Research Association.

teeth in his study tended towards greenish yellow and 4.3 percent towards reddish yellow. *Clark* found that, as tooth colours grow darker (lower in Value or Brightness), they weaken in Saturation (Chroma); this is opposite to the trend seen in *Sproull's* study in 1973. However, both studies agreed that, as teeth become redder, they become darker.

Sproull (1973) stated that an acceptable tooth shade guide, based on the volume of colour space of the natural teeth must

1. embrace the coordinates established by natural teeth,
2. be logically arranged, and
3. have sufficient data points to fill the total volume.

He criticised the modern shade guides and cited the following defects:

1. Available guides do not extend through the volume of colour space required;

2. an orderly or systematic arrangement or relationship between tabs is usually lacking;
3. there will be clustering or duplication of colours in certain areas of colour space and voids in other regions.

Sproull recommended that a single guide should be developed that is composed of the proper materials and arranged according to the *Munsell* System. It should have sufficient volume and detail to permit free travel within the "envelope of colour" of the natural tooth.

There is little doubt that the dental porcelain manufacturers would endorse the comments of *Sproull* and, indeed, the *Clark* Tooth Colour Selector of the 1930's was a classical example of the manufacturer attempting to come to terms with a logical colour system. Although Dr. *Clark* favoured the *Munsell* System as an overall or reference standard, his statistical measurements of natural tooth colour showed a scatter-

145

ing of tooth shades predominantly in a small part of the light yellow area, relatively fewer in the band above, and no occurrence over more than 99 percent of the *Munsell* range. Thus the *Clark* Tooth Colour Selector focussed on the 1 percent of the total range which was important to teeth and covered it in a grid of equal size units (*Semmelman,* 1973). This was eminently logical for that period but the elapse of time has revealed very definite practical and commercial objections. The extreme edges of the *Clark* grid were oversupplied with seldom-used commercial shades, while the target centre was not covered with fine enough shade distinctions for the often-found tooth colours. Meanwhile, hand-mixing of laboratory tooth shades became almost extinct, as previously described on page 131 and pre-mixed shades became the order of the day. These shades evolved gradually but not in a standard grid (*Semmelman,* 1973). The tendency was towards intense coverage of the most popular range and relatively sparse coverage of the less-frequent fringes. This trend has resulted in the production of our modern shade guides which, although being open to the criticisms outlined above, have been developed on a more logical and practical basis than the dental profession might be prepared to acknowledge. The high cost of manufacture of porcelain teeth and shade guides must place limitations on the range of Hue that can be offered, and it is doubtful whether any manufacturer could afford to stock all the colours that may be indicated by scientific colour measurement of teeth. However, providing the dentist selects a guide with a range of Hue that suits his own individual requirements and has mastered the basics of colour matching, then his shade selection must improve. To do this, the clinician must understand the principles of colour as described under Hue, Value (Brightness) and Chroma (Saturation). In addition, if he can recognise metameric defects in crowns in the mouth, he is well on the road to success. The latter depending on his ability to recognise changes in colour under artificial lighting.

There is little doubt that all ceramists can extend any shade guide range if they are prepared to custom build their shade guides and to blend colours. In particular, the mixing of pre-blended shades is reasonably accurate providing the ceramist uses large fractions during mixing. Such a procedure must enhance the possibilities of increasing the range of Hue and provide a more logical sequence of colour space within the boundaries of the manufacturer's original colour bands. It is doubtful whether any manufacturer will ever provide a manufactured tooth shade guide that will meet all clinical requirements. The keen ceramist must, therefore, be prepared to extend the manufacturer's range of tooth shades if he wishes to master all variations in tooth colours.

Shade Matching

The Custom-Built Shade Guide

Optimum shade matching for the construction of porcelain veneer crowns can only be achieved by the use of custom-built shade guides. Ideally the keen ceramist should fabricate a custom-built shade guide of porcelain or metal-ceramic crowns and use these in conjunction with shade buttons or wedges of fused porcelain.

The construction of a porcelain jacket crown shade guide is time-consuming but quite simple. In the case of the regular or aluminous porcelains, a typodont model may be used on which an individual typical preparation is prepared. The ceramist will then be able to control the thickness of each crown by reference to the adjoining teeth. Added refinement may be given to the guide by duplicating each tooth shade, one with a distinct gingival or neck dentine in position and one without. By eliminating

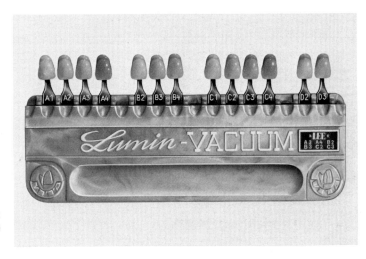

Fig. 3-21 Photograph of the Vita Porcelain Tooth Shade Guide showing grouping of colours.

the neck dentine on one set, the problem of matching younger teeth, where no root is exposed, is made easier.

The blending of colours may follow the shades selected by the manufacturer for his vacuum-fired production teeth. However, by blending equal parts of two colours, intermediate shades can be made which are often of great value. The manufacturer who groups his colours in definite ranges of hue will materially assist the dentist, as explained earlier in this monograph. Once the hue of the tooth is established, it is much easier to select the correct shade according to chroma and luminance or value.

For example, the Vita Tooth Company has divided its tooth shades into four main groups (Fig. 3-21) which correspond to the following colours:

Group	Hue
A	Brownish tones
B	Yellowish tones
C	Grey tones
D	Reddish tones

Construction of a custom-built porcelain jacket crown shade guide to match these colours may

then be made, and any intermediate shades of porcelain can be introduced according to the operator's choice. In this case, intermediate shades and shades darker than the manufacturer's teeth may be included. However, the guide should still adhere firmly to the principle of grouping the colours under their correct ranges of hue. The crowns should be mounted in parallel so that each colour grouping can be quickly assessed and the range of hue determined. If teeth are mounted on a key-ring guide, the dentist will find shade-matching much more difficult. Each tooth has to be held individually and this does not allow the clinician to compare the differences in hue between each group of teeth. In addition, he is much more likely to suffer from the effects of "successive contrast" which are discussed later.

The Custom-Built Metal-Ceramic Shade Guide

Metal-ceramic crowns present greater problems in shade-matching than the all-porcelain restoration. *Bazola* and *Malone* (1967) have described a technique for building a shade guide for metal-ceramic crowns to facilitate colour determination for the clinician and to aid in the eval-

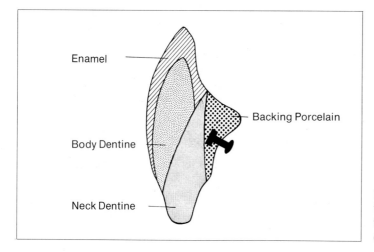

Enamel

Backing Porcelain

Body Dentine

Neck Dentine

Fig. 3-22 Diagram of a section through a modern porcelain pin tooth showing the various blends of colour.

uation of the vacuum-fired porcelain technique. Wax templates were made on a convex anterior die which simulated the area normally covered by the metal coping. The templates were cast in metal-ceramic gold and the porcelain veneer baked to position by standard technique. *Bazola* and *Malone* concluded that when matching an anterior vital tooth as a single restoration, more problems were presented in matching selected colours than "off shades" or stained teeth. Equally, posterior teeth were easier to match in comparison with anterior teeth, probably due to less light reflection during shade matching.

There is little doubt that a custom-built metal-ceramic shade guide can materially assist the clinician in his shade selection. However, the construction of such a shade guide can be expensive and very time-consuming and few ceramists are prepared to hand-make their shade guides. In view of this fact, the next best procedure is to use a factory-made vacuum-fired porcelain tooth shade guide.

Vacuum-Fired Porcelain Tooth Shade Guides

The large laboratory owner is generally presented with a specific shade, selected by the dentist from a modern multi-blended vacuum-fired tooth shade guide. Modern dental porcelains and, in particular, the aluminous porcelains, have been formulated with this situation in mind. A description of the blending of a vacuum-fired shade tooth guide is most pertinent to any discussion on shade selection since, without a knowledge of its construction, the ceramist will find it very difficult to duplicate.

An examination of a modern multi-blended vacuum-fired tooth reveals that it comprises four basic colours (Fig. 3-22). These colours consist of a dense backing porcelain containing the pin anchorage, a darker dentine colour that is carried up into the gingival of the tooth to create a dense neck area, and the body or dentine porcelain overlaid by a translucent enamel. This enamel porcelain covers the labial and lingual aspects of the incisal edge and generally overlays the dentine on the entire labial surface. Various concentrated body and surface stains are applied as "effect masses". Many manufacturers extend the enamel porcelain around the approximal areas to give the "wrap-around" effect of natural tooth enamel, with the result that modern vacuum-fired teeth simulate the human dentition extremely well. For this reason, the ceramist is strongly advised to study the construction of several kinds of manufactured teeth since he will find much to learn from the art of porcelain tooth construction.

In order to duplicate a vacuum-fired shade guide tooth, jacket crown porcelains must be fired in layers corresponding to that of the shade guide tooth enamel and dentines. For example, an aluminous core porcelain or regular opaque will correspond with the dense backing porcelain (Fig. 3-22). The gingival or neck dentines, although being much thinner, can give a similar effect to that of the tooth guide gingival porcelain. The body dentine containing the "effect colours" should be covered with enamel porcelain to produce the classical "wrap-a-round" effect in a natural tooth. In this way a much closer simulation of the shade guide tooth may be obtained.

The Eye and Colour Perception

The eye is an excellent colour-perceiving mechanism. The light sensitive nerve cells, or rods, which are located in the retina, are close together in the periphery but are more widely spaced in the central field of vision. Rods are sensitive to light but not to colour, i.e. they only give a perception of light.

The colour receptors or cones are especially closely-packed in the central area of vision, which is a rod-free area known as the fovea. Because the cones are very closely packed in the fovea, reliable colour discrimination by the observer subtends a very small angle of about two degrees. At wider angles, critical judgement of colour declines as more and more rods are brought into action. It has been accepted as an international convention that precise colour measurement shall be done using a field of vision that subtends two degrees (*Heath*, 1968). The important conclusions which the clinician must draw from these facts about the eye are as follows:

1. Since the cones only operate at relatively high levels of illumination, there must be ample light for correct colour matching.
2. For precise colour perception, the clinician should use a small angular field. This can be achieved by concentrating on one tooth at a time, or covering the adjoining teeth with a cardboard mask.

A prolonged scrutiny of a given area will produce increasing strain upon the cones until eventually the original colour is perceived more as a grey than as a given hue. One way of helping to compensate for this physiological weakness is to use the technique of looking intermittently at a blue card after each shade selection, as suggested in the Trubyte Bioform shade selection booklet. If another comparison is then to be made with a different shade, the clinician should look at the card again before glancing at the new shade.

It is essential to make a rigid rule never to select a shade after prolonged and fatiguing operative surgery. The best time to select a shade is when the clinician is fresh; such a time could be during examination and treatment planning. At a subsequent date, this shade can then be checked for accuracy.

The natural dentition should be kept dry during shade selection but once the decision on shade has been taken, it is extremely useful to reassess the colour under wet conditions. Although this may increase the surface gloss of the tooth, it should be remembered that the patient is viewing his teeth under wet conditions in the natural state.

Recommended Procedures for Shade Matching

The patient should be viewed so that his head is at the operator's eye-level. It is often convenient to have the patient standing near to the office window or, alternatively, sitting on an operating stool. Whichever method is used, it is important to use the maximum amount of daylight. Ideally the light source should be a northern exposure and shades should preferably be taken in the middle of the day. Early morning and late afternoon lights have a large yellow component in the spectrum and can affect colour judgement. Very bright sunlight and blue skies will also accentuate the blue component of the spectrum, and teeth must never be matched under direct sunlight. Daylight will, of course, be modified by its surroundings. Reflection from the walls, ceilings, curtains, windows and even clothing can all influence the colour rendering. However, it has been the author's experience that providing the patient is standing or sitting as close as possible to the window then the influence of surrounding objects is markedly reduced. Whenever and wherever possible natural daylight should be used for assessing colour and artificial lighting should then be employed as a double check as will be described. In cases where this is impossible, then a standard light source developed specifically for colour work should be used. These are rated in terms of the *Kelvin* (symbol K) temperature scale. Average northern daylight would correspond to a temperature of 6700 °K and new standard light sources have been developed averaging 6500 °K which is a useful compromise in duplicating average daylight conditions. These new lights use a small filtered incandescent source.

The surgery walls should not be painted in brilliant colours, since these, too, can affect the colour rendering and cause metameric effects to develop. In general, neutral colours such as grey provide by far the best medium for colour matching, even thought the clinician may find his surgery more drab than he would desire.

It has already been shown that, for precise colour matching, the clinician should use a small angular field. In addition, he must be careful not to become influenced by apparent changes in colour due to "successive contrast" effects. An apparent change in colour may occur due to the clinician having viewed another colour previously. The eye becomes adapted to one colour and will then tend to memorize this colour for a short period. This is why it is not advisable to view colours for long periods. In addition, the receptors for the particular colour being observed can tire and lose their ability to differentiate.

The natural dentition should always be kept dry during final shade selection and the teeth viewed from several different angles.

At this stage it is better to concentrate on the middle third of the tooth since the body shade is the most important basic colour in the tooth.

With these basic principles in mind, the clinician is recommended to adopt the following detailed procedures when matching a specific tooth colour.

Determing Hue

1. Orientate the shade guide so that each tooth colour can be passed in parallel across the tooth to be matched. Key-ring guides are not recommended and the clinician should use a metal slotted type fixed in plastic holders, such as the Vita or Trubyte Bioform guides. Whether a custom-built or factory-made guide is being used, it is essential for the clinician to be able to view all the groups of colours simultaneously. In this way the tooth shade will fall into a specific range of hue or group of colours. A note should be made of this hue; it may be reddish-yellow, bluish-yellow, grey, or orange-yellow, etc.

   Three basic shades must be determined as previously described on page 132 − 133.

The Incisal Third – composed mainly of enamel, can be extremely varied in colour. The shade may be light or dark grey in highly translucent teeth or opalescent and milky in the more opaque tooth. The colour may vary from one area to another and is generally greyer or bluer in the approximal region because of the higher enamel content (see Fig. 3-11).

The Middle Third – composed mainly of dentine, is the area normally termed "the body colour". This colour may again be influenced by the overlying enamel but will generally fall into the orange-red, blue-yellow, grey or grey-yellow areas of colours.

The Cervical Third – this area is termed "the gingival colour" and will often be a quite distinct colour, particularly if part of the root area has to be duplicated in the crown. The colour will be much closer to that of pure dentine and can vary from yellow-orange to deep red-browns.

Variations in shades of teeth

Teeth can vary greatly in colour and generally the maxillary incisors and premolars are closest to the same shade. The following guide is given of variations in shade:

a) Maxillary incisors and premolars are similar in shade with the central incisors often being the lightest.

b) Mandibular incisors are generally one shade lighter than maxillary incisors.

c) Canine teeth are at least two shades darker than the maxillary incisors, and this will apply particularly to the body shade.

The above general rules are particularly important when constructing a full mouth rehabilitation in dental porcelain.

2. Select the group of colours that most closely match the tooth and these should match the general hue of the natural tooth. For ex-ample, in the Vita tooth range, the colour may be brownish and in the Vita A range of colour or hue. Selection of the correct range of hue will eliminate a great many of the variables in colour matching.

The decision on basic hue having been made, it is important to concentrate on the incisal third or enamel colour. This colour may vary from the shade guide tooth and a separate selection must be made from tabs of enamel porcelain which most porcelain manufacturers will supply.

Determining Chroma

Once the basic hue has been determined, it should now be possible to concentrate on the correctly matching group of tooth colours and eliminate those with the poorest match in colour saturation or chroma.

3. Concentrate on the selected group of colours and decide which colour matches the tooth in saturation or purity of colour. When in doubt, the clinician is advised to select a shade that is fractionally darker in hue, since too light a shade can be very obvious in the mouth. It should now be possible to select a single tooth from the shade guide. If a shade button or wedge of porcelain is available, this too should be used to confirm the earlier decision on hue.

4. The effect of reflected light on the natural tooth must now be observed and compared with the shade guide tooth to see whether high-lighting the surface markedly alters shade. The colour should now be checked from arm's length, and at this stage it is useful to check whether the brightness or luminance of the two teeth matches.

Determining Value

The brightness or value of natural teeth depends upon the relative presence or absence of white in the body and incisal shades (*Granger, 1975*). As explained on page 121, young patient's teeth are "whiter and brighter" because of the absence of secondary dentine. On such occasions it may sometimes be necessary to use white modifiers in the dentine porcelains. However, many porcelain crowns are too bright or highly light reflective so that the use of white modifiers should seldom be necessary. By contrast, brightness can be decreased by increasing the depth of translucency, i.e. increasing the enamel thickness. Orange and brown colour, when added to the basic dentine colour, will reduce the brightness or value. Pure yellow will enhance it.

The ceramist is advised not to introduce pure colour into the porcelain without studying the effect of colour neutralisation and the use of complementary colours. For this reason the dentist who asks the ceramist to alter the brightness or value of his tooth shade may find that he is creating more trouble for himself than attempting to stay within the tooth manufacturer's body shade as supplied. It is easier to alter the value of a tooth by increasing the enamel depth than by attempting to alter the basic dentine shade.

After completion of the shade selection, a further observation should be made for any metameric differences between the shade guide tooth and the natural dentition.

Determining Metameric Effects

The surgery curtains must be drawn and a tungsten filament operating lamp only is left switched on. The shade guide tooth is now held alongside the natural tooth and the operating lamp gradually swung up from the patient's chest until the light source just starts to illuminate the tooth. If there is no apparent change in colour, the light is swung up further until the full beam strikes the teeth. If no marked changes in colour are apparent, it is almost certain that the selected tooth colour is very accurate since, in this situation, metameric effects will be obvious. Subdued tungsten light is the most critical of all lighting for revealing metameric changes in colour. In particular, an opaque porcelain in a metal-crown will be placed under the severest test by this procedure. Further checks can be made using colour-corrected lamps but the author favours the extremes of changing from natural daylight to tungsten filament light as the severest test for colour matching. If this is correct the crown should appear very natural in normal overhead surgery lighting.

Blending of Colours

The blending of the selected shade guide tooth may not match that of the tooth and corrections can now be made. A drawing of the tooth is made to indicate to the technician the exact blending required (Fig. 3-23). The gingival, dentine and enamel colours are marked and a tracing of the enamel blend is important since it may be longer or shorter than the shade guide tooth or even more acute in angle. If additional depth of translucency is required, it is often

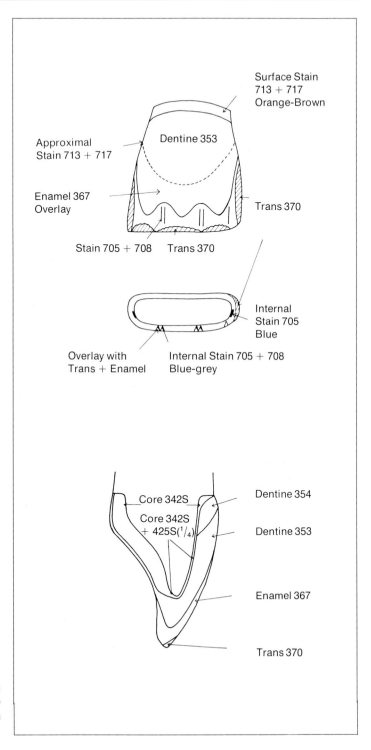

Surface Stain
713 + 717
Orange-Brown

Dentine 353

Approximal
Stain 713 + 717

Enamel 367
Overlay

Trans 370

Stain 705 + 708   Trans 370

Internal
Stain 705
Blue

Overlay with
Trans + Enamel

Internal Stain 705 + 708
Blue-grey

Core 342S

Dentine 354

Core 342S
+ 425S($^1/_4$)

Dentine 353

Enamel 367

Trans 370

Fig. 3-23 Diagram illustrating the shade prescription given to the dental ceramist for a crown matching Vita Shade A2.

better to mark in an overlay of transparent porcelain over the enamel. If the enamel is increased in thickness, it can alter the shade, whereas a thin veneer of a clear glassy porcelain will increase the depth of translucency with only a slight alteration of the shade to the grey side. This is often desirable in highly translucent teeth. The translucency of the incisal tip of the tooth can be accentuated by placing translucent porcelain behind the incisal edge, or in grooves cut in the labial surface.

"Effect" colours may now be marked in to simulate the areas of variation of dentine calcification. Enamel check lines can be marked and a note made of variations in surface contour and the type of glaze finish indicated. For example, some teeth may have smooth, highly-polished surfaces, whilst others may be heavily imbricated with deep groove lines.

If the laboratory work is carried out away from the surgery, the technician is completely dependent on the information sent to him. Accurate study casts and detailed information on the colour blending and surface anatomy of the tooth will greatly assist his work.

Custom staining

Custom staining of teeth should be confined to creating surface defects or colours that are present only on the natural tooth surface. Custom staining should never be used for altering incorrect colours except in very marginal cases. Far too many porcelain crowns and bridges are inserted with colour correction made by surface staining. These crowns often appear too bright and lack the natural depth of translucency of human teeth. Colour in porcelain crowns should be built in depth as explained on page 125. Surface colour is always highly reflective and must be used sparingly. The most useful areas to use surface staining will be in the approximal and cervical areas of the tooth. In particular, failure to use approximal staining can cause a crown or

series of crowns to look highly artificial since the contact areas will appear too bright.

The Study Cast

A natural tooth in its unworn state does not present an absolutely smooth labial or lingual surface. In general, it may be seen as a gentle, undulating surface, traversed horizontally with very fine grooves (Fig. 3-24). These are the perikymata, and accurate simulation of these surface irregularities is as important as the matching of shade and shape to the overall labial harmony. If light should reflect off a restoration in a different way from the neighbouring teeth, even if shade and form matching are accurate, it will give the effect of being artificial. In consequence, the technician should be supplied with an accurate impression, so that these characteristics may be reproduced in the model without loss of detail.

Some stone model materials, whilst reproducing surface detail very accurately, may prove unsuitable because of their colouring, which does nothing to assist the ceramist to see these very fine markings. Yellows and greyish-whites have this effect, whilst pinks and blues show up more clearly. Newly copper and silver-plated models are clearly seen, but deteriorate rapidly when tarnishing occurs. Plastics of the epimine type* when filled with materials such as copper filings, can often produce the best surfaces (Fig. 3-25).

A perfect replica of the tooth can often give more information to the ceramist than the most detailed written prescription.

The use of sealants and varnishes on stone models should be kept away from the buccal surfaces, and only applied to the immediate contact area. The liberal use of these materials

---

* Scutan – ESPE, West Germany.

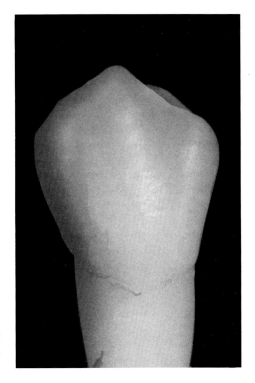

Fig. 3-24 Photograph of a human tooth showing the typical undulating surface produced by the perikymata and developmental grooves.

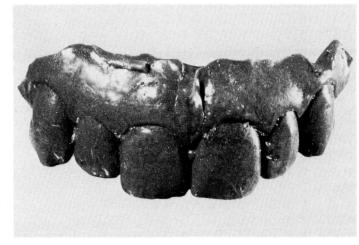

Fig. 3-25 Photograph of a replica of anterior teeth made in Scutan resin (epimine resin) containing copper filings.

will give the impression of smoothness which may not be a true representation of the surface in the mouth. Very worn surfaces which appear flat and characterless are not necessarily easier to reproduce. In general, a natural tooth does not have the same high surface reflectivity of glazed porcelain, and whilst it may appear highly reflective on a good model, it may not be so in the mouth. Information should be supplied to the ceramist if matting of the surface will be necessary. This may be done with a polishing wheel of the silicon carbide rubber bonded type running under water, with the laboratory hand piece at slow speed (900 to 1000 r.p.m.).

Worn teeth invariably wear in different directions, and where two worn surfaces meet, sharp angles occur, particularly at the labio-incisal angle where much of the character of a tooth can be seen and reproduced. The rounding and smoothing of these edges when matting down, can lose the natural character, but a compromise must be made as thin exposed edges will be very prone to chipping.

The Influence of Tooth Contour on Aesthetics

The response of gingival tissue to alterations in tooth contour can be quite marked and even where improvements in the patient's appearance are desired, these improvements should not be made at the expense of periodontal health. An increase in the labio-lingual or approximal width of tooth crowns can provoke a gingival response, and subsequent periodontal

therapy will never alleviate this inflammation. When aesthetic improvements in tooth contour are to be made, the general condition of the surrounding periodontium should be assessed before commencing any treatment. Gross destruction of supporting tissue can be very easily achieved in the name of cosmetic dentistry and the patient may be left with a permanent and ugly blue gingivae. (Fig. 3-26).

Cosmetic correction of dentitions with porcelain veneer crowns may be divided into two categories:

1. Restoration of original tooth contour which has been destroyed by caries, fillings, abrasion or trauma.
2. Alteration of original tooth contour in order to improve the aesthetic appeal of the dentition.

The restoration of original tooth contour may be undertaken without disturbance of the gingival tissue, and the general outline, form and colour of the teeth may be improved. Alteration of the original tooth contour requires considerably more clinical judgment, since sudden changes in contour can provoke an immediate response from the gingiva. Alteration of the original tooth contour should be made to improve the general outline of the teeth when viewed against the dark oral background, or to eliminate undesirable shadows or highlights produced by mal-aligned teeth.

Vertical correction

The general outline of the teeth can often be improved by restoring their original vertical form with porcelain veneer crowns. The porcelain veneer crown lends itself very well to the correction of vertical abnormalities since it involves no alteration of labial or buccal thickness of porcelain. Adequate thickness of porcelain may be provided and the restoration will still possess depth of translucency.

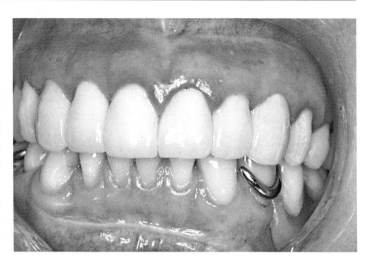

Fig. 3-26 Photograph of a patients upper dentition restored with metal-ceramic crowns. Note the over-contouring and severe gingival response around 11 and 21. The break-up of light on the crowns is also poor and the porcelain work is highly light reflective and metameric. The distal surface of 23 is also visible which spoils the effect of a natural front-to-back progression.

Lengthening of short teeth with porcelain veneer crowns should be undertaken with great care since encroachment upon the interocclusal space may cause severe damage to the dentition or fracture of the porcelain. Vertical correction of teeth is better confined to the restoration of irregular incisal angles, or the improvement of cervical contour, unless a full mouth reconstructions is contemplated and a complete analysis has been made of the effects of lengthening incisor teeth (Figs. 3-27 a to 3-27 d).

Horizontal correction

When any form of directional lighting, other than flat frontal lighting is being used, any tooth not in antero-posterior alignment with its neighbour will cast a shadow, either on itself if placed lingually, or on adjacent teeth if placed labially (Fig. 3-28). (Kurland, 1970). This type of shadowing can be particularly unpleasant under studio conditions of film or television lighting. Horizontal abnormalities in tooth contour or position are frequent and often difficult to correct. Horizontal abnormalities may be grouped as follows:

Instanding or outstanding teeth

Rotated teeth

Spaced teeth

Teeth inclined mesially or distally

Instanding and Outstanding Teeth

It is technically possible to alter the position of a tooth with a porcelain veneer crown. However, it is essential to recognise that although the labial or lingual surfaces may be altered in contour, the tooth stump is in a fixed position. If the crown has to be reduced in labial thickness in order to correct an outstanding incisor, then aesthetic problems are created in the labio-incisal third of the preparation (Fig. 3-29). This situation is so common that every ceramist has at some time become involved with attempts to disguise the cement or opaque layers at the incisal one-third. As noted previously, grey or grey-blue cements and opaque porcelains will improve translucency in these cases. By contrast, an instanding incisor may be corrected more easily by increasing the labial thickness of

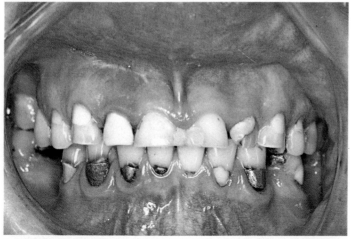

Fig. 3-27a   Photograph of a worn dentition in a young girl aged 26 years prior to full mouth rehabilitation for correction of loss of vertical height.

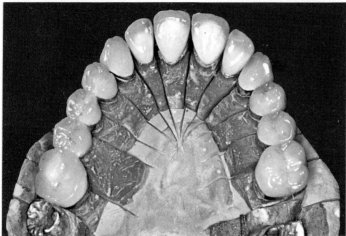

Fig. 3-27b Completed upper crowns and bridges on model. Note occlusal carving of porcelain and high alumina sheet backings on 12, 11, 21, 22.

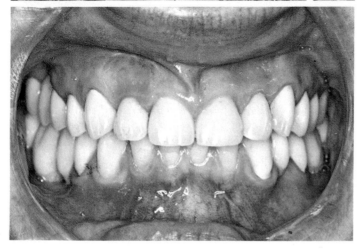

Fig. 3-27c Completed case in mouth. Upper incisors restored with aluminous porcelain crowns (Vitadur). Posterior teeth restored with metal-ceramic crowns and bridgework (VMK 68). Lower incisors restored with composite fillings.

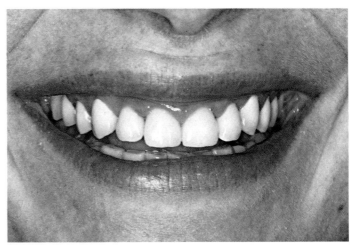

Fig. 3-27 d Completed case cemented with glass-ionomer cement. Note the dominant role of upper central incisors and the correct placement of the canines showing only the mesial aspects. The posterior teeth are also correctly contoured giving the correct front-to-back progression. Horizontal and vertical space allocation of the dentition is also pleasing.

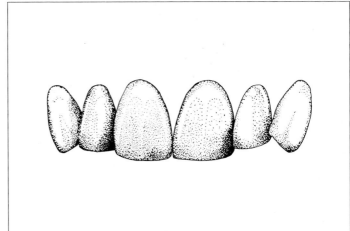

Fig. 3-28 Diagram illustrating the effect of frontal lighting on lingually and labially placed incisors. The lingually placed incisor 12 is particularly susceptible to being placed in shadow on the mesial aspect.

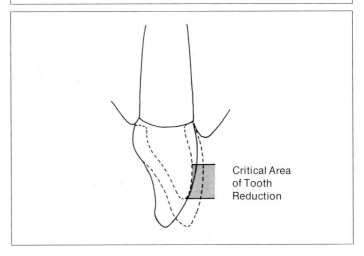

Critical Area of Tooth Reduction

Fig. 3-29 Diagram of the possible result obtained when correcting a labially displaced incisor. Unless the labioincisal third of the preparation is severely reduced the aesthetics of the crown can be very poor. Dotted line indicates the difference in position of the tooth.

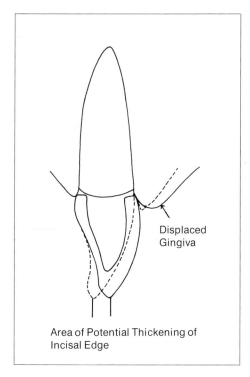

Area of Potential Thickening of
Incisal Edge

Fig. 3-30a   Effect on the gingival tissue of moving a lingually placed incisor too far labially. Although the crown may improve the aesthetics of the patient, the gingival response can be acute and prolonged.

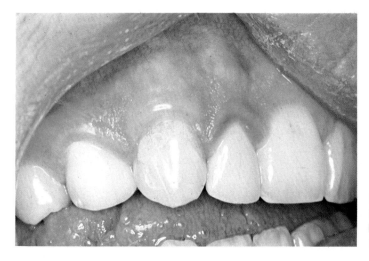

Fig. 3-30b   Clinical case illustrating inflammation around a labially corrected porcelain crown on 12.

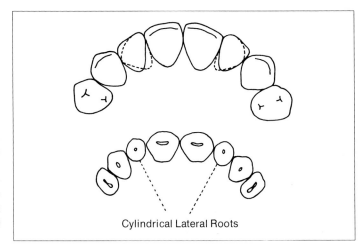

Fig. 3-31 Diagram illustrating the differences in diametral form between the upper incisors, canines and premolars. The upper lateral incisor being the nearest tooth to a cylindrical form is clearly the easiest tooth to rotate to a new position.

Cylindrical Lateral Roots

the porcelain veneer crown. In this case, the clinician often overlooks the fact that this increase in thickness can have a devastating effect on the gingival tissue. If the labial contour is increased by over 1 mm, then a cervical stagnation area must be created and the gingival tissue may even become displaced (Fig. 3-30a and b). In cases where the tooth has to be moved by more than 1 mm then, where possible, orthodontic correction should be advised.

Labial movement of a tooth in a horizontal plane will inevitably result in a thicker incisal edge being created in the porcelain veneer crown (see Fig. 3-30). By contrast, lingual movement of a tooth (i.e. reduction of the labial surface) can result in a reduction in thickness of the incisal edge (see Fig. 3-29). If the relationship of the incisal edge of the porcelain crown to the tooth preparation is altered in order to compensate for the reduction in thickness, then increased leverage forces will be incurred and fracture of the crown may occur. The clinician must take care not to make significant alterations in incisal guidance without a careful occlusal analysis.

Rotated Teeth

The correction of rotated teeth by insertion of porcelain veneer crowns is dependent upon the intra-arch space available and the maximum width of the mal-aligned tooth. It is obvious that if all teeth were cylindrical, then no problems would arise since the intra-arch space would remain constant. Unfortunately, all teeth are elliptical and considerable variation in both labio-lingual and mesio-distal diameters are encountered. The maxillary lateral incisor is the nearest tooth to a cylindrical form and its mesio-distal and labio-lingual diameters at the cervix are very similar. For this reason it is easier to rotate a lateral incisor porcelain veneer crown than it is a maxillary central incisor (Fig. 3-31).

Significance of intra-arch space

Providing there is sufficient intra-arch space, it is easier to correct a rotated tooth than one which is instanding or outstanding. In the latter case the position of the dental pulp exercises a stern discipline on the operator. Where the intra-arch space is limited, the insertion of individual porcelain crowns can be a waste of

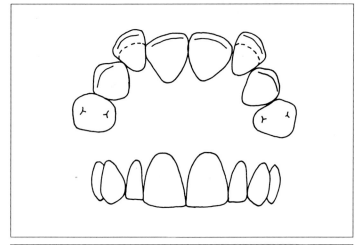

Fig. 3-32 Diagram illustrating a theoretical case where an attempt might be made to correct two outstanding lateral incisors where the intra-arch space is insufficient to accommodate them. This will result in the production of two peg-top lateral incisors of bizarre appearance with the central incisors dominating the mouth.

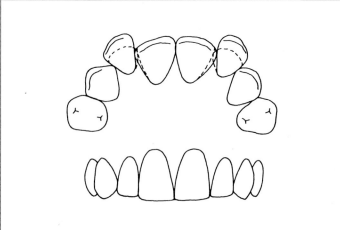

Fig. 3-33 Diagram illustrating the more preferable treatment for the case in Fig. 3-32. Here the central incisors are crowned and their mesio-distal diameters reduced slightly to accommodate the lateral incisors which can now be widened to improve the front-to-back progression from the central incisors. The reduction in tooth widths is indicated by the dotted lines.

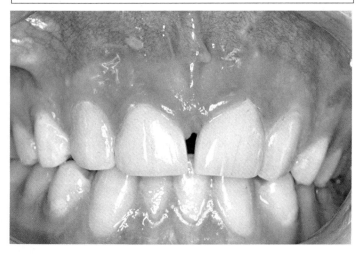

Fig. 3-34 Clinical photograph of aluminous porcelain jackets made for 11 and 22 to close space and simulate the missing 21 central incisor.

time and may often make matters worse. For example, attempts to move a lateral incisor into a normal relationship could produce a bizarre effect. A theoretical case is illustrated in Fig. 3-32 where there are two outstanding incisors with insufficient intra-arch space. Assuming both teeth could be corrected by the insertion of porcelain veneer crowns, the mesio-distal width of the finished crowns could produce an aesthetic effect even worse than the originals. Where the intra-arch space loss is much greater than 1 mm, it is far better to construct porcelain veneer crowns for all the incisor teeth and borrow a little of the central incisors' space (Fig. 3-33). In this way, the lateral incisor space can often be increased by as much as 1 mm.

Spaced teeth

A diastema between the upper central incisors is probably the most frequently encountered space to which patients will object. Closure of these gaps by insertion of porcelain veneer crowns is possible, providing the gap is no wider than 2 mm. Once the gap exceeds this distance, not only will the central incisor crowns look abnormally large, but there is a grave danger of compressing the interdental papilla. Inflammation in this area can become chronic and a constant source of irritation to the patient. Equally, attempts to correct spaced lateral incisors can also damage the interdental tissue. At the same time, it is very easy to enlarge the lateral incisor porcelain veneer crown to a degree where the patient can look grotesque. Correction of spaced teeth must be undertaken with the greatest circumspection and it is advisable to construct a mock-up in the mouth of the proposed teeth. This may be done rapidly by filling the approximal spaces with a self-curing acrylic such as "Sevriton".* When the

* A. D. International. London. W.I.

acrylic is set, it may be carved quickly to shape with a suitable bur. The patient may then decide that the end-result is not aesthetically pleasing and much labour and controversy can be avoided.

A case in which two maxillary incisors have been crowned to simulate a congenitally missing central incisor is illustrated in Fig. 3-34. This case represents the maximum type of space closure and the contouring of the Vitadur aluminous porcelain crowns has been carried out artistically by the ceramic technician.

Mesial or distal inclination of teeth

The problems of the inclined tooth are in many ways similar to the spaced tooth. Alteration of alignment can be made by altering the angle of the crown preparation. However, if the gap between the teeth at the cervical margin is too great, then increasing the width of the crowns will again cause an impingement on the gingiva. Correction of inclined teeth may only be undertaken where minor discrepancies in alignment are present.

Outline form and Size

The outline form and size of a porcelain veneer crown should duplicate the original tooth contour unless a definite alteration in shape is required. Even where alterations in size have been made, the general outline form should conform to the original.

Accurate reproduction of the original tooth anatomy in a porcelain veneer crown will often compensate for minor discrepancies in colour matching. By contrast, any mismatches in colour will be enhanced if the tooth anatomy does not harmonise with the adjoining teeth (Fig. 3-35).

Making a tooth look wider or narrower

When illusions of size or position are desired, subtle variations in the mesial and distal angles or variations in the contact areas of the crown can be made. For example, a tooth can be made to look wider by flattening the mesial and distal angles and moving the contact areas labially and incisally (Fig. 3-36). The resultant longer straight line along the incisal edge will make the tooth look wider (*Johnson* et al., 1967). Conversely, teeth can be made to look narrower by reversing the above procedures. The mesial and distal angles of the tooth may be made more convex, the contact areas can be set lingually and cervically, and the line angles can be moved toward the centre of the tooth, with the surface angled in a plane towards the contacts.

Making a tooth look shorter or longer

A very long tooth may be made to look shorter by moving the level of the cervical line incisally and creating an artificial root effect in the porcelain crown with deeper yellow, orange or brown "effect" powders (Fig. 3-37). Conversely, a tooth may be made to appear longer by moving the labial cervical line gingivally, if the anatomical crown is above the gingival margin. Alternatively, vertical developmental grooves may be carved in the labial surface and the approximal line angles kept nearer to parallelism.

Orthodontic Correction

Correction of occlusal deformities by orthodontic means has, in recent years, become more widely practised on adults (*Halden*, 1974). It is often wiser to seek the advice of an orthodontist before attempting the correction of grossly malformed dentitions with porcelain veneer crowns. The orthodontist is in a position to move teeth much further than can be achieved by minor corrections with porcelain jacket crowns. Attempts to correct malformed dentitions with porcelain veneer crowns may appeal to the clinician's heroic instincts but this can soon be tempered by the patient's disappointment with the result. The student must be advised that the indiscriminate cutting of human enamel without careful treatment planning is a sure way to a patient-dentist conflict.

Reproducing Tooth Anatomy in Dental Porcelain

It is essential that the dental ceramist has a detailed knowledge of tooth anatomy. To achieve this he must continually examine human teeth and study their anatomy. He is strongly advised to read Wheeler's textbook of dental anatomy and physiology and familiarise himself with the outline form, occlusal tables and surface characteristics of every tooth in the dental arch. The skilled ceramist must have a good working knowledge of occlusion and be able to recognise quickly the faults he makes in constructing a full arch of dental porcelain crowns and pontics. Errors in pontic design, width of occlusal tables, or position of the enamel supra-bulge should be instantly recognised.

The most important feature to recognise in tooth anatomy is that every tooth is formed by the combination of four lobes or more. Each lobe represents a primary centre of formation. As *Wheeler* (1969) points out, "the multiplication and fusion of lobes during tooth development are demonstrated graphically when teeth are viewed from the mesial or distal aspects." All anterior teeth show traces of four lobes, three labially and one lingually, the lingual lobe

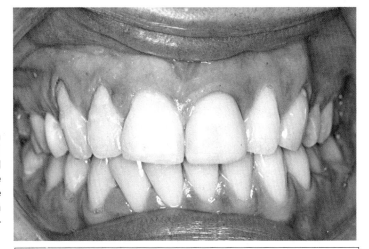

Fig. 3-35 Clinical photograph of a single jacket crown on 21 showing poor anatomy caused by over-glazing. All surfaces are rounded and the incisal line angles have been lost. The tooth does not harmonize with the upper right incisor.

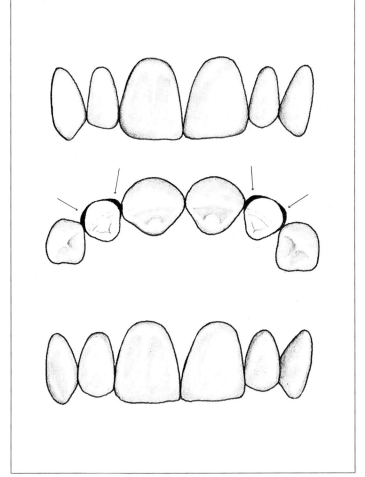

Fig. 3-36 Diagram illustrating how to create the illusion of 12 and 22 looking wider. By moving the contact areas labially and incisally, as indicated by arrows, the visible mesiodistal is increased.

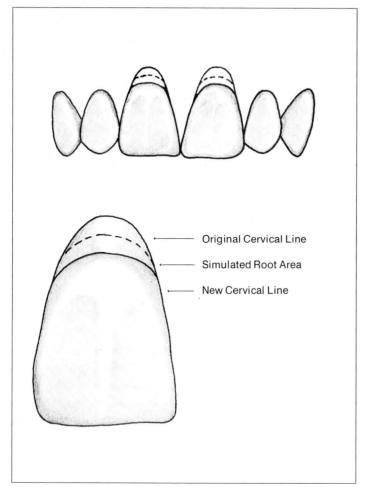

Original Cervical Line

Simulated Root Area

New Cervical Line

Fig. 3-37 Diagram showing how to make a tooth look shorter by moving the cervical line incisally. The original dentino-enamel junction is indicated by the dotted line.

being represented by the cingulum (Fig. 3-38). Each labial lobe of the incisor terminates incisally in rounded eminences known as mamelons. The junction between the three lobes in the incisors accounts for the labial grooves which are clearly seen in most teeth.

In the case of the premolars and molars the lobes are easily distinguished since each one corresponds with a cusp (Fig. 3-39). Although at first sight the premolars may only appear to have two cusps, the buccal cusp is the result of the fusion of three lobes.

Another important aspect of tooth anatomy which the ceramist must understand is the geometric form of crown outlines. This may be summarised as follows:

Facial and lingual aspects	– trapezoidal
Mesial and distal aspects of anterior teeth	– triangular
Mesial and distal aspects of maxillary posterior teeth	– trapezoidal
Mesial and distal aspects of mandibular posterior teeth	– rhomboidal

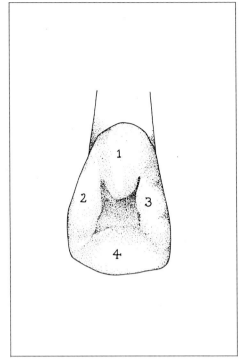

Fig. 3-38 Diagram of the lingual aspect of an upper lateral incisor showing the developmental lobes. The ceramist should build his porcelain in this fashion so as to simulate these important anatomical features.

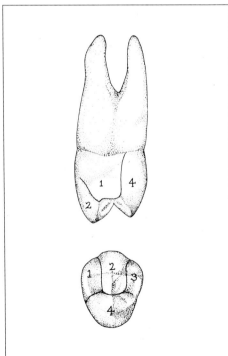

Fig. 3-39 Outline form of the four developmental lobes in a maxillary premolar. Ceramists often fail to imitate lobes 1 and 3 with the result that the tooth looks too square. In addition, failure to build up lobe 2 as a distinct prominence will flatten the occlusal table and produce very poor aesthetics on the buccal surface.

In addition the outline form of the occlusal tables is equally important. The maxillary molars are nearly always rhomboidal in form whereas the mandibular molars are trapezoidal.

Failure to recognise these main anatomical features in teeth will result in the production of ceramic work which is flat and uninteresting. To capture the beauty of natural teeth the ceramist must build each lobe or cusp individually. Even when building an upper incisor he must still duplicate the undulating form of the labial surface produced by the fusion of the three facial lobes. Natural teeth in the unworn state are rounded in form. It is only during masticatory wear that sharp line angles are created.

Common faults in porcelain tooth anatomy

The two most common faults in porcelain crown construction are firstly, a tendency to flatten the labial face of upper incisors and, secondly, to widen the occlusal tables of the posterior teeth (Fig. 3-40).

The incisors are easily flattened due to a tendency to over-brush or carve the labial face of the "green" or unfired porcelain. Widening of occlusal tables is a natural tendency since the ceramist may often be struggling to establish enough buccolingual space for aesthetics. In addition, the dentist may not have provided sufficient depth in his tooth preparation to allow the ceramist space for both metal and porcelain (Fig. 3-41). Widening of occlusal tables frequently results in mandibular molars and premolars looking like maxillary teeth and the whole effect of a full mouth rehabilitation can be ruined (Fig. 3-40).

The Central Incisors

The central incisors should dominate the anterior tooth arrangement and the maxillary central incisors are the widest mesiodistally of any of the anterior teeth. Although the labial face of the central incisor is less convex than the maxillary lateral incisor or canine, it must not be given a too-square or rectangular appearance. It is essential to make the distal outline of the crown more convex than the mesial outline. In this way the whole tooth will appear rounded and avoid an undesirable flat appearance.

The labial face of the mandibular incisors should be smooth and flat at the incisal third. The middle third is more convex and narrows to the convexity of the root at the cervical portion. A common fault when duplicating these teeth in porcelain is to make them too rectangular. Incisal edges can also look unnatural if too thick and blunt. (See frontispiece Vitadur maxillary incisors).

Lateral Incisors

Reproduction of the shape of the lateral maxillary incisor is vital when a full mouth reconstruction in porcelain is carried out. Although these teeth can vary in development more than any other tooth in the mouth, there are certain anatomical features which, if omitted can make these teeth look very artificial. The maxillary lateral incisor has more curvature than the central incisors. The labial face must not be flattened and the incisal ridge and point angles should be rounded mesially and distally. The crest of contour mesially is usually at the point of junction of the middle and incisal thirds. The distal outline of the crown should be more rounded than the mesial and the crest of contour carved more cervically, usually in the centre of the middle third. The ceramist should aim at making the lateral incisor more cylindrical in form so that the central incisors can continue to play their dominant aesthetic role (see Fig. 3-27 and 3-50).

The Canine Teeth

Few teeth can present such a challenge to the ceramist as the maxillary and mandibular ca-

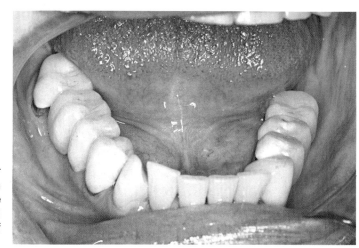

Fig. 3-40 Photograph of a lower metal-ceramic rehabilitation in which all the posterior teeth have flattened and widened occlusal tables due to over-contouring of the buccal and lingual surfaces.

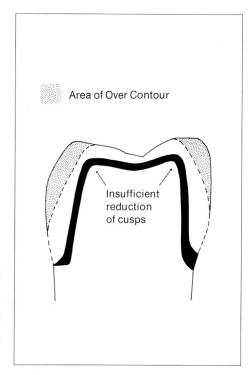

Fig. 3-41 Diagram illustrating how the occlusal tables of a mandibular molar may become widened as in Fig. 3-40. Invariably this widening occurs on the bucco-occlusal and linguo-occlusal surfaces. A study of the over-contoured area will reveal how easy it is to convert these teeth into maxillary molars, where reduction of cusps has been inadequate.

nines. *Wheeler* (1969) describes the anatomy of the maxillary canine in detail and the most difficult area to reproduce in porcelain is the labial face. "The labial surface of the crown is smooth, with no developmental lines of note except shallow depressions mesially and distally, dividing the three labial lobes. This produces a ridge on the labial surface of the crown. A line drawn over the crest of this ridge from the cervical line to the tip of the cusp is a curved one, inclined mesially at its centre. All areas mesial to the crest of this ridge exhibit convexity except for insignificant lines in the enamel. Distally to the labial ridge there is a tendency towards concavity at the cervical third of the crown, although convexity is noted elsewhere in all areas approaching the labial ridge."

A common fault in reproducing the maxillary canine tooth in porcelain is to make the labial face too flat and to lose the effect of the concavity in the distal area from the labial ridge. The mesio-labial aspect of the canine will also look unnatural if it is not kept convex. An accurate piece of carving in dental porcelain of a maxillary canine is illustrated in Fig. 3-42.

The Posterior Teeth

Classical carvings in dental porcelain of a selection of posterior teeth are illustrated in Figs. 3-43. It will be noted that once again the principle of lobe development is followed and each tooth has clearly defined cusps, suprabulges and occlusal tables. By contrast, a maxillary first molar is illustrated in Fig. 3-44 which shows many features that the ceramist has failed to reproduce. The occlusal table is too wide and the mesial and distal profiles are incorrect. In particular the incisal third of the buccal surface does not slope inwards sufficiently. The tooth looks square and unnatural and no attempt has been made to produce supplemental grooves or other refinements present in the natural tooth.

Full Mouth Reconstruction

When building a full mouth reconstruction, the ceramist must be familiar with the correct placement of teeth in relation to factors such as proportion, front-to-back progression, and horizontal and vertical space allocation.

Lombardi (1973) has given an excellent account of the principles of visual perception and their clinical application to denture aesthetics which can be of great value to the dental ceramist in correcting faults in tooth orientation even when making fixed restorations.

The repeated ratio

This is accomplished by the use of a continued proportion or repeated ratio which can be applied to the width of the central and lateral incisor. This ratio can be continued in the placement of the remaining teeth and spaces. If the same ratio between the width of the central incisor and lateral incisor is repeated between the lateral incisor and the amount of canine shown, and between the canine and premolar etc., each tooth size will be different (variety) but related (unity) because of the repetition of the same ratio. In the extremely wide mouth, the premolar may be the tooth that "turns the corner". As Lombardi states, "the first premolar is one of the most common sinners against both perception and reality, and is often placed without adequate consideration to its explosive effect on an otherwise attractive set-up." He therefore recommended that the first premolar should be considered as one of the eight anterior teeth from an aesthetic standpoint.

Front-to-back progression

The front-to-back progression is a critical factor because the illusion of arch shape and depth must be provided in the composition. The prin-

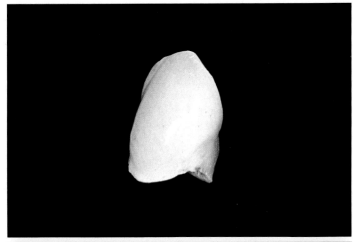

Fig. 3-42a Labial view of left maxillary canine showing correct position of distal lobe.

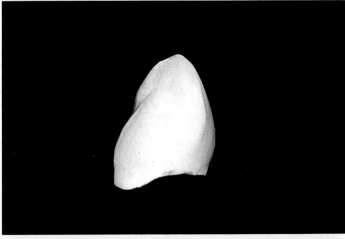

Fig. 3-42b Lingual view of left maxillary canine showing the positioning of the lingual lobe forming the cingulum area.

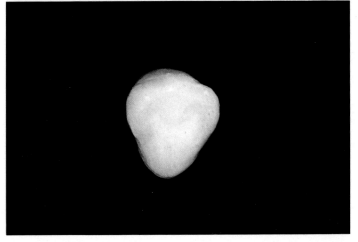

Fig. 3-42c Incisal view of left maxillary canine showing correct outline form and placement of the three labial lobes.

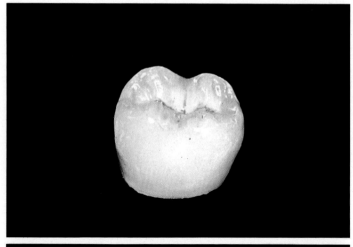

Fig. 3-43a   Buccal view of a left mandibular molar showing correct occlusal outline and positioning of buccal and lingual cusps.

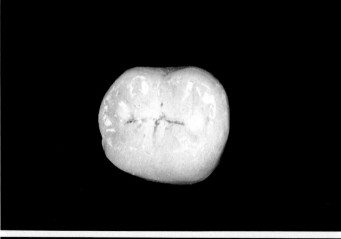

Fig. 3-43b   Occlusal view of a left mandibular molar. Note that the occlusal table has not been widened nor the buccal surface over-contoured.

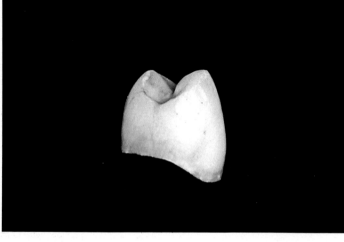

Fig. 3-43c   Mesial view of right maxillary premolar showing correct buccal and lingual contour.

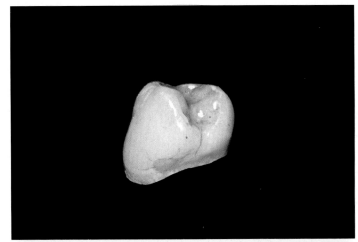

Fig. 3-43d Distal view of right maxillary premolar showing the correct degree of buccal supra-bulge and cervical contour.

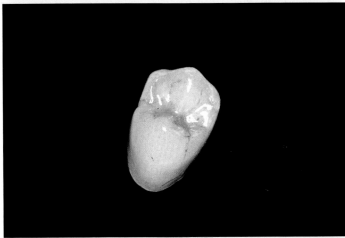

Fig. 3-43e Occlusal view of right maxillary premolar showing the three buccal lobes forming the correct cusp form.

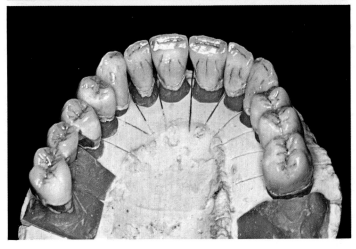

Fig. 3-43f Maxillary rehabilitation in Vita porcelain. Vita-Pt crowns.

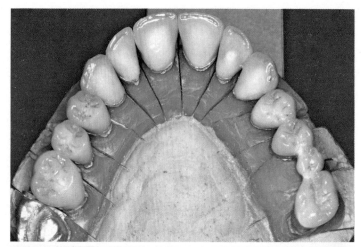

Fig. 3-43g and h Full mouth rehabilitation in Vita Porcelain. All individual crowns made in Vita-Pt porcelain and the bridges in VMK 68. Occlusal tables have not been widened and the teeth exhibit the correct lobe formation.

Figure 3-43g

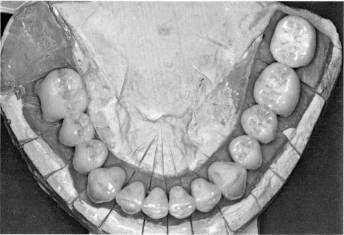

Figure 3-43h

Fig. 3-43i and j Full mouth rehabilitation in Vita-Pt and VMK 68 porcelain showing the excellent aesthetics at the gingival margin produced by the porcelain butt fit of the Vita-Pt crowns on 13, 12, 11, 21, 22, 23.

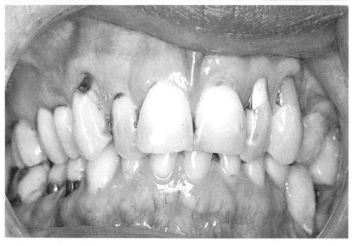

Fig. 3-43i Case before treatment.

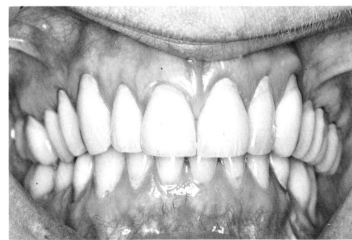

Fig. 3-43 j   Case after treatment.

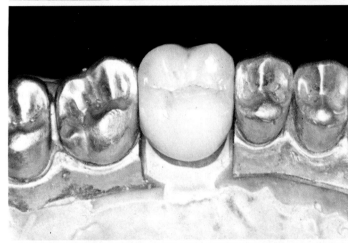

Fig. 3-44 a Incorrect reproduction of a maxillary first molar showing widening of occlusal table.

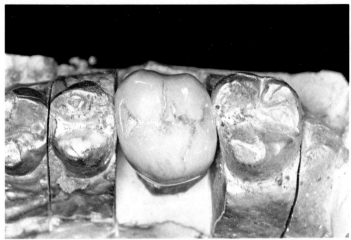

Fig. 3-44 b   Correct reproduction of a maxillary first molar.

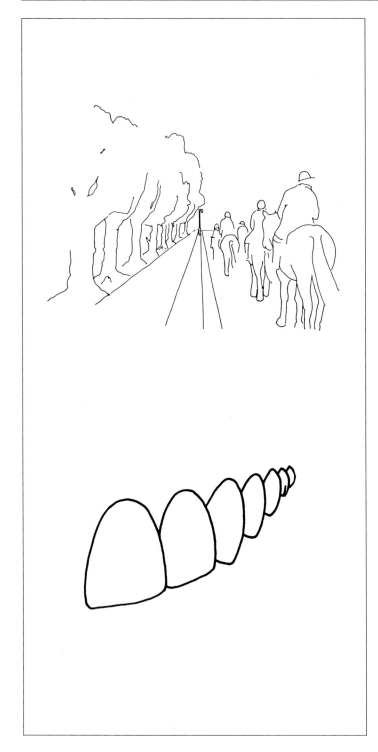

Fig. 3-45 Correct front-to-back progression in a dentition giving the same effect of harmony as the horse-riders in the picture above.

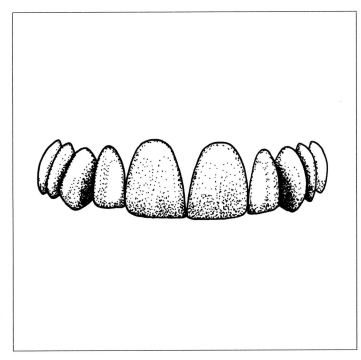

Fig. 3-46 Diagram illustrating how the maxillary canine teeth will not harmonise with the arch if their distal aspects are visible from the labial aspect. The mesial aspect can be placed in shadow and the distal aspect highlighted by the incorrect inversion.

ciple of gradation must be observed. If two like structures are placed at different distances on a line from the viewer, the closest one to the viewer will appear longer. If other like structures are interposed between these two, the size reduction will appear to be a gradual one from the size of that of the closest one to that of the furthest (Fig. 3-45). The use of a premolar with a short buccal cusp violates this principle and is a common sight in full mouth reconstruction. In particular the maxillary canine tooth can look very artificial if the distal surface is not "turned round the corner" (Fig. 3-46). Only the mesial aspect of the canine must be seen and in this way the premolars will then fade into the distance. As light falls on the dental arch, it will be seen that on the more distal teeth, the light is reduced and this gives a gradually darker shade and therefore a smaller appearance. It also blurs the detailed features, which increases the illusion of distance and therefore depth. This is why the anterior teeth are much more difficult to

reproduce in porcelain and achieve a good colour match and natural contour.

Horizontal and Vertical space allocation

Lombardi (1973) has illustrated the importance of both horizontal and vertical space allocation when constructing a new dentition. Important features to be considered are width and height, and the location of commissures when the mouth is in a smiling position. When the entire upper arch is to be restored in dental porcelain, the mouth should be regarded as a blank space of irregular outline into which the porcelain crowns will be made. It is therefore very easy for the ceramist to fail to allocate the correct vertical and, to a lesser extent, horizontal space to his reconstruction. This can often result in a "static denture" or "piano-key smile" (Fig. 3-47). Correct allocation of space is illus-

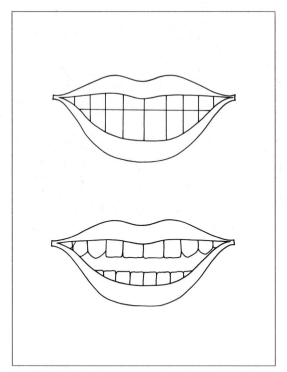

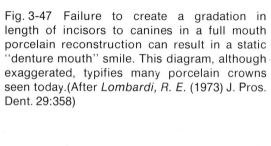

Fig. 3-47 Failure to create a gradation in length of incisors to canines in a full mouth porcelain reconstruction can result in a static "denture mouth" smile. This diagram, although exaggerated, typifies many porcelain crowns seen today.(After *Lombardi, R. E.* (1973) J. Pros. Dent. 29:358)

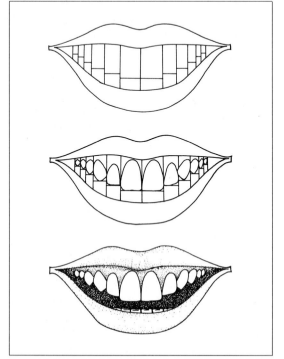

Fig. 3-48 Correct allocation of space in a full mouth porcelain reconstruction. (After *Lombardi, R. E.* (1973) J. Pros. Dent. 29:358)

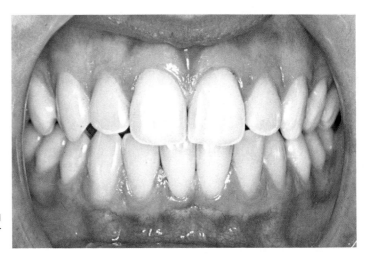

Fig. 3-49 Photograph of a young natural dentition, showing similar space allocation as in Fig. 3-48.

trated in Figs. 3-48, where the upper central incisors dominate the lip space and the canines are perfectly placed so as to maintain the proportion between lateral incisors and the premolars. A study of the natural dentition, illustrated in Fig. 3-49 will reveal that the ceramist's work in Figs. 3-50, 3-51 compares very favourably with the natural set-up (see also Fig. 3-27).

It is also important to note in Figs. 3-50, 3-51 that the teeth are in balance with the midline. Deviation from this normal arrangement can result in very ugly results, in particular bad alignment of the central incisors or canines can be very unaesthetic, as illustrated in Fig. 3-52.

The rebuilding of natural dentitions in dental porcelain is the most challenging area of restorative dentistry.

The reproduction of tooth contour, surface finish, built-in colour and occlusal harmony, taxes the skill of the best dentists and technicians. Indifferent results in porcelain stem from a number of causes. In particular, bulk build-up of porcelain with a spatula and then carving it back is frequently a cause for producing poor anatomy and colour. Subtle anatomy and built-in colour giving depth to the crown can only be achieved with an incremental brush build-up. Other poor results often result from the inability of the ceramist to see incorrect contour and occlusal disharmony. This again stems from a lack of knowledge of tooth anatomy. Perfection in the art of dental ceramics can only be developed by constant practice and self-criticism. Both dentist and technician must be willing to accept this criticism.

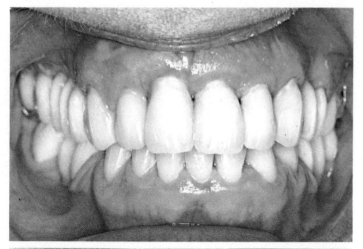

Fig. 3-50 Photograph of a patient with advanced periodontal disease in which a full mouth reconstruction has been carried out in dental porcelain. Note the attractive appearance of the lateral incisors in which the labial faces are not too flattened, and the harmonious relationship between the central incisors and the canine teeth. The ceramist has also correctly simulated the neck area of 11 where tissue loss has been severe. All the teeth were splinted with VMK 68 metal-ceramic crowns. The creation of the approximal spaces in the upper incisors has been done with subtlety.

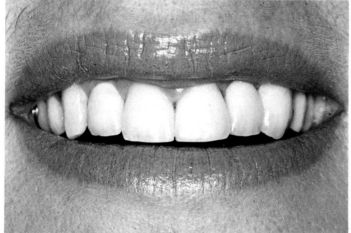

Fig. 3-51 A further case of full mouth reconstruction in dental porcelain. 12, 11 and 21, 22 were restored with Vita-Pt Porcelain. Front-to-back progression in this case is very pleasing.

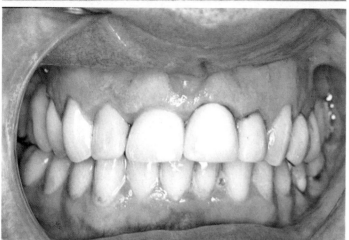

Fig. 3-52 Photograph of badly aligned incisor porcelain crowns which are sloping sideways and unbalancing the whole dentition.

Monograph III

References

Bazola, F. N., and *Malone, W. F.* (1967). Shade Guide for Vacuum-Fired Porcelain-Gold Crowns. J. Am. Dent. Assoc. 74:114.

Clark, E. B. (1933). The Clark Tooth Colour System, Parts I and II. Dent. Mag. Oral Top. 50:139.

Culpepper, W. D. (1970). A Comparison of Shade-Matching Procedures. J. Pros. Dent. 24:166.

Dinsdale, A., and *Malkin, F.* (1955). The Measurement of Gloss with Special Reference to Ceramic Materials. Trans. Brit. Ceram. Soc. 54:94.

Granger, R. G. (1974). Esthetics in Porcelain-Veneered Fixed Prostheses. J. Pros. Dent. 32:534.

Halden, J. R. (1974). Orthodontics in Relation to Restorative Dentistry. In: Restorative Procedures for the Practising Dentist. Ed. Harty, F. J. and Roberts, D. H. John Wright and Sons Ltd., Bristol.

Heath, F. J. (1968). Colour. The Tintometer Ltd., Salisbury, England.

Hefferen, J. J., Hefferen, S. M., Hoerman, K. C., and *Balekjian, A. Y.* (1967). Phosphoresence of Enamel Treated with Stannous Salts. J. Dent. Res. 46:1368.

Herzberg, T. W., Gettleman, L., Webber, R. L., and *Moffa, J. P.* (1972). Effect of Metal Surface Treatment on the Masking Power of Opaque Porcelain. J. Dent. Res. 51:468.

Horsley, H. J. (1967). Isolation of Fluorescent Material Present in Calcified Tissues. J. Dent. Res. 46:106.

Judd, D. B., and *Wyszecki, G.* (1963). Colour in Business, Science and Industry. Ed. 2. John Wiley and Sons Inc., New York.

Kingery, W. D. (1960). Introduction to Ceramics. John Wiley and Sons Inc., New York.

Kubelka, P., and *Munk, F.* (1931). "Ein Beitrag zur Optik der Farbanstriche." Z. tech. Physik. 12: 593.

Kurland, P. (1970). Cosmetic Correction with Jacket Crowns. Brit. Dent. J. 129:378.

Lombardi, R. E. (1973). The Principles of Visual Perception and their Clinical Application to Denture Aesthetics. J. Pros. Dent. 29:358.

McDevitt, C. A., and *Armstrong, W. G.* (1969). Investigations into the Nature of the Fluorescent Material in Calcified Tissues. J. dent. Res. 48: 1108.

McLean, J. W., and *Hughes, T. H.* (1965). The Reinforcement of Dental Porcelain with Ceramic Oxides. Brit. Dent. J. 119:251.

McLean, J. W. (1966). The Development of Ceramic Oxide Reinforced Dental Porcelains with an Appraisal of their Physical and Clinical Properties. M.D.S. Thesis, University of London.

Moore, J. E., and *MacCulloch, W. T.* (1974). The Inclusion of Radioactive Compounds in Dental Porcelains. Brit. Dent. J. 136:101.

Munsell, A. H. (1961). A Colour Notation. Ed. II. Munsell Colour Company, Baltimore.

Nickerson, D. (1946). Colour Measurement. U.S. Dept. of Agriculture. Misc. Pub. 58. March p. 9.

Semmelman, J. O. (1973). Personal Communication.

Sproull, R. C. (1973). Colour Matching in Dentistry, Part II. Practical Application of the Organisation of Colour. J. Pros. Dent. 29:556.

Wilson, H. J. (1969). Restorative Materials and Ultra-Violet Radiation. Brit. Dent. J. 126:345.

Monograph III

Selected Reading

Allen, E. (1969). Some New Advances in the Study of Metamerism. Colour Eng. 7:35.

Billmeyer, F. W. Jr., and *Saltzman, M.* (1966). Principles of Colour Technology. John Wiley and Sons Inc., New York.

HMSO (1972). 3rd. edition. Code of practice for the protection of persons against ionizing radiations arising from medical and dental use.

Hyashi, T. (1967). Medical Colour Standard V. Tooth Crown. Japan Colour Research Institute, Tokyo.

Lee, J. H. (1962). Dental Aesthetics. John Wright and Sons Ltd., Bristol.

Nimeroff, I. (1969). A Survey of Papers on Degree of Metamerism. Colour Eng. 6:44.

O'Riordan, M. C., and *Hunt, G. J.* (1974). Radioactive Fluorescers in Dental Porcelain. National Radiological Protection Board Report No. 25. HMSO.

Wright, W. D. (1964). The Measurement of Colour. Ed. 3. Hilgar and Watts Ltd., London.

Dental Porcelain. The State of the Art. Edit. Yamada. H.N. and Grenoble P.B. University of Southern California, 1977.

Alternatives to Gold Alloys in Dentistry. Conference Proceedings. N.I.H. 1977.

Monograph IV

Porcelain as a Restorative Material

Porcelain as a Restorative Material

What is the role of the porcelain veneer crown in restorative dentistry? To understand this problem it is essential, firstly, to consider the properties of porcelain in relation to resistance to plaque formation, ease of fabrication and maintenance of fit and occlusal stability. Only then can the clinician use this material to its best advantage. The excellent chemical resistance and stability of dental porcelain has already been described in Monograph I (The Nature of Dental Ceramics). This monograph is more concerned with the biological implications when using this material.

The role of dental plaque in causing periodontal disease and dental caries will probably be the most significant area of research in the next decade. This research will not only be confined to the hard and soft tissues in the mouth but also to the restorative materials used to replace these tissues. The susceptibility of various dental materials to accumulation of bacterial plaque is receiving increasing attention and a greater knowledge of these processes must enable the clinician to use his materials to better effect in combating dental disease.

The correct design of bridge pontics, the significance of tooth contour, surface integrity, and marginal seal of restorations in preserving the health of gingival tissue as well as tooth structure cannot be over-emphasized.

In addition, the study of occlusion and its greater understanding in the teaching schools will also offer the future graduate the opportunity of constructing restorations of a much higher standard than has been possible in the past.

Plaque Accumulation on Restorative Materials

Rough surfaces on any restorative material will increase the accumulation and retention of dental plaque (*Swartz,* and *Phillips,* 1957). It has also been shown that accumulation of dental plaque on tooth surfaces will produce an inflammatory response from gingival tissue (*Loe* et al., 1965). The degree of plaque formation on fixed restorations is therefore of paramount importance.

Glazed dental porcelain is the most easily cleansed material that is used in dentistry today. Although it has been shown that plaque can accumulate on dental porcelain in areas where it is not self-cleansing, these studies have perhaps confused the issue as to the material's easy cleansability. Studies carried out on plaque formation occurring on the polished surfaces of pontics constructed of cast gold, acrylic resin and glazed porcelain showed no significant difference between any of the materials (*Clayton* and *Green,* 1970). It was also shown that all these materials may produce an inflammatory response in the residual ridge mucosa (*Stein,* 1966; *Podshadley,* 1968). There seems little doubt that there is no dental material available today that will actually resist plaque formation, and until such a material is produced it is of

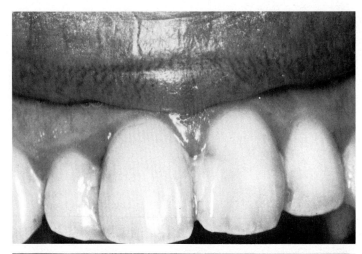

Fig. 4-1   12, 11 and 21, 22 prior to crowning. Gingival inflammation present particularly in the interdental papillae.

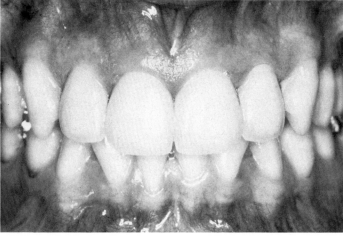

Fig. 4-2   12, 11 and 21, 22 after insertion of aluminous porcelain jacket crowns (Vitadur). Gingival condition shows a marked improvement after 5 years.

greater interest to the clinician to know what degrees of plaque accumulation are to be found on current restorative materials, where some cleansing action can be effective.

Newcomb (1974) found that plaque indices for porcelain were lower than those for homogeneous uncrowned teeth. The improvement in gingival condition of a patient's teeth after crowning with aluminous porcelain jacket crowns is illustrated in Figs. 4-1 and 4-2 and supports Newcomb's findings.

An earlier interesting study carried out by *Kaqueler* and *Weiss* (1970) on plaque accumula-tion on dental restorative materials revealed that in experiments performed, in vivo, on dogs, that significant differences did exist between various restorative materials. After periods of up to 19 days on a soft diet, the dogs' teeth were painted with basic fuschine 1 percent and magnified colour pictures were taken. The staining reaction of the plaque showed consistently that plaque accumulation was greatest on the surface of unpolished amalgam, zinc phosphate cement, silicate cement, and finally glazed porcelain, which showed almost no accumulation except at the margin where it increased with time. This study confirms what many clinicians observe, that dental porcelain is the most self-cleansing of all our restorative materials. A simple example can often be seen where a single porcelain crown will appear lighter in shade than the surrounding teeth until these teeth are cleaned. By contrast an acrylic crown can often appear darker due to accumulation of plaque and surface stain.

However, in a recent study, *Wise* and *Dykema* (1975) showed that there was no statistical difference between the plaque-retaining capacities of freshly-polished acrylic resin and porcelain, but that porcelain had a statistically significant lower plaque-retaining capacity than for a ceramic high-fusing gold alloy. It is likely that the gingival inflammation often seen around acrylic resin crowns could be caused by rapid loss of polish due to wear, and also to marginal leakage, which is not improved by the low modulus of elasticity of acrylic resin and its high water absorption and thermal expansion.

Marginal Fit

A criticism levelled at the complete porcelain veneer crown (the porcelain jacket crown) is that it generally has "open margins". By contrast the porcelain veneer metal-ceramic crown is often claimed to produce a better fit. However, it is possible by careful control of the porcelain build-up, to minimize the firing shrinkage and produce remarkably accurate fitting crowns. A technique for doing this has been described (*McLean*, 1970). Crowns made by this technique were cemented to jacket crown preparations in vivo using a polyether rubber* as the cementing medium (*McLean*, and *von Fraunhofer*, 1971). This rubber produced a film thickness of 22 μm when tested according to B.S. 3364 and simulated the performance of zinc phosphate or zinc polycarboxylate ce-

---

* Impregum, ESPE GmbH, Seefeld, West Germany.

ments. The rubber film was removed from the crown and embedded in an epimine resin prior to sectioning and measuring the rubber's thickness. A typical film thickness of rubber under one of the aluminous porcelain jacket crowns is illustrated in Fig. 4-3 and it may be seen that a maximum film thickness of 60 μm was recorded.

This study showed that a well-made aluminous porcelain jacket crown could be made to fit the tooth as well as a metal-ceramic crown, and that the space created by removal of the platinum foil shim may make a greater contribution to accuracy of seating than hitherto thought.

The clinician might be tempted to think that a gap under a metal-ceramic crown is less than is actually present, since fit is often assessed by probing at the wrong angle (Fig. 4-4). By contrast, any inaccuracy in the fit of a porcelain jacket crown made to a butt joint is much more easily detected (Fig. 4-5).

The merits of the bevel, deep chamfer and flat shoulder will be discussed later in this monograph, and the rationale behind them explained in scientific terms (see page 276).

Micro-leakage under Porcelain Crowns

Clinicians who have been in practice for long periods are often struck by the fact that seldom do they ever see secondary caries under a complete porcelain veneer crown. Many times these crowns can be quite an indifferent fit and yet the cement lute is intact. By contrast a gold crown can be of vastly superior fit and yet show signs of micro-leakage and secondary decay. What is the explanantion for this?

It is generally agreed that micro-leakage is caused by the following factors:

1. Solubility of the cement under dental plaque.
2. Changes in dimension of the restoration or cement due to thermal or occlusal stressing.

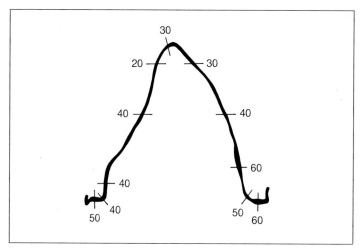

Fig. 4-3 Tracing of a typical Impregum "replica" of a cement film beneath an aluminous porcelain jacket crown in the labiolingual plane, film thickness in microns. (After *McLean, J. W.,* and *von Fraunhofer, J. A.* (1971) Brit. dent. J. 131:107.)

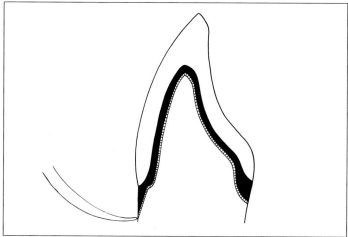

Fig. 4-4 Diagram showing incorrect angle of explorer tip when assessing the fit of a metal-ceramic crown made with a long-bevel collar. Exploration of a finely bevelled margin may suggest only a minor defect when in fact the discrepancy is quite substantial.

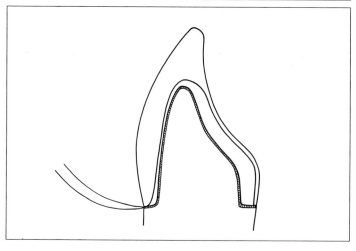

Fig. 4-5 Diagram showing the easier application of an explorer to a butt fitting aluminous porcelain jacket crown.

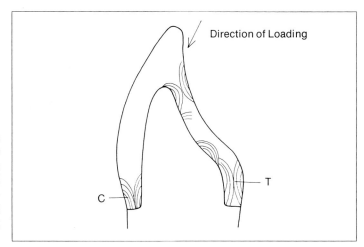

Direction of Loading

C

T

Fig. 4-6 Diagram showing the development of tensile stresses at the margins of a porcelain jacket crown. These stresses will not cause permanent deformation at the margin until the crown fractures. C = Compression; T = Tension.

3. Lack of adhesion between the tooth and cement or between the cement and crown material.

The solubility of cement rapidly increases when the seal between restoration and tooth is broken. It is likely that thermal or occlusal stressing of a restoration could be a major cause of microleakage in the full crown restoration. Dental porcelain is an excellent material to resist such changes since it has the following properties:

High modulus of elasticity (stiffness)

Low thermal conductivity

Minimal solubility in water or weak acids

High creep resistance

All the above properties stem from the nature of the atomic bonding of ceramics described in Monograph I.

In clinical terms, dental porcelain is a rigid and chemically resistant material so that any forces applied to it are likely to break the material before it deforms. Because of the rigid nature of porcelain the cement seal is unlikely to be broken unless the crown fractures (Fig. 4-6). In addition, because the material accumulates minimal plaque, the chances of acid dis-

integration of the cement at the margins are also small.

Failures in metal-ceramic crowns are often produced when thin gold bevels are used which distort on firing or lift under occlusal stress during function (Fig. 4-7). In addition, if gold collars are used they may oxidise on the surface and collect plaque more easily. For this reason a more hygienic result can be produced if the metal is finished to a knife edge and the porcelain butted onto the cervical margin of the tooth.

Although the porcelain jacket crown requires more skill from both operator and ceramist, from a biological standpoint, it is still the best material to use on the front teeth where the occlusion is favourable for the following reasons:

1. Conservative tooth preparations can be made.
2. Less risk of over-contouring.
3. Improved aesthetics (see Monograph III).
4. More resistant to plaque formation.
5. Lower cost.

The metal-ceramic crown also has three great advantages. The preparation can be done with less attention to the effect of stress on the

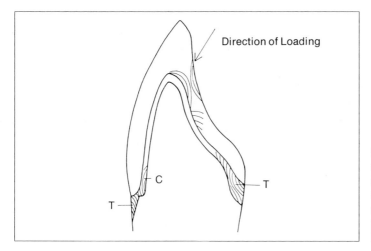

Fig. 4-7 Diagram showing the development of tensile stresses at the margins of a metal-ceramic crown. Thin or long gold bevels could lift and cause leakage patterns to develop in the cement lute.

crown, and if a gold collar is used, the fit of the crown is easier to obtain. The strength of the metal-ceramic crown is also greatly superior to the complete porcelain restoration.

Occlusion and Dental Porcelain

Dental Porcelain is the most difficult of all restorative materials with which to develop accurate occlusal surfaces. Not only has the ceramist to contend with high firing shrinkages, but also the hardness of dental porcelain makes the carving of occlusal surfaces more difficult. There is little doubt that cast gold is a more satisfactory material for reconstructing occlusal surfaces. The lost wax process facilitates the accurate duplication of occlusal anatomy produced by methods such as the "add-on" functional waxing techniques (*Payne*, 1970; *Thomas*, 1976). In addition, the sand-blasting of the surfaces of cast gold occlusal surfaces enables the clinician to detect any prematurities more easily than with porcelain. Cast gold is also better tolerated by opposing human enamel and will exhibit some ductility.

The demand by the dental profession for stronger porcelains has largely been met with the introduction of metal-ceramics. However, a price has been paid for this development. Occlusal inaccuracies do not always cause fracture of the crowns, and premature contacts, incorrect centric relationships and heavy balancing side contacts may go undetected. Inevitable the stresses placed upon the supporting periodontium are too great and these tissues will often react vigorously. It is not an infrequent sight to see both the porcelain-covered teeth and the opposing natural teeth drift or loosen and the dentition deteriorate rapidly. The ceramist is therefore required to exercise even greater care with his occlusal anatomy than when using any other restorative material.

The demand by patients for more aesthetic dentistry is increasing and the dental profession is being placed under increasing pressure to fulfill this demand. It is therefore not surprising that the use of porcelain restorations is increasing each year.

It is outside the scope of these monographs to discuss the principles involved in restoring occlusion to natural teeth, but it is important to recognize what types of occlusion are most destructive to dental porcelain. Crack propagation in dental porcelain has been

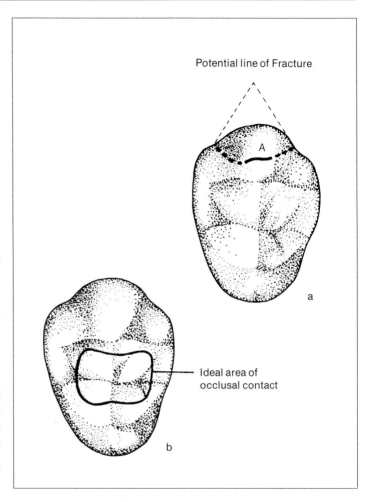

Potential line of Fracture

A

a

Ideal area of
occlusal contact

b

Fig. 4-8a and b (a) Diagram illustrating the overloading of the
flaw system in dental porcelain.
Assuming the deepest microcrack in the surface is at point A,
if this area is contacted by an
opposing tooth then the microcrack can be deepened to the
point of brittle fracture. Avoid-
ance of the tooth area at A reduces this risk. The optimum
type of occlusion which can resist
these destructive forces should
provide minimal tooth contact
outside centric relationship. The
ideal area for tooth contact in
centric relationship is illustrated
in Fig. 4-8 (b).

discussed in Monograph II, and evidence presented to illustrate the damage that can be
caused by overloading the flaw-system which is
always present in the surface of dental porcelain.

It is well known that functional movements of
the mandible produce less destructive forces
than para-functional movements such as
bruxism, clenching or habitual biting of pipes,
pencils, etc. (*Huffman* et al., 1969). Functional
movements exercised during chewing, swallow-
ing or speaking minimize the duration of tooth
contact per day and the magnitude of the forces

applied. Functional movements of the mandible
are therefore much less likely to overload the
flaw system in dental porcelain. By contrast,
para-functional movements can be very destructive, and when the occlusal surfaces of the
porcelain are not in harmony with the mandibular movement, a sudden premature contact
on a cusp of porcelain can very easily propagate a surface micro-crack. This is probably the
most common cause of fracture or chipping of
porcelain crowns (Fig. 4-8 a and b).

The optimum type of occlusion which can resist these destructive forces would therefore

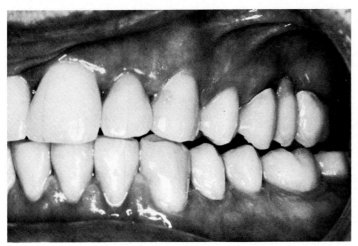

Fig. 4-9 Full mouth porcelain reconstruction showing "cuspid disclusion". Upper buccal shearing cusps of the posterior teeth should not be in contact once the patient moves from centric relationship. All upper and lower teeth made in Vitadur bonded platinum crowns except for VMK 68 bridge on 25, 26, 27.

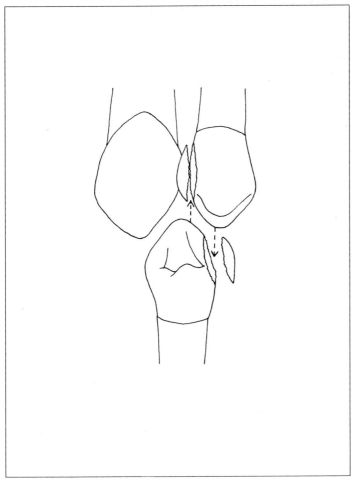

Fig. 4-10 Diagram showing possible lines of fracture in the occlusal surfaces of porcelain when lower buccal cusps occlude on upper marginal ridge areas.

conform to one that provides minimal tooth contact outside centric relationship. Bilateral balanced occlusion should be avoided and flat-cusped teeth, often seen in bruxists, are much more prone to excessive and continuous exposure to overloading of the flaw system in the dental porcelain. Ideally, porcelain will suffer the least damage if the maximum intercuspation of the teeth coincides with centric relationship. In eccentric positions of the mandible there should be no tooth contact on the balancing side or the orbiting condyle side, and no posterior teeth should contact once the mandible leaves centric. This type of occlusion is often referred to as "Disclusion" and forms the basis of much of the current thinking in the field of gnathology.

The controversy surrounding many occlusal concepts is too well-known to need repetition but there seems little doubt that many of the thoughts expressed by *Stallard* and *Stuart* (1963) and others, on mutually protected occlusions, certainly mitigate the risk of over-stressing porcelain restorations. If the canine tooth is used as a discluding mechanism in any eccentric movements of the mandible, i.e. "cuspid disclusion", then the three groups of teeth, incisors, posterior teeth and canines can function independently of each other (Fig. 4-9). At no time can large numbers of teeth be subject to sudden premature contact with the resultant over-stressing of the porcelain flaw system. In complete rehabilitation of an occlusion in porcelain, to assure mandibular freedom, the cusp tips should be set and shaped to run in grooves without contacts in the eccentric excursive movements. The eminences in front of the condyles should compel disclusion of the rear teeth. Attention should be paid to ensuring that stamp cusps occlude in fossae and the occlusal marginal ridges of shearing cusps should have no occlusion (*Stuart*, 1964).

Wherever possible, lower buccal cusps should never occlude on upper marginal ridges. In the case of porcelain this is an easy way of causing chipping of fine edges on the occlusal tables (Fig. 4-10).

Achieving these objects is very difficult when working porcelain and it is important to avoid sharp line angles which can also increase stress concentration.

In the majority of cases treated for full porcelain coverage it is impossible to make any major alterations in the occlusal pattern since only small groups of teeth may need restoring. In these cases it is essential to establish correct centric relationship by occlusal adjustment prior to commencing work and under no circumstances should the fossae be over-reduced or cusps flattened to "free" the occlusion. The stamp cusp must nestle in the fossae and maintain correct vertical relationship, otherwise over-eruption of the opposing teeth may occur and a premature contact will develop during eccentric excursive movements. This is a very common fault in porcelain work, particularly in cases of bilateral balanced occlusion, and will result in either fracture of the porcelain or damage to the periodontium.

The insertion of porcelain or metal-ceramic crowns in cases of bruxism should also be done with great circumspection. The metal-ceramic crowns will function quite well in these cases and the incidence of fracture is very low. However, it is vital that the original occlusal table is not widened and thus increase the area of flaw size in the porcelain (Fig. 4-11). Not only may the porcelain chip but the opposing natural teeth will also be subject to excessive wear and trauma. In all cases of this type, periodic checks should be made to see whether the occlusal surfaces are still in harmony. Complete-porcelain veneer crowns are not indicated in cases of bruxism or severe para-functional activity, the incidence of fracture being too high.

The restoration of the incisor teeth with porcelain veneer crowns is the most widely-practised procedure. Often crowns are placed upon these teeth with little thought given to the existing

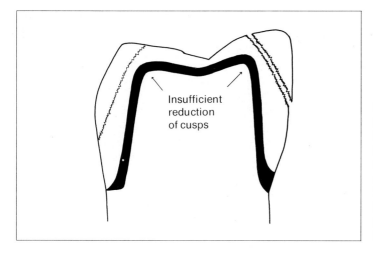

Insufficient
reduction
of cusps

Fig. 4-11 Diagram illustrating the effect of an incorrect preparation causing widening of occlusal tables. The fracture resistance of the metal-ceramic crown is reduced and the wider the table the further the porcelain edge is from its metal support. Fracture lines may easily develop from the extended occlusal table.

occlusion and subsequent failure is attributed to the technician. It is essential for the clinician to examine the whole occlusion prior to inserting porcelain veneer crowns in the anterior region and recognize any abnormalities. Deflective malocclusions may be present and typical examples are to be found where heavy balancing contacts occur in the molar region. In protrusive movements of the mandible a pattern of occlusion may develop which results in a Class I lever arrangement. As the jaw opens, protrudes, and attempts to close in the incisal edge to edge position, if a heavy molar contact should exist, thereby preventing the anterior teeth from contacting for stability, the molars will overpower the condyles which act as the fulcrum. The power is supplied by the muscles behind these teeth and the work load is transmitted to the anterior teeth, creating the more powerful Class I lever as opposed to the normal Class III jaw lever (Fig. 4-12a and b) (*Huffman* et al., 1967).

A Class I lever system may be seen when the anterior teeth are severely worn, with only moderate wear of the posterior teeth (Fig. 4-13 a and b). Attempts to restore such teeth with porcelain veneer crowns is doomed to failure unless the heavy balancing molar contacts are eliminated. Although these anterior teeth might

be restored with metal-ceramic crowns without actual failure of the porcelain, something must give, and invariably it will be the surrounding periodontium.

Wear facets on teeth are therefore good indicators of the stresses that might be applied to the porcelain surface. The use of thin plastic shims to check occlusal contacts prior to cutting the teeth can also aid the clinician in his diagnosis. In general it might be stated that anterior porcelain jackets are much more likely to fracture where excessively tight occlusal contacts exist in the anterior region and heavy wear facets are apparent on the incisal edges of both upper and lower incisors and the lingual concavities of the uppers.

For example, wear facets are often visible on the linguo-cervical one-fifth of the upper incisors where a deep incisal overlap occurs. This type of occlusion is highly unfavourable to dental porcelain, and metal or high alumina reinforcement of the lingual surface should be employed. Lingually inclined incisors may show considerable wear facets at the linguo-incisal one-third, and leverage forces in this area will be high. If the tooth preparation only allows a thin labio-cervical thickness of porcelain, a classical labial crescent-shaped fracture may occur. This defect will be even further exacer-

Fig. 4-12a and b (a) Diagram of the normal Class III lever system occurring in mandibular hinge movements. (b) A Class I lever system may develop when premature molar contacts occur.

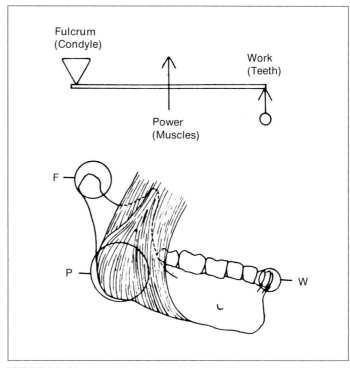

Figure 4-12a

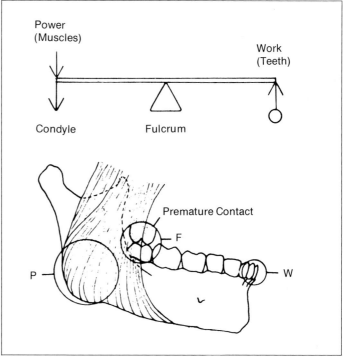

Figure 4-12b

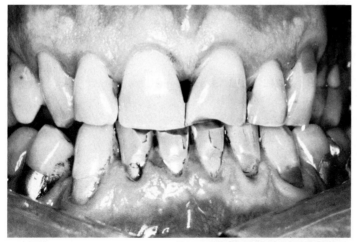

Fig. 4-13a and b (a) Clinical case illustrating severe wear of the lower anterior teeth. (b) Heavy balancing contact seen in the molar region.

Figure 4-13a

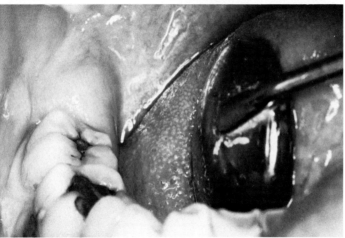

Figure 4-13b

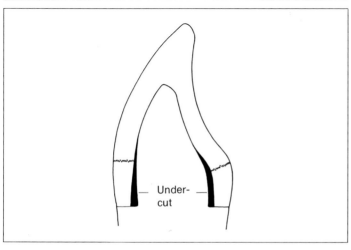

Fig. 4-14 Diagram illustrating the type of fracture occurring when a small undercut is present at the labio-cervical or linguo-cervical margin of lingually inclined incisors.

bated if a small undercut is present at the labio-cervical margin (Fig. 4-14).

There are so many patterns of occlusion that it is impossible to make hard and fast rules as to the suitability of porcelain as a restoration in all cases. The clinician must recognize that he is dealing with an unyielding and brittle material, capable in the case of metal-ceramics, of causing infinite damage to a dentition where occlusal morphology has been ignored. However, the pressure from the general public for more aesthetic dentistry is inexorable. Occlusal coverage in gold, particularly in the lower teeth, is meeting with more and more resistance. The future graduate in dentistry will probably be forced to develop his skills in dental porcelain despite the physiological criticisms of this material. A mastery of porcelain technique and occlusal carving can surprise even the most devoted student of the gold occlusal surface.

Gold versus Porcelain Occlusion

Questions are frequently asked about the desirability of inserting full porcelain occlusions against gold or natural teeth. There is little doubt that if the abrasion resistance of these three materials is considered then porcelain must be regarded as a material that will cause wear facets in any gold or natural tooth surface, particularly where premature contacts occur. As explained previously, where a mutually protected occlusion has been developed, i.e. cuspid disclusion, then opposing teeth should not make contact once the mandible leaves centric. This ensures minimal wear on teeth and in these cases there should be no faceting on gold surfaces opposed by porcelain. The answer to the problem of deciding on whether to insert full porcelain veneer crowns against opposing gold restorations must lie in the assessment of the patient's occlusion. If the patient exhibits a "group function" occlusion with fairly massive occlusal contacts during chewing, then a gold surface must wear faster than the porcelain or, alternatively, the porcelain will cause faceting of opposing natural teeth. In particular, if premature contacts occur on lower lingual or upper buccal cusps then the softer material will abrade more quickly.

The optimum type of occlusion which can resist differences in abrasion rate between metal and porcelain surfaces must conform to one that provides minimal tooth contact outside centric relationship.

Indications for use

Despite the above remarks, the indiscriminate use of full porcelain coverage should not be used as an easy way out of more difficult operative procedures. Tooth preparations involving removal of healthy and often aesthetically-pleasing buccal or labial enamel are undertaken since a metal-ceramic crown can compensate for any deficiencies in preparation. The fact that these crowns may make a violent intrusion into the gingival crevice is sometimes ignored and there is little doubt that whatever work the periodontist may subsequently perform, many mouths are condemned to permanent gingival inflammation. A healthy periodontium is a prerequisite before any full coverage restorations are even contemplated.

Human enamel is still our best restorative material and the clinician must always be conscious of the fact that unless he can replace it with accurately fitting and properly contoured porcelain crowns which are in harmonious relationship with the gingiva, then other methods of restoring these teeth are biologically preferable.

Although the clinician may embark on full porcelain coverage with the best of intentions to fulfill the patient's desire for improved aesthetics, the final result may produce a conflict of

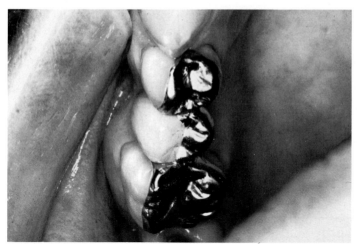

Fig. 4-15a and b   Alumina tube pontic bridge using three-quarter crowns as retainers on 16 and 14.

Figure 4-15a

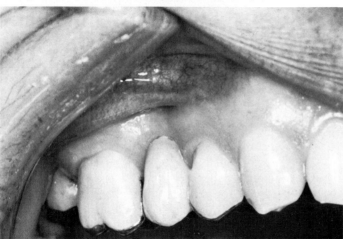

Figure 4-15b

interest in what is aesthetically possible. Unfortunately there is a world-wide shortage of skilled ceramic technicians and it is more common to see over-contoured and aesthetically displeasing crowns than the converse. It is for this reason that many clinicians who show high regard for the health of gingival tissue are questioning the results that are achieved in full porcelain coverage.

Kahn (1965) has summarized these views succinctly and drawn attention to the fact that the degree of gingival irritation is directly proportional to the amount of restorative material in contact with the gingival tissue, and to the accuracy of marginal fit. Whenever and wherever it is possible to keep margins away from gingival tissue, the more favourable will be the opportunity for periodontal health. There is little doubt that the use of full coverage in cases of advanced periodontal disease is good practice, since the splinting of teeth requires maximum support. The important consideration in this category is not the preservation of tooth structure per se, but rather the preservation of the periodontium. In cases where the periodontal involvement is only moderately advanced and the labial and buccal enamel of the teeth are intact and aesthetically pleasing, partial coverage becomes a practical proposition and biologically desirable.

The use of three-quarter crowns as bridge retainers is still preferable in many cases and the occlusal re-surfacing of posterior teeth may be done by using MOD onlays with or without accessory anchorage. Although these types of restorations place a heavy demand on the operator's skill, they often provide a better service to the patient from a biological point of view. The author makes frequent use of these retainers on teeth where the enamel crown length is adequate for retention. Three-quarter crowns combined with porcelain pontics can provide a bridge with excellent aesthetics (Fig. 4-15).

Indications for the use of porcelain veneer crowns have been admirably summarized by *Johnston* et al. (1967). They advocated their use "to return the coronal portion of a tooth to form, function and aesthetic desirability when generally accepted operative procedures will not suffice." The requirements of the tooth preparation such as adequate bulk of dentine and coronal length to support the porcelain crown will be discussed later in this monograph. However, at this stage it is useful to consider the specific situations where porcelain or metal-ceramic crowns may be used. They may be summarized as follows:

1. Gross carious lesions.
2. Heavily restored teeth where splitting of the cusps may eventually occur.
3. Traumatic fractures of incisal angles or buccal cusps of teeth.
4. Badly discoloured teeth.
5. Occlusal corrections and improvements of function and alignment.
6. Congenital abnormalities.
7. Splinting of mobile teeth (with metal substructure).
8. Abutment retainers in fixed and removable partial prosthodontics.

The decision as to whether complete porcelain or metal ceramic veneer crowns should be used in these situations is mainly related to strength, aesthetics, and biological requirements.

Indications for Use of Porcelain Jacket Crowns

1. Conservation of tooth structure and maintenance of periodontal health.
2. All anterior teeth where aesthetics is of prime importance.
3. Lower incisors where space is available.
4. Limited use on the premolar teeth where the occlusion allows some protection of the buccal shearing cusps e.g. cuspid disclusion. In these cases the posterior teeth will generally have the cusps remaining relatively intact.

Contra-Indications for Use of the Porcelain Jacket Crown

1. In cases of parafunctional activity of the mandible, e.g. bruxism, or where deflective malocclusions remain uncorrected.
2. Where occlusal clearance after tooth preparation is less than 0.8 millimeters e.g. very thin teeth, deep incisal overjets with lingual wear facets.
3. Insufficient tooth support or where the preparation design causes sudden changes of thickness in the porcelain (cleavage lines).
4. Molar teeth.

199

Indications for use of the Metal-Ceramic Crown

1. In cases of parafunctional mandibular activity where an aesthetic restoration is essential.
2. Where lingual clearance of less than 0.8 millimeters is present after tooth preparation (e.g. the metal-backed crown).
3. Teeth requiring fixed splinting or being used as bridge abutments.
4. In all posterior teeth where full coverage is necessary for aesthetic reasons.
5. Where deep chamfer preparations are desirable, e.g. lingual shoulder areas or periodontally involved teeth.
6. Where gold occlusal surfaces are required.

Contra-Indications for use of the Metal-Ceramic Crown

1. Adolescent teeth where minimal tooth preparation is essential.
2. Adult teeth where enamel wear is high and there is insufficient bulk of tooth structure to allow room for metal and porcelain, e.g. 1.5 millimeters.
3. Anterior teeth where aesthetics is of prime importance, e.g. light shades or very translucent teeth.

Aluminous Porcelain Compared with Metal-Ceramics

Aluminous Porcelain

Advantages

1. Good aesthetics easily obtained if the core porcelain is correctly placed (see Monograph III).
2. Full lingual core porcelains protect the crown against impact shock from opposing incisors.
3. The resistance to pyroplastic flow or slump of the core porcelain can produce better fits when compared with regular porcelain. This property also allows staining of the crown without the platinum foil.
4. May be used in thicknesses of not greater than 0.8 mm and still provide good aesthetics.
5. Greater depth of translucency obtainable (see Monograph III).
6. Less expensive to construct than metal-ceramic crowns.

Disadvantages

1. Crowns are still not strong enough to resist fracture in the posterior region or in cases of bruxism or inadequate occlusal clearance.
2. Preparation of the tooth requires more attention to detail than the metal-ceramic crown if proper support is to be given to the porcelain.
3. Cannot be used in long span bridgework or for multiple splinting.

Metal-Ceramics

Advantages

1. Very high strength due to prevention of crack propagation from the internal surfaces of crowns by the metal reinforcement.

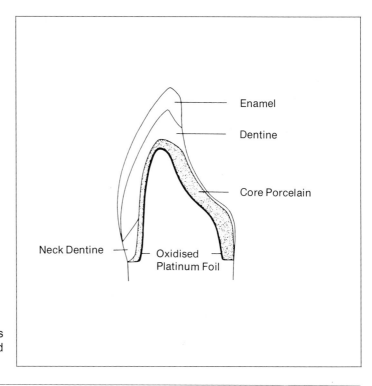

Fig. 4-16 Diagram of the various layers of porcelain in a Bonded Alumina Crown.

2. Improved fit on individual crowns provided by cast gold collar.
3. The only porcelain material that can be used in fixed bridgework and for splinting teeth.

Disadvantages

1. Increased opacity and light reflectivity, particularly in tungsten filament light.
2. May only be used in thickness of 1.5 mm or more, due to the necessity of providing room for 0.5 mm of metal. This restricts their use for individual crowns if there is a risk of over-contouring.
3. More difficult to create depth of translucency in the crown due to the "mirror" effect of the dense opaque masking porcelains. If enamels or dentine powders are used which are too translucent, then there is a danger of the opaque porcelain showing through.

4. The fit of long span bridges or splints may be affected by the creep of the metal during successive bakes of porcelain.
5. More difficult to obtain good aesthetics than regular or aluminous porcelain.
6. Porcelains used in the metal-ceramic technique are more liable to devitrification which can produce cloudiness.

The Platinum bonded Alumina Crown

A study of the advantages and disadvantages of the aluminous porcelain and metal-ceramic crown will reveal that no solution has yet been found to the problem of making high strength

201

porcelain veneer crowns of 1 millimetre average thickness which are also aesthetically pleasing. The development of the platinum bonded alumina crown has, to a large extent, solved this problem since it combines the best properties of both aluminous porcelain and metal reinforcement (*McLean,* and *Sced,* 1976). The bonding of aluminous porcelain to a thin platinum foil coping allows a much greater depth of porcelain to be used on the labial surface of the crown (Fig. 4-16). In addition, the "Twin Foil" technique described by *McLean* et al. (1976) gives the ceramist the opportunity to achieve a porcelain butt fit at the critical labio-cervical area.

The bonded alumina crown derives its strength from the internal platinum bonded surface since micro-cracks, which are normally present in an aluminous porcelain core are largely eliminated. The elimination of these micro-cracks enables the glassy porcelain to reach more closely to its theoretical strength, which can be very high in a "flaw-free" surface.

Indications for use of the Bonded Alumina Crown

1. Porcelain veneer crowning of adolescent teeth where minimal tooth preparation is necessary.
2. Porcelain crowning of all anterior adult teeth where space is at a premium, e.g. heavily worn teeth, thin or short teeth, minimal occlusal clearance but not less than 0.8 mm.
3. Anterior teeth where metal reinforcement is essential.
4. Complete porcelain cantilever bridges on anterior teeth, e.g. replacing lateral incisors.
5. Coping jacket crowns on unit built bridgework.
6. Repair of fractured metal-ceramic bridges where removal of the bridge or splint is undesirable.
7. Pre-molar teeth where space is limited.

Contra-indications

1. Periodontally involved teeth where preparations extend deeply into root-face and no shoulder preparations are possible.
2. Where gold collars are considered desirable for reinforcing teeth.
3. Posterior teeth where large areas of tooth are missing and uneven bulk of porcelain is inevitable i.e. porcelain must cover platinum in even thickness for maximum strength.
4. Where lingual shoulder preparations are impossible particularly in the molar region.
5. Where occlusal clearance is less than 1 mm in the posterior teeth.

Clinical Cases

In order to illustrate the use of porcelain in restorative dentistry, the following cases have been selected.

Case 1: A typical example of the value of full porcelain coverage is illustrated in Fig. 4-17. The patient (female, aged 28 years) presented with a classical picture of the ravages of uncontrolled bacterial plaque formation on all her teeth. The amalgam restorations in the posterior teeth had corroded due to anodic attack via oxygen concentration cells forming in the amalgam surface under the plaque. The y_2 phase (tin-mercury) had leached out and her teeth were heavily discoloured. Acrylic and silicate restorations have eroded and discoloured in the anterior teeth and in particular some of the approximal silicates have suffered from acid attack via the plaque. Her gingival condition is also poor but without severe bone loss. A dehiscence has formed on 23 due to loss of the thin cortical plate of bone.

All the posterior teeth were restored with metal-ceramic crowns (VMK 68) and metal-ceramic bridgework on the lower left side. Aluminous porcelain crowns (Vitadur S) were inserted on the upper anterior teeth due to their better aesthetics and depth of translucency. Great care was taken with the crown contours and occlusal tables to ensure that over-contouring was avoided. Fig. 4-18 illustrates the case four years later where it may be seen that the gingival tissue has responded well to improved oral hygiene combined with the easy cleansability of the porcelain crowns. Fig. 4-19 a and b illustrates the centric and eccentric relationships and it will be noted that the "cuspid protected occlusion" allows the patient to disclude on the posterior teeth. All the preparations were designed so that they only encroached into the gingival crevice to a depth of 1.0 mm and it is the author's opinion that such a procedure contributes greatly to the longivity of multiple crownwork. It is interesting to note that the gingival cleft on 23 has improved considerably without surgical intervention, although a flap operation may be indicated at a later date.

Case 2: Although porcelain crowns have been advocated in cases of congenital abnormality or badly aligned teeth, it should be noted that there is a limitation to the amount of correction that can be achieved (see Monograph III). It is rarely possible to reduce the labial thickness of a malaligned tooth to any degree since the thickness of porcelain left for aesthetics and strength is too small. A rotated tooth may be corrected more easily and approximal correction can be made. In addition to the difficulty of combining aesthetics with strength, the response of the gingival tissue to corrections of contour are often quite noticeable. A case illustrating the reaction of the tissues under a porcelain jacket crown replacing a "peg-top" lateral incisor is shown in Fig. 4-20. The new contour

of the tooth has produced a severe gingival response.

Case 3: Patient male, age 55 years. Premature contacts detected on lingual cusps of lower molar teeth causing a lateral deflection to the right (Fig. 4-21 a and b). The collapse of the posterior occlusion has resulted in a major discrepancy between centric relationship and the patient's centric occlusion (maximum intercuspation). This patient was treated by inserting bonded alumina crowns on all the teeth, except for those missing teeth which were bridged with VMK 68. Maximum intercuspation of the teeth now coincides with centric relationship.

The completed case is shown in Fig. 4-22 and the left and right-handed excursion in Figs. 4-23 and 4-24. Particular attention should be paid to the effect of correct contour on the gingival tissue after only six weeks. The tissues, although not perfect, have responded very well to the porcelain butt fit of the bonded alumina crowns. In the case of 43 a flap operation could be performed at a later date to increase the attached gingival thickness. Note the good "front to back progression" of the teeth and correct placement of the canine teeth. All the teeth have been characterised to suit the patient's age group.

Case 4: Patient female, age 13 years. Administration of tetracycline as a child has caused heavy staining of all the anterior teeth (Fig. 4-25). This case could have been treated by the use of aluminous porcelain crowns but in view of the thinness of the teeth, even alumina reinforced crowns could fracture. It was therefore decided to use bonded alumina crowns. The lower preparations and completed case are shown in Figs. 4-26, 4-27 and 4-28. Because of the minimal thickness of metal used (0.025 mm) the bonded alumina crowns have been kept well within the original contour of the natural teeth.

Case 5: Patient male, age 52 years. Severe bone loss around all the upper teeth with considerable mobility patterns present. Fixed splinting using metal-ceramic crowns was undertaken and the preparations carried up the root face. In this case it was impossible to use a classical right angle shoulder since space would not permit. Long chamfer preparations were prepared and the porcelain finished to the metal edge. The preparations and completed case are illustrated in Figs. 4-29 and 4-30.

The above cases, illustrating the use of dental porcelain, serve to show its versatility in clinical dentistry and despite the deficiencies of dental porcelain outlined in this monograph, it is still our most permanent and aesthetic material. In the foreseeable future it is doubtful whether materials' scientists will find an organic plastic or composite material that can replace ceramics. The nature of dental alumino-silicate glasses discussed in Monograph I, provides the dentist with a material that can closely simulate human enamel. However the brittleness and hardness of glass still present a major problem. The composite structure of human enamel is unique and the bonding of the hydroxy-apatite crystals in their collagenous matrix will continue to fascinate the best brains in the materials science world.

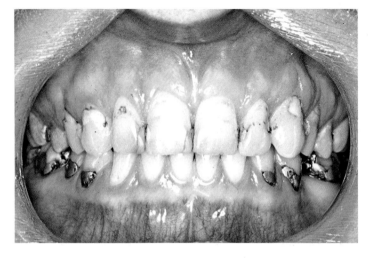

Case 1

Fig. 4-17 Case before treatment with porcelain veneer crowns. Female age 28 years.

Fig. 4-18a and b   (a) Completed case. 13, 12, 11 and 21, 22, 23 Aluminous porcelain crowns. (b) All posterior crowns and bridges metal-ceramic VMK 68.

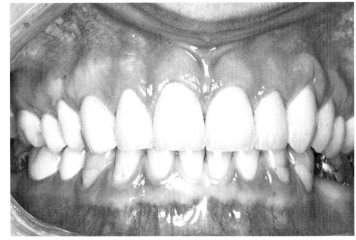

Figure 4-18a

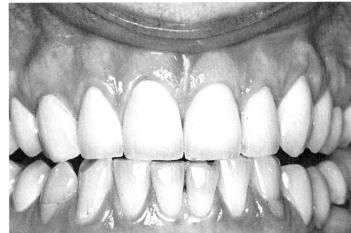

Figure 4-18b

Fig. 4-19a and b   (a) Completed case in centric occlusion. (b) Completed case in right lateral excursion.

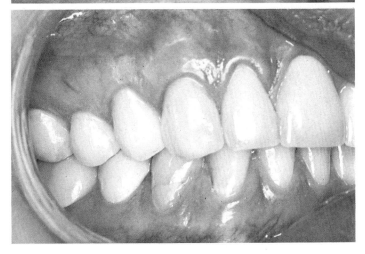

Figure 4-19a

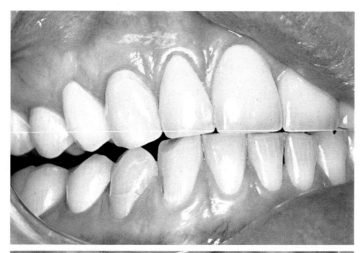

Figure 4-19 b
Case 2

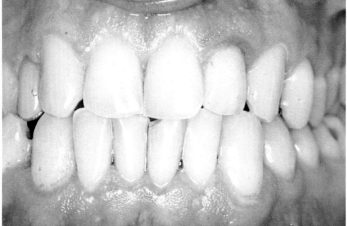

Fig. 4-20 Severe gingival response under a crowned "peg-top" 22 lateral incisor.

Case 3

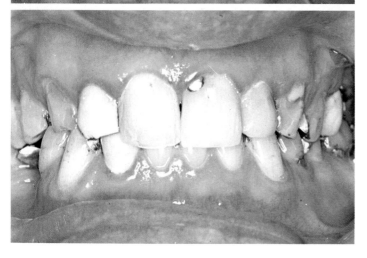

Fig. 4-21 a and b Case before treatment showing heavy wear of 43 and 33 and collapse of posterior occlusion. Male age 55 years. (a) Anterior view; (b) Palatal view.

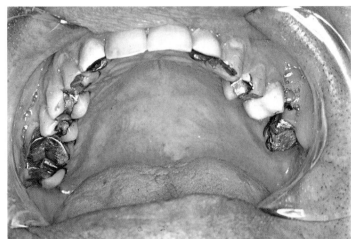

Figure 4-21 b

Fig. 4-22 a and b Completed case with all teeth restored in porcelain (original 4-21). (a) Anterior view; (b) Palatal view.

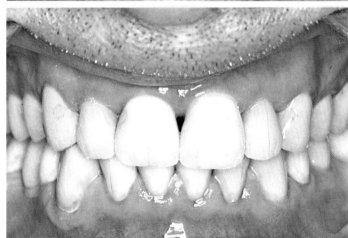

Figure 4-22 a

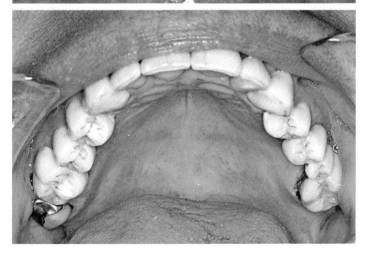

Figure 4-22 b

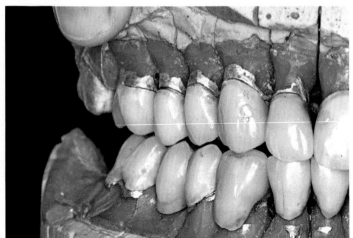

Fig. 4-23a to c (a) Right lateral completed case on articulator (b) completed case in centric relation (c) in right lateral excursion showing an ideal cuspid disclusion.

Figure 4-23 a

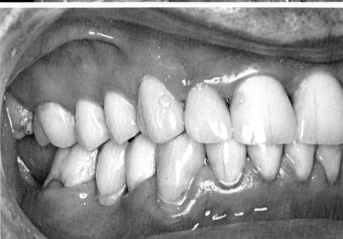

Figure 4-23 b

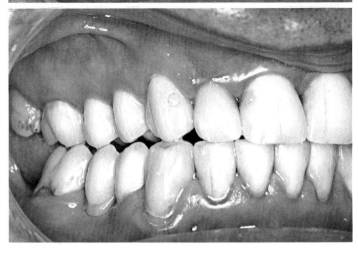

Figure 4-23 c

Fig. 4-24 a to c (a) Left lateral completed case on articulator (b) completed case in centric relation (c) in left lateral excursion.

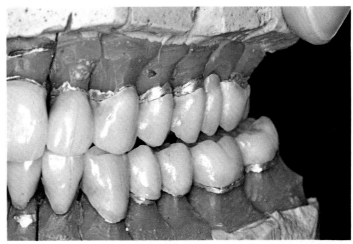

Figure 4-24 a

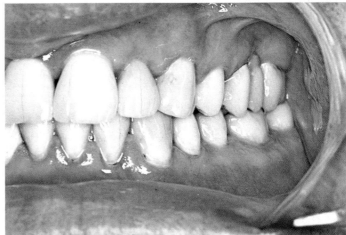

Figure 4-24 b

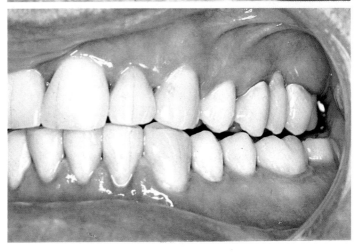

Figure 4-24 c

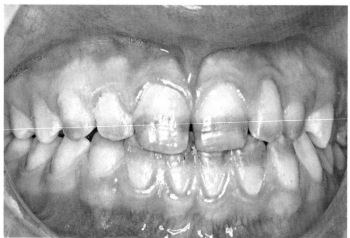

Case 4

Fig. 4-25 Patient aged 13 years showing heavy staining of teeth due to tetracycline administration.

Fig. 4-26 a to c Lower incisor preparations with upper bonded alumina crowns in position.

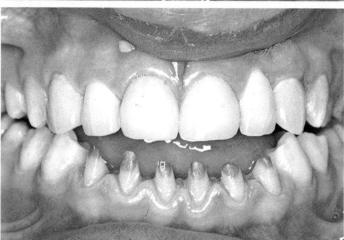

Figure 4-26 a

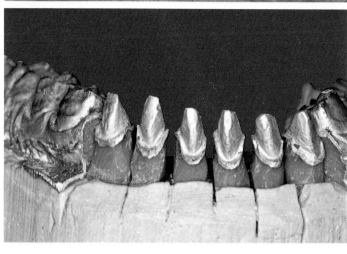

Figure 4-26 b

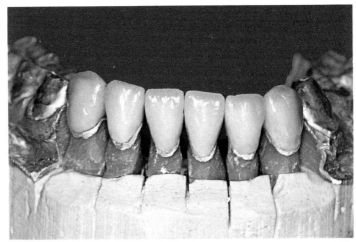

Figure 4-26 c

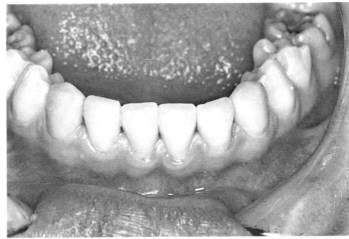

Fig. 4-27 Completed case with 43, 42, 41 and 31, 32, 33 bonded alumina crowns cemented Labial view.

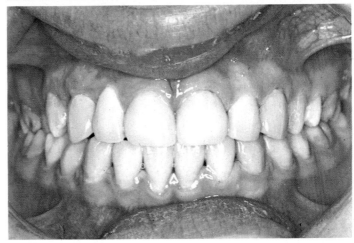

Fig. 4-28 Completed case from Fig. 4-25. Bonded alumina crowns inserted on 13, 12, 11, 21, 22, 23 and 43, 42, 41, 31, 32, 33.

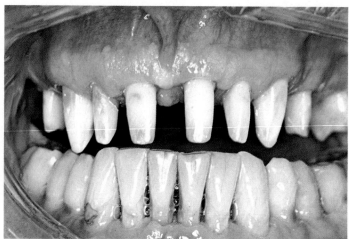

Case 5

Fig. 4-29 a Periodontal splinting. Completed preparations with long chamfer preparations extending up root face.

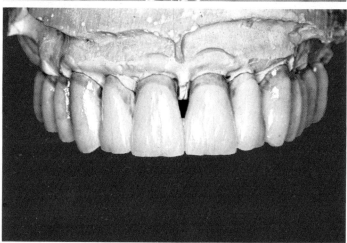

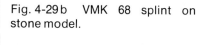
Fig. 4-29 b VMK 68 splint on stone model.

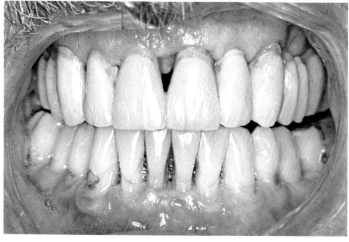

Fig. 4-30 Metal-ceramic splint (VMK 68) cemented to position showing the difficulty in obtaining colour at the thin cervical margins.

The Complete Porcelain Veneer Crown and the Platinum Bonded Alumina Crown

The success of a porcelain veneer crown is dependent upon four main factors:

1. Aesthetics
2. Strength
3. Maintenance of periodontal health and occlusal stability.
4. Preservation of the vitality of the dental pulp.

Aesthetics

In order to achieve optimum aesthetics, sufficient tooth structure must be removed to allow for at least 0.8 mm labial thickness of porcelain. This represents the minimum thickness of porcelain that will provide depth of translucency and avoid the risk of cement linings or opaque layers of porcelain having a marked influence on colour (see Monograph III).

Strength

The strength of a porcelain veneer crown will depend upon the amount of remaining tooth structure which can support the porcelain, the design of the preparation, the mechanical strength of the porcelain and the film thickness and strength of the cement.

Uneven thicknesses of porcelain are inevitable in all porcelain jacket crowns, but preparations which cause sudden changes in thickness of any section of porcelain are by far the least satisfactory. The junction between a thick and thin section is the weakest point and a potential cleavage line can then develop.

Periodontal Health and Occlusion

The maintenance of gingival health will depend upon the contour of the crown, the depth of shoulder in relation to the gingival crevice, the marginal fit and the amount of injury inflicted on the tissues during preparation and impression-taking. The construction and fit of the temporary restoration will also play a significant role in preserving gingival health.

A healthy periodontium is a pre-requisite prior to any porcelain veneer crown work being contemplated. The vital part played by periodontal therapy cannot be over-emphasised. Healthy gingival tissue will resolve many of the clinician's problems during preparation and impression-taking. In addition the aesthetic appeal of the crown to the patient will be enhanced. The correct contour of the crown can only be established by providing the technician with accurate diagnostic study casts. Further methods of ensuring the accuracy of this information, which should also include a prescription for the shade, have been discussed in Monograph III.

Diagnostic study casts are also invaluable aids in assessing the pattern of occlusion. In the case of multiple jacket crowns, the casts may be mounted on an adjustable articulator in order to detect any prematurities or deflective malocclusions. The importance of assessing the pattern of occlusion in vivo should also be emphasised since no articulator can reproduce mandibular movements to the accuracy that is often required. The types of occlusion least favourable to porcelain veneer crowns have been discussed at the beginning of this monograph.

Health of the Pulp

The preservation of the pulp will depend not only on the condition of the existing pulp tissue but also on the relationship of the pulp horns to the tooth surface. Radiographic evidence will

213

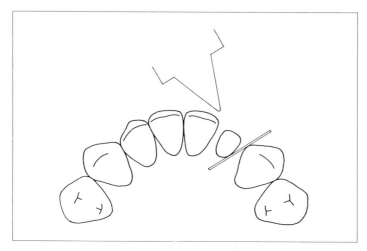

Fig. 4-31 Diagram illustrating a method of taking a radiograph of a porcelain jacket crown preparation to establish cross-sectional anatomy of the dental pulp in a mesio-distal plane.

assist in revealing any marked abnormalities and, in the case of the younger patient, the size of the pulp chamber can also be partially established. It should be noted that radiographs of the pulp will only be taken in one plane and a study of the anatomy of pulp chambers can benefit the student. *Wheeler* (1969) states that when anterior teeth, in young persons, have well-marked developmental lobes, accentuated pulp horns may be expected, especially in the labial portion, as extensions into the three labial lobes. These are always most marked in young teeth and they usually disappear as age advances. A study of the labio- or bucco-lingual section is most important since it is in this direction that the pulp chambers show the greatest number of variations. *Wheeler* has drawn the clinician's attention to the fact that he may be less familiar with the root canal anatomy from the mesial and distal aspects.

Routine radiographs only show the cross-sectional anatomy from the labial and buccal aspects. The outline of the pulp chambers vary little from these aspects, since they tend to conform generally to the crown and root outlines. Because of technical difficulties it is impossible to take radiographs of the teeth in situ showing the cross-sectional anat-

omy mesially or distally. Once tr‚ and distal cuts have been made in the preparation it is possible with some teeth to insert a film between the teeth and obtain a picture (Fig. 4-31), and this is a useful aid where doubt remains in the clinician's mind.

It is clear that the critical areas of injury to the pulp lie in the incisal one-half of the tooth and the labial surface demands the greatest respect. By contrast the cingulum area and lingual fossa of the tooth presents fewer problems and this is an area where removal of tooth structure can provide invaluable reinforcement to a porcelain jacket crown.

Preserving Pulp Vitality

Although vitality tests of the pulp may assist the clinician in assessing the prognosis of the prepared tooth, the author has never placed great reliance on these methods. There is always an element of clinical judgement and good luck in deciding whether a tooth pulp will continue to remain healthy. The clinician can assist nature by avoiding over-healing or drying of the tooth during cutting, and the judicious use of high-speed instruments has been frequently emphasized in the literature.

Morrant (1963) has given an excellent survey of the effect of operative procedures on the pulp, in which he has drawn attention to the many variables encountered both in clinical techniques and their interpretation during histological investigations of the cut tooth. Of considerable importance is the state of the tooth which is being cut. Owing to carious attack, or erosion, attrition etc., there may already be present a degree of sclerosis and secondary dentine formation, which will, to a certain extent, protect the underlying pulp from injury. On the other hand, this sclerosis is most likely to occur in the older tooth which may be less able to react and recover from any damage which does affect the pulp. By contrast, the young pulp may be less protected by reason of its more permeable dentine and yet able to react more vigorously and effect repair rapidly. *Morrant* concluded that in trying to assess the effects of a traumatic stimulus, the clinician cannot afford to hope that any tooth will automatically recover from injury which could have been avoided, and therefore the only possible course is to take every reasonable precaution against damage. In the light of present knowledge it can be categorically stated that an adequate coolant should always be used with higher operating speeds. Prolonged drying of the cut tooth surface may also cause damage to the odontoblasts even when low speeds are used.

The insertion of porcelain veneer crowns for teenage patients has been a hazardous procedure. If sufficient tooth structure is removed to allow construction of a strong porcelain crown, then the pulp may die. If insufficient tooth is removed then the incidence of fracture of porcelain crowns is also high since they are generally too thin. With the introduction of the platinum bonded alumina crown this problem has largely been overcome since very conservative preparations can be made (see Figs. 4-25 to 4-28).

The Devitalised Tooth

Porcelain jacket crowns should not be inserted on devitalised anterior teeth unless the tooth is reinforced with a post and cast gold core. Posterior teeth may be built up with pins and either an amalgam, glass-ionomer cement or composite filling core. A platinum bonded alumina crown may then be inserted on the premolars or a cast metal-ceramic crown on the molars (Figs. 4-32 and 4-33).

Composite filling materials and glass-ionomer cements exhibit low tensile and shear strengths and should not be used to restore missing areas of incisal dentine where lateral stresses can be high. A cast metal core must be used in the anterior post crown preparation. Preservation of the maximum amount of dentine is mandatory in these cases and the crown preparation should involve both metal and dentine if maximum support and retention is to be obtained for the crown and post. Where all the coronal dentine is missing, stabilising pins or boxes in the post hole should be provided and provision made for fitting a gold collar to prevent root fracture.

The Preparation

The Typical Preparation

In order to understand the basic principles involved in preparing teeth for porcelain veneer crowns it is essential to consider the normal or typical preparation. Such a preparation would be suitable for teeth which conform in dimensions to an average anatomical size. *Wheeler* (1969) has suggested dimensions for carving teeth of average anatomical size and these dimensions correspond very closely to those given by *G. V. Black* in his study of human teeth. Typical measurements of an incisor tooth with average anatomical dimensions would be as follows:

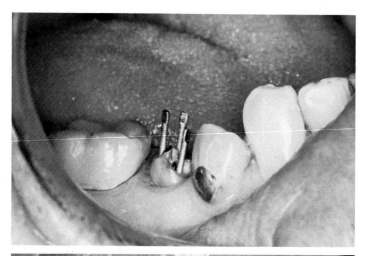

Fig. 4-32 TMS pins inserted into tooth prior to build-up of core.

Fig. 4-33 a and b Composite filling core built up on tooth and re-prepared for a veneer crown (a). Completed bonded alumina crown cemented (b).

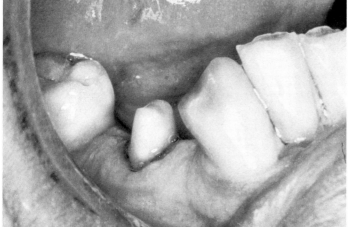

Figure 4-33 a

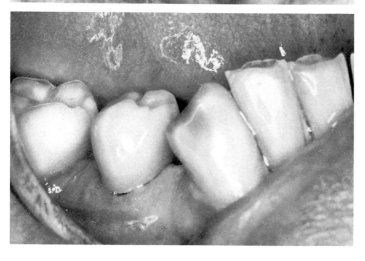

Figure 4-33 b

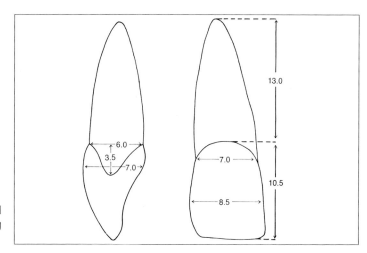

Fig. 4-34 Diagram of a typical maxillary central incisor showing dimensions in millimetres.

Maxillary Central Incisor (Dimension in Millimetres)

Cervico-incisal length of crown	Length of root	Mesio-distal diameter of crown	Mesio-distal diameter of crown at cervix
10.5	13.0	8.5	7.0
Labio lingual diameter of crown	Labio lingual diameter at cervix	Curvature cervical line – mesial	Curvature cervical line – distal
7.0	6.0	3.5	2.5

If the clinician masters the outline form for preparing such a tooth (Fig. 4-34) then he is better equipped to deal with the atypical preparation. Teeth that deviate from the anatomical average will be classified as atypical, but this is purely for convenience when discussing porcelain veneer crown preparations, since normality is hard to define. In addition, teeth that have suffered from carious attack, erosion or traumatic injury, sufficient to destroy their original outline form, will be classified as a-typical.

Design Factors

Application to the Metal-Ceramic Crown

Although the following principles on the design of porcelain crown preparations refer to the complete porcelain or platinum bonded alumina veneer crown, the design factors still apply to the metal-ceramic crown. With the exception of the shoulder finishing lines, the principles outlined in relation to length of preparation and retention form are important to the success of a metal-ceramic crown. Although these crowns will still function on less than adequate preparations, failures, particularly in bridge-work, can be traced to faulty design of the preparation. In addition, if the design of the coping in a metal-ceramic crown follows the principles outlined for the veneer crown preparation, greater support will be given to the porcelain veneer.

The Porcelain Veneer Crown

The preparation for the complete porcelain or platinum bonded alumina veneer crown should follow principles well known in engineering. *Heywood* (1952) has stated that the theoretical aim in designing structures is to achieve a uniform stress at all points in the surface of the part, with the magnitude of the surface stress such that failure is just avoided in service. The practical designing of structures involves safety factors in which the stress required for failure is rarely reached. Unfortunately these aims are difficult to achieve with dental porcelain but adherence to these principles can improve the resistance of the crown to fracture. Occlusal stresses will only be resisted if the finished preparation has planes at right angles to these stresses (*Tylman,* 1970) and that there is sufficient bulk of tooth structure left to protect the dental pulp.

The thickness of the dental porcelain is also of considerable importance and *Craig* et al. (1967) have drawn attention to the importance of the dimensions of a restoration. The improvement of engineering designs is accomplished by two methods:

1. The cross-sectional area of low-stressed regions may be reduced.
2. The cross-sectional areas in the region of maximum stress may be increased, allowing the concentration of stress to be distributed over a greater area. The latter statement is of considerable importance when the atypical preparation is discussed.

In addition to these engineering design recommendations, the tooth preparation must also provide maximum retention for the porcelain veneer crown. Dominating all these requirements is the aesthetic factor, since patients are demanding higher standards in appearance.

Porcelain is weak in thin sections (0.5 mm) and obtaining natural enamel effects and depth of translucency is not possible practically within these tolerances. The author considers that 0.8 to 1.0 mm of porcelain is the minimum thickness with which to develop optimum aesthetics on the labial surface. For this reason the tooth preparation should ideally provide this thickness and it must be regarded as the minimum requirement. In the case of the typical maxillary central incisor this thickness can safely be increased to 1.3 mm except at the shoulder.

If we accept the aesthetic demands for a minimum thickness of 0.8 to 1 mm of porcelain it is now possible to consider the occlusal stresses which are most frequently applied to a porcelain veneer crown and relate these stresses to optimum design factors. For purposes of illustration the preparations will closely conform to that described by *Conod* (1937) and *Tylman* (1970). This preparation, in general, is a miniature reproduction of the tooth that is being restored and has clearly defined shoulders.

Stress Analysis and Design Factors

Cervical area and shoulder requirements – Maxillary central incisor

The stresses most likely to develop in a typical maxillary central incisor porcelain veneer crown during protrusive movements of the mandibular incisors are illustrated in Fig. 4-35. Two points of rotation occur at A and B and tensile stresses

Fig. 4-35 Diagram illustrating the two points of rotation at A and B which will occur in a porcelain veneer crown during incisive movements of the mandible. Crescent-shaped fractures may occur on the lingual or labial surfaces if the cement lute is broken under stress. In the case of the metal-ceramic crown, if the metal coping is too thin the same type of fracture can occur in the veneer porcelain.

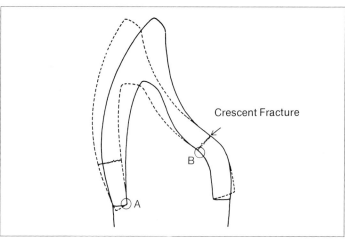

Fig. 4-36 Diagram illustrating the reflection of cement through a porcelain jacket crown made to a chisel edge.

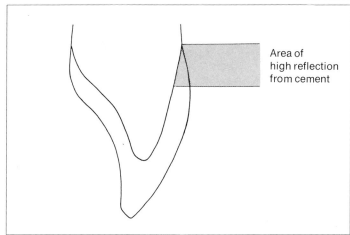

will develop in these areas. *Walton* and *Leven* (1955) have demonstrated that significant tensile strain will also occur on the outer portion of the lingual surface. *Lehman* and *Hampson* (1962) have calculated the stresses near the gingival margin to be as high as 42.3 N/mm^2 (6,042 p.s.i.). It is therefore not surprising that this is an area of frequent breakage, and crescent-shaped fractures may develop on either the labial or lingual surfaces (Fig. 4-35). These areas of high stress must be reinforced with the maximum thickness of porcelain permitted by the biological requirements of the tooth preparation. On these grounds alone the shoulderless preparation is the weakest type of construction that can be used. In addition the fit of porcelain to a chisel edge is extremely variable and the cervical aesthetics of the crown can be marred by cement or opaque layers reflecting through the thin layer of enamel veneer (Fig. 4-36).

Design Factor – Cervical and Shoulder area – Maxillary central incisor

A porcelain veneer crown preparation should have clearly-defined shoulders

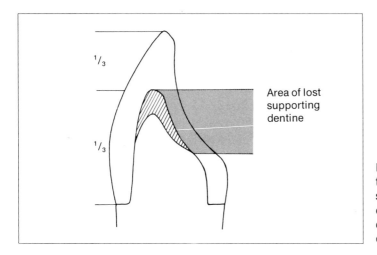

Area of lost
supporting
dentine

Fig. 4-37 Diagram illustrating the area of lost tooth support in a short preparation. The reduction of supporting dentine will increase the stress on the mid-cervical area of porcelain.

which allow the maximum thickness of porcelain at the cervical one-third commensurate with the biological requirements of tooth preservation and dentinal support of the crown. This cervical portion should be regarded as a reinforcing ring which forms a near-parallel encirclement of the tooth.

The lingual and labial surfaces and length of preparation – Maxillary central incisor

The length of the preparation will have a considerable influence on the stresses developing both on the lingual and labial surfaces. A short preparation as opposed to the typical preparation is illustrated in Fig. 4-37. When force is applied in a linguo-labial direction, the labial shoulder porcelain will be placed under considerable compression, *Walton* and *Leven* (1955). Tension will develop higher up on the lingual and labial surfaces of the crown and will only be resisted by the surface-bearing area of dentine that is present, and by the thickness of the porcelain itself. These factors are of much greater importance than the actual shoulder in resisting occlusal stresses. The shoulder is mainly useful in increasing the thickness

of porcelain and obtaining good colour values. It is unlikely that it can support the jacket against a "wedging effect" since the underlying cement at the shoulder and incisal areas would give way first. Porcelain jacket crowns rely on maximum surface area support combined with adequate porcelain thickness if high stresses are to be resisted. The short preparation decreases this area and will also increase the amount of leverage on the porcelain crown. If the distance between the tip of the preparation and the incisal edge of the crown is increased, the effective leverage at the labial and lingual surfaces of the porcelain are increased, as illustrated by *Conod* (Fig. 4-38). It is also important that the incisal edge of the porcelain veneer crown should correspond, in a vertical direction, with the incisal edge of the preparation.

If the latter edge is moved labially, the leverage forces are increased when a linguo-labial thrust is incurred (Fig. 4-39). Fortunately these incisal edges will generally be in alignment providing the clinician maintains an even depth of preparation on both labial and lingual. In addition the technician has the responsibility of ensuring that the porcelain tooth contour corresponds with the original tooth, and on no account must the incisal edge be moved lingually, since the

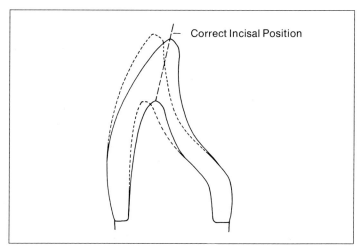

Fig. 4-38 (After *Conod, H.*) Diagram illustrating effect of force on triangle abc. A lingual thrust at point **a** will force angle **b** gingivally. Point **c** will rise incisally and pull away from lingual shoulder. Labial pressure will be resisted by surface area of preparation (see Fig. 4-37). In lower series of drawings, if the lever **a-o** is lengthened (dotted line) No. 1. The forces at **b** and **c** are increased No. 2. If **a-o** is shortened, the forces at **b** and **c** are reduced No. 3. If the line **b-o** is shortened by moving **o** towards **b,** the force is increased at **b** and traction is lessened at **c** No. 4. Incisal edge of tooth preparation **o** should be as close as possible to incisal edge **a**, in order to reduce stresses on the crown.

Fig. 4-39 Over-reduction of the lingual surface will cause the incisal edge of the veneer crown preparation to be moved labially in relation to the tooth's original incisal edge. In protrusive movements of the mandible the leverage forces on the labial porcelain shoulder will be increased. Incorrect position of the incisal edge of the preparation is indicated by the dotted line.

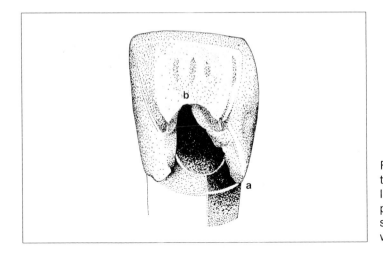

Fig. 4-40 Diagram illustrating a typical fracture caused by sharp lingual line angles. The fracture path travels along the thinnest section a-b until it finds another weak cleavage plane.

incisal guidance will be changed. In the case of the metal-ceramic crown, although fracture may not occur, severe damage could be inflicted on the periodontium.

Uneven or thin sections of porcelain are also highly detrimental to the strength of the lingual surface. If the lingual surface porcelain is too thin (<0.8 mm) and the line angles between the axial walls and the lingual surface are sharp, then a plane of weakness is created. *Pettrow* (1961) has clearly demonstrated the stresses that develop at sharp line angles, and these areas are one of the most common causes of weakness. *Pettrow* considered that rupture usually pursues the cleavage line and travels along the thinnest section in a source of least resistance to another weak part (Fig. 4-40). Rounding of internal line or point angles produces more even bulk in the crown and eliminates specific lines of cleavage. The design of the coping in a metal-ceramic crown should also follow these principles.

The necessity for even and adequate thickness of porcelain on both labial and lingual surfaces of the jacket crown is well established. It is also demonstrably clear that the preparation must have sufficient length to resist occlusal stresses. The main question that must now be answered is "What length does the preparation require?"

Dominating this discussion must be the aesthetic requirements of the porcelain jacket crown. If the preparation is too long there will be inadequate thickness of labio-incisal porcelain for aesthetics and the lingual porcelain may be weakened by a cleavage line. A long preparation will inevitably introduce the risk of light travelling through the thin labial porcelain being reflected back by cement or opaque core porcelains. This will result in the disappearance of much of the enamel translucency at the incisal one-third of the crown. If the aesthetic requirements of the typical maxillary central incisor are considered, the preparation must allow at least 1 mm thickness of porcelain at the blend line between enamel and dentine porcelain if depth of translucency is to be achieved. A typical maxillary central incisor will only provide this thickness at a depth of approximately 3.0−3.5 mm from the incisal edge and this will correspond to a length of preparation of two-thirds the height of the original anatomical crown (Fig. 4-41). Although some clinicians state that three-quarters of the anatomical crown is desirable, the author considers that this length provides too delicate a balance between aesthetics and strength. A preparation cut to the two-thirds level of the anatomical

Fig. 4-41 Diagram illustrating the correct length of the preparation in relation to the aesthetic appeal of a porcelain veneer crown. Preparation finished at a level of $^3/_4$ the height of the original anatomical crown may leave too sharp an incisal edge on the preparation to give adequate support to the porcelain and reduce the area required for enamel porcelain. Extending the coping in a metal-ceramic crown to this level will create considerable problems in achieving good aesthetics in the veneer porcelain.

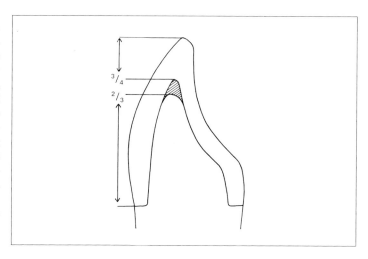

crown will also provide adequate thickness of dentine at the incisal level. This thickness will be approximately 1.5 mm and provide a wider area of stress distribution which can assist in reducing the "wedging actions" that occurs in complete porcelain crowns. The importance of the angle of the incisal bevel has probably been over-emphasized since the more essential requirement is that the junction between the lingual plate of the porcelain jacket and the incisal porcelain should not create a potential cleavage line. If the bevel is inclined lingually at an angle of approximately 45° to a vertical line drawn through the centre of the tooth then a reasonable compromise has been made. The rounding of the incisal line and point angles of the preparation will make a far greater contribution to strength and decrease stress concentration at the critical linguo-incisal edge of the preparation. The length of the metal-ceramic coping should also be not more than two thirds the length of the anatomical crown and should give the same support to the porcelain as if it was a jacket crown preparation.

Design factor – Lingual and labial surfaces – Maxillary central incisor

The preparation should be two-thirds the length of the anatomical crown of the tooth. The labial and lingual surfaces should be covered with an even thickness of porcelain of not less than 1 mm. The junction between these surfaces and the axial walls and incisal edge should be rounded and provide no sudden changes in thickness of porcelain. The incisal edge of the preparation should be in alignment with the incisal edge of the porcelain jacket, and with that of the original tooth.

Approximal axial walls – Maxillary central incisor

The occlusal stresses which may develop in a typical maxillary central incisor during incisal edge-to-edge contact are illustrated in Fig. 4-42. Providing the dentine or cement support does not give way, the fit surface of the porcelain will not be placed under sufficient tension to cause fracture. If the stresses are too great or there is insufficient supporting dentine then fracture

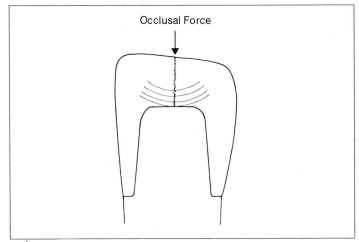

Occlusal Force

Fig. 4-42 Diagram illustrating the stresses that may occur in a typical maxillary incisor porcelain jacket crown during incisal edge-to-edge contact.

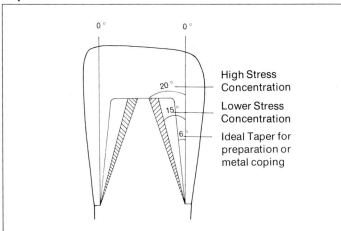

0°   0°

20° — High Stress Concentration

15° — Lower Stress Concentration

6° — Ideal Taper for preparation or metal coping

Fig. 4-43 Diagram illustrating the sharp increase in stress concentration when convergence angles increase from 15° to 20°.

Fig. 4-44 Diagram illustrating the various stress concentration factors with different types of shoulder geometry in descending order of magnitude.

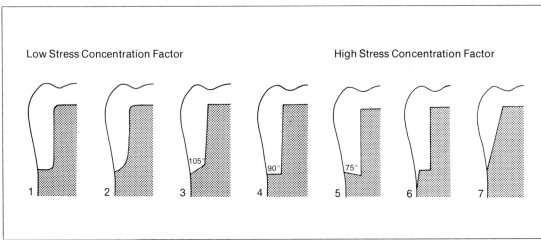

Low Stress Concentration Factor   High Stress Concentration Factor

1   2   3   105°   4   90°   5   75°   6   7

may occur as shown in Fig. 4-42. Commonest faults in preparation which may induce longitudinal fracture are leaving the top of the preparation too thin labio-lingually and reducing the width of the preparation by over-tapering the axial walls. *El-Ebrashi* et al. (1969) have demonstrated that sloping of these axial walls can increase the stress concentration factor. The optimum convergence angle was between 2.5° and 6.5°. They found that the stress concentration factor increased slightly from 0° to 15°, and increased sharply at 20° (Fig. 4-43). The mesial and distal walls of a jacket crown preparation should therefore be nearly parallel and a taper of 5° to 10° will assure minimum stress concentration in the approximal areas. The width of the approximal shoulders should be less than the labial or lingual shoulders, since the bulk of porcelain in the approximal spaces is always greater than the labial or lingual surfaces due to the tooth flaring out to the contact areas. A typical maxillary central incisor should not require shoulders much greater than 0.5 mm wide at the mesial and distal and 0.8 mm wide at the labial and lingual.

Application to the Metal-Ceramic Crown

The convergence angle and its relation to stress concentration applies equally to the design of a metal coping for porcelain bonding. Many metal-ceramic crowns fracture because the porcelain is unsupported in a vertical direction. Occlusal loading on a 20° tapered coping will be vastly greater than where the porcelain is supported by a 6° taper angle. Attempts to save gold by reducing the width of a metal coping in broken-down teeth are doomed to failure.

Design factor – Approximal Axial Walls – Maxillary central incisor

The preparation should have maximum width and near parallelism (5° to 10°) of

the mesial and distal axial walls. The approximal shoulders should only be 0.5 mm wide to provide this width.

Shoulder geometry

El-Ebrashi et al. (1969) have investigated the stresses developing at the approximal margins of dental restorations and analysed the degrees of stress occurring with various types of shoulder geometry. Although these studies were carried out on occluso-mesial restorations, the results are pertinent to any discussion on the shoulder geometry of porcelain veneer crowns. Seven types of shoulder preparation were analyed and it was found that when the approximal shoulders were loaded occlusally (vertically) on the same approximal marginal ridge, the stresses at the shoulder were compressive in nature. The various types of shoulder preparation are illustrated in Fig. 4-44 and these are arranged in order of their stress concentration.

Definitions

Shoulder angle is defined as the angle formed between the axial wall and the line of the shoulder. Thus, a flat shoulder subtends an angle of 90° with a vertical axial wall.
The angle of bevel α is taken as the angle formes by the created bevel surface with the surface which has been bevelled i.e. when there is no bevel $\alpha = 0$.

Model 1   represents a flat shoulder with rounded internal line angles (no sharp angle between the axial wall and gingival floor).

Model 2   represents the deep chamfer.

Model 3   represents a minus 15 degree angulation to a 90° shoulder. Angle at axial wall 105°.

225

Model 4   represents a flat shoulder (axial wall is at 90° to the gingival floor).

Model 5   represents a plus 15 degree angulation to a 90° shoulder. Angle at axial wall 75°.

Model 6   is the same as Model 4 except for an extended bevel at the cervical margin.

Model 7   represents the chisel edge margin (shoulderless).

The optimum type of shoulder preparation recommended in these studies is Model 1. The shoulder is very slightly rounded at the angle between the axial wall and the gingival floor, with a sharp line angle at the external cervical margin. The author supports these views and always avoids forming any sharp line or point angles on all the internal surfaces of a veneer crown preparation. Sharp line angles will be of even greater significance in increasing stress concentration in a brittle material such as dental porcelain. The brittleness of this material will not permit the clinician to take many liberties.

It should be noted that when the taper of the axial wall is increased to 15° in a jacket crown preparation, it has been thought necessary to increase the angulation of the shoulder to +15°. This would then ensure a 90° angle at the gingival floor. It is safer to increase this angle, Model 3, rather than decrease it, Model 5. If an acute angle is created the stress concentration will increase. This finding contradicts the recommendations of *Conod* (1937).

The curvature of the mesial and distal cervical line is also most important since it represents approximately the extent of curvature of the periodontal attachment. If the curvature is in excess of the average 2.5 mm to 3.5 mm (see Fig. 3-34) then it will present an atypical situation. Normal cervical line curvatures are unlikely to present a great problem with regard to stress concentration at the shoulder. However when this curvature is excessive there is a tend-

ency for V-shaped approximal notches to be created in the porcelain and stress concentrations will be high. A longitudinal fracture may easily occur with the labial face of the crown splitting off the lingual plate (Fig.4-45). *Derand* (1974) considers that the maximum tensile stresses occur in the approximal region of a porcelain veneer crown.

Design factor – Shoulder geometry

Shoulders should be cut at a 90° angle to the axial walls of the preparation but never at an acute angle. All internal line angles should be slightly rounded. The height of the approximal shoulders should conform to the cervical line but a smooth roll should be created labiolingually. Approximal V-shaped notches in the porcelain shoulder must be avoided.

Retention

The retention of all dental restorations is directly related to the parallelism of axial walls and the diameter and length of the tooth. The retention of crowns was analysed as a function of geometric form by *Rosenstiel* (1957) and *Jorgensen* (1955). *Rosenstiel* advocated that a full crown preparation should be designed so that it only had one path of insertion and he showed that multiple paths of insertion reduced the retention form. Geometry and mechanics were used by *Lewis* and *Owen* (1959) to evaluate the degree of convergence of axial walls. They reported that, as the slope of axial walls increases, their length increased and the retentivity decreases. They assumed in their hypothesis that both crown and the tooth were rigid, i.e. the distance between every pair of points remained fixed and that the adjoining sides of the crown and the prepared tooth were frictionless.

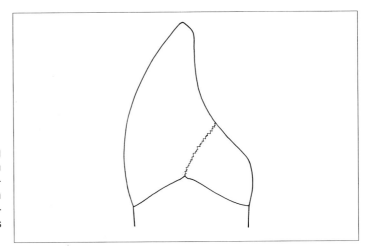

Fig. 4-45 Diagram illustrating the possible line of fracture which may occur from V-shaped approximal notches in a porcelain veneer crown. The highest stresses during function occur at this approximal area (*Derand*, 1974).

In the light of this work and the subsequent results on stress analysis by *Craig, Peyton* and *El-Ebrashi* at the University of Michigan, the recommended convergence angles for axial walls is well defined. Ideally an angle of 5° to 6°, would appear to be the optimum, but taper angles of up to 10° would satisfy both the requirements for minimal stress concentration and maximum retention. In the case of the maxillary central incisor preparation, retention is greatly improved and one path of insertion secured if the cervical area of the labial and lingual surfaces, up to the level of the cingulum, has the same taper or near parallelism as the mesial and distal walls.

Design factor – Retention

The retention of porcelain veneer crowns will be improved by maintaining near parallelism (5° to 10°) of the mesial and distal axial walls, and the cervical one-third or quarter of the labial and lingual surfaces according to the position of the cingulum. This area of near parallelism will ensure that the crown has only one path of insertion.

Cement film thickness

The analysis of stress concentration in porcelain jacket crowns has been carried out by photo-elastic stress studies on simulated models and plastic crowns. In addition, intelligent observation of fracture paths in porcelain crowns by clinicians has compiled a wealth of information over the years. The clinical fit of the porcelain jacket crown has received little attention since the assessment of accuracy in the mouth presents a number of problems. More recently *McLean* and *von Fraunhofer* (1971) have devised a method of assessing the film thickness of cement under dental restorations in vivo. A brief description of the technique has been given on page 187. It was found that the cement film thickness of a well-fitting aluminous porcelain jacket crown compared favourably with other types of dental restorations but there were still definite discrepancies from one area of the fitting surface of the crown to another. *Jorgensen* and *Holst* (1967) have investigated the relationship between the retention of cemented veneer crowns and the crushing strength of cements and concluded that by increasing the crushing strength of the cement there was an almost proportional increase in retention. Variations in the film thickness of cement could also affect the retention and strength of a porcelain crown (see Fig. 4-3).

An evaluation of the strength and physical properties of dental cements is given at the end of this monograph.

The Bonded Alumina Crown and the Complete Porcelain Veneer Crown or Aluminous Porcelain Crown

Recommended dimensions for tooth preparation

Tooth preparation for the platinum bonded alumina crown should not differ from that of the regular or aluminous porcelain veneer crown preparation. Since the bonded alumina crown only requires 0.025 to 0.05 mm thickness of metal, the effect on the total thickness of porcelain veneer is negligible.

The following recommendations for the thickness of porcelain, and design of preparations for full veneer porcelain restorations will therefore cover all types of porcelain crowns with the exception of the cast metal-ceramic crown.

Recommended dimensions for the typical maxillary central incisor preparation

The optimum design factors for a porcelain veneer crown preparation have been evaluated and it is now possible to specify the ideal thickness of porcelain which will make the greatest contribution to the resistance of occlusal stresses in the typical maxillary central incisor.

The longitudinal and horizontal sections of porcelain that should be provided are illustrated in Fig. 4-46. The lingual section of the porcelain

crown is the most important area on which the clinician should concentrate since it is here that the majority of errors occur. In addition, it should again be emphasised that the preparation must have sufficient width and length to support the veneer crown.

Recommended dimensions for the typical maxillary lateral incisor preparation

The dimensions suggested for the typical lateral incisor are illustrated in Fig. 4-47. It will be seen that in this case the thickness of the porcelain is scaled down to conform to the tooth dimensions. The recommended porcelain thickness on the labial and lingual surfaces is 0.8 mm, thus providing sufficient room for the development of aesthetics and strength.

Recommended dimensions for the typical maxillary canine porcelain veneer crown preparation

The same basic principles of preparation design will apply to the maxillary canine as have already been described for the typical maxillary central incisor. However, the author has found that certain modifications to the lingual surface can be made with advantage, and increase both the retention and strength of the canine porcelain veneer crown.

The standard type of maxillary canine porcelain veneer crown preparation will conform to the outline form illustrated in Fig. 4-48. In this case the lingual surface of the preparation will tend to incline rather sharply towards the labial once the cingulum region has been reached, since the anatomy of the canine tooth dictates this path. A canine preparation will therefore tend to be more conical when viewed from the mesial or distal aspects. When the opposing lower canine tooth strikes the lingual surface of an upper canine porcelain veneer crown there is a tendency for the crown

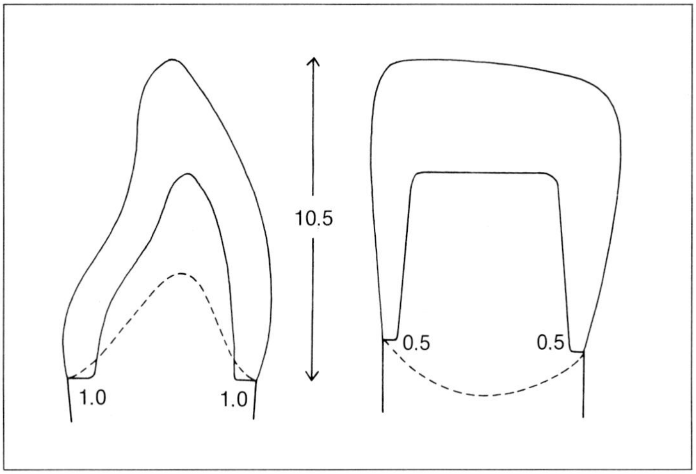

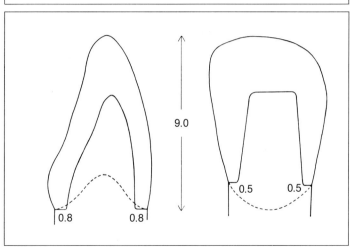

Fig. 4-46 Longitudinal section through the ideal maxillary central incisor crown preparation showing the dimensions of the porcelain crown in millimetres.

Fig. 4-47 Longitudinal section through the ideal maxillary lateral incisor crown preparation showing the dimensions of the porcelain crown in millimetres.

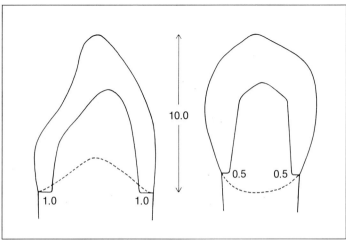

Fig. 4-48 Diagram of a typical maxillary canine jacket crown preparation.

229

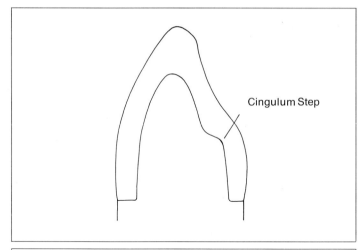

Fig. 4-49 Diagram illustrating the cingulum step prepared in the lingual surface of a maxillary canine. This step permits a greater degree of parallelism between the labial and lingual axial walls. It is most important that all internal point and line angles are slightly rounded to avoid stress concentration.

Cingulum Step

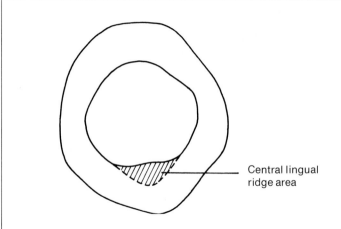

Central lingual ridge area

Fig. 4-50 Horizontal section through a maxillary canine jacket crown preparation showing the importance of creating one lingual surface plane which avoids a plane of weakness if a central lingual ridge is present. The area to be removed is indicated by the dotted line.

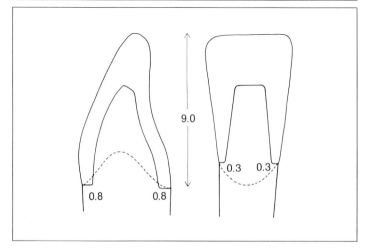

9.0

0.8   0.8

0.3   0.3

Fig. 4-51 Diagram of the recommended porcelain thickness for a mandibular incisor crown.

to slide up this sloping lingual surface and fracture may then occur. If for some reason the mesial and distal axial walls have also been cut at an excessive taper angle (>15°), the whole preparation will become conical. This situation is probably the commonest cause of fracture in the maxillary canines, and frequently these porcelain veneer crowns will have several paths of insertion.

In order to reduce this effect the author creates a cingulum step in the lingual surface of the preparation (Fig. 4-49). This step may be cut with safety since the pulp horns do not generally encroach into this area. The cingulum step permits a greater degree of parallelism to be achieved between the labial and lingual axial walls. If the lingual surface is reinforced with aluminous core porcelain a thick cingulum strut of porcelain is created without causing any thinning of other critical sections. It should be emphasised that the lingual shoulder and axial line angles should be rounded and under no circumstance should the cingulum line angle be sharp.

The lingual surfaces of a maxillary canine tooth may be quite varied even when the anatomical dimensions conform to the average. *Wheeler* (1969) has drawn attention to the large cingulum which may be pointed like a small cusp. In the latter types, definite ridges are found on the lingual surface of the crown below the cingulum and between strongly developed marginal ridges. Very often a well-developed lingual ridge is seen which is confluent with the cusp tip; this extends to a point near the cingulum. There may be shallow concavities between this ridge and the marginal ridges. These mesial and distal lingual fossae create two inclined planes which are often duplicated in the standard maxillary canine porcelain veneer crown preparation. The author avoids this procedure, since by using the cingulum step technique and reducing the lingual ridge so that the entire lingual surface only has one surface plane, the lingual section of porcelain is increased in the critical cleavage path areas (Fig. 4-50).

The curvature at the cervical line of the typical maxillary canine is less than the incisor teeth, varying between 2.5 mm on the mesial and 1.5 mm on the distal (*Wheeler,* 1969). This small curvature can be of great advantage when preparing the approximal axial walls since maximum supporting width may be provided for the porcelain without incurring the risk of creating V-shaped notches.

The principles outlined above are very useful when preparing canine teeth for metal-ceramic crowns. In particular the retention of bridgework can be greatly improved when the tooth preparation is increased in parallelism.

Recommended dimensions for the Typical Mandibular Incisor Preparation

The crown of the mandibular incisor has little more than half the mesio-distal diameter of the maxillary central incisor (*Wheeler,* 1969). However when preparing this tooth for a porcelain veneer crown it is fortunate that the labio-lingual diameter is only 1.0 mm less. Occlusal stresses on the mandibular incisors are greatest in a labio-lingual direction so that it is important to cover the labial and lingual surfaces of the crown with the maximum thickness of porcelain. The recommended porcelain thicknesses for the typical mandibular incisor are illustrated in Fig. 4-51 and attention should be drawn to the width of shoulder (0.8 mm) that can be provided on the labial and lingual surfaces. The approximal shoulders should be as narrow as possible since even a small increase in shoulder dimensions will reduce the mesio-distal supporting width. Conical preparations on the mandibular incisors should be avoided, since the bulk of supporting dentine is severely limited.

In view of the fact that the mandibular incisor is the smallest tooth in the dental arch, metal-ceramic crowns are seldom indicated. If such a restoration is placed, it will invariably be over-contoured and cause a cervical stagnation area.

Gingival health will be more easily maintained by the use of bonded alumina or aluminous porcelain veneer crowns. (Fig. 4-27 platinum bonded alumina crowns.) The author has found that the use of high fusing aluminous core porcelains on the lingual surfaces of the mandibular incisor crown to be of great value in providing extra strength.

Recommended dimensions for the Typical Mandibular Canine Preparation

The mandibular canine crown may be as long or even longer than the maxillary canine so that support for a porcelain veneer crown is good. The mesio-distal diameter is less than the maxillary canine but the labio-lingual diameter is only a fraction of a millimetre less (*Wheeler*, 1969). The shoulder preparation of the mandibular canine must therefore take account of these anatomical variations and approximal shoulders should be considerably narrower than the labial and lingual shoulders. The lingual surface of the mandibular canine is flatter and comparable with the mandibular incisors. The cingulum is smooth and poorly developed and the lingual ridge is not very distinct. Because of these anatomical features the preparation of the lingual surface may conform closely to that of the mandibular incisors and no special precautions are necessary as described for the maxillary canine. The optimum design for a mandibular canine preparation is illustrated in Fig. 4-52.

Stress Analysis of the Posterior Molar Crown

Craig et al. (1967) have investigated the general stress distribution in full crown restorations using a two-dimensional photoelastic stress analysis method. Crowns on tipped molar abutments as well as on normally aligned molars were analysed. The maximum compressive stresses on the interior of crowns was generally found to be on the reduced cusp surface of restorations. Maximum tensile stresses were observed in the central fossa and along the axis of symmetry of the crown, when the crowns were loaded bilaterally to simulate oral conditions.

Stresses were also investigated at the free boundaries of a full molar crown, and tensile stresses were observed at the cervical margin of the restoration with compressive loads of 60.2 kgf (133 pounds) and at a cusp angle of 39 degrees.

Craig and his co-workers concluded that the stress distribution in the crown which they analysed could be made more uniform by the following modification.

1. It is desirable to have multiple point contact when a antagonistic tooth occludes with the abutment crown, to reduce stress concentrations near the central fossa of the restored tooth.
2. Full shoulders on complete crowns are recommended in order to increase the bulk in the critical cervical margin, thus redistributing the tensile stresses developed.
3. Reduced cusps should be rounded on the preparation, to avoid the development of high compressive stresses on the interior surface of the crown, which may induce post-operative pain.
4. Deep developmental grooves carved near the centre of the tooth should be avoided, as they will tend to produce deleterious stress concentrations.

These conclusions are highly important when considering the preparation of posterior teeth for full porcelain coverage. The author considers the use of full shoulders or chamfers on metal-ceramic or complete porcelain veneer crowns to be essential if maximum cervical support for the crown is to be achieved. In addition, the creation of occlusal planes which follow the cusp angles is essential if proper thickness of porcelain is to be obtained. The impor-

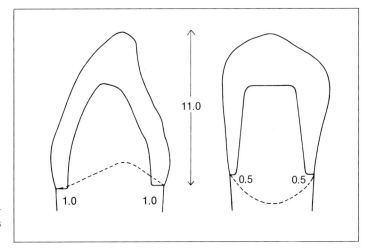

Fig. 4-52 Diagram of the recommended porcelain thickness for a mandibular canine crown.

tance of providing sufficient space for porcelain in the occlusal surface has been emphasised on page 194 (Fig. 4-11).

The Premolar Porcelain Veneer Crown

Although cast metal-ceramic crowns have virtually displaced the porcelain jacket crown in the premolar region, the introduction of the platinum bonded alumina crown will probably reverse this situation (*McLean* et al., 1976). The premolar teeth are difficult to prepare for full porcelain coverage if 1.5 mm of tooth structure has to be removed for a metal-ceramic restoration. The risk of pulpal damage during metal-ceramic crown preparation is therefore greater. If the premolar teeth are not reduced sufficiently to provide room for both metal coping and ceramic then there is a tendency for technicians to over-contour the crown. Gingival stagnation areas will be created and occlusal tables may be increased in surface area.

In the case of the platinum bonded alumina crown the tooth preparation is more conservative. Tooth removal in these cases may conform to regular porcelain jacket crown preparations with the exception that the lingual surface may be reduced even less than in the con-

ventional preparation, since a direct bonded platinum collar may be used (Fig. 3-43g and h).

Recommended dimensions for the Typical Maxillary First Premolar Preparation

The width of the crown of the maxillary first premolar mesio-distally is about 2 mm less at the cervix than its width at the point of its greatest mesio-distal measurement (*Wheeler*, 1969). The average diameter at the cervix is 5 mm and for this reason this tooth is one of the most difficult to prepare for a porcelain veneer crown. Not only may the pulp be endangered by cutting back the mesial and distal axial walls but the area of the occlusal surface may be so reduced that insufficient support will be left for the porcelain. The bucco-lingual section presents fewer problems since the difference between the diameter of the crown and cervix is only 1 mm. The preparation must provide for these differences and there must be a marked change in shoulder thickness from the bucco-lingual to the mesio-distal surfaces. The mesial and distal shoulder should only be reduced by 0.3 mm, sufficient to provide a definite finishing line, whereas the buccal and lingual shoulder can increased to 0.8 mm (Fig. 4-53). The narrow

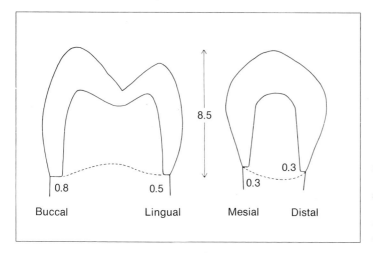

Fig. 4-53 Diagram of the recommended porcelain thickness for a maxillary first premolar preparation. Undercut preparations may easily occur with over-reduction of the approximal shoulders.

mesial and distal shoulders will still provide sufficient cervical thickness of porcelain since the tooth will flare out sharply towards the contact area. The cervico-occlusal length of the crown will generally allow a 1.5mm reduction of the occlusal surface and this will provide the optimum thickness of porcelain which can resist occlusal stresses. Fortunately the curvature at the cervical line in the maxillary first premolar is minimal and provides one of the few useful anatomical features in this tooth for porcelain veneer crown preparation. The maxillary second premolar closely resembles the first premolar, therefore, the preparation of these teeth should be similar to the dimensions suggested in Fig. 4-53.

Recommended dimensions for the Typical Mandibular First Premolar Preparation

The dimensions of the mandibular first premolar closely resemble those for the maxillary first premolar except for a reduction in the bucco-lingual diameters. Their occlusal anatomy is different, but basically both teeth present similar problems in full crown preparation. The mesial and distal shoulders once again present the greatest problem and should be considerab-

ly narrower than the buccal and lingual shoulders.

The suggested dimensions for a porcelain veneer crown are illustrated in Fig. 4-54.

Recommended dimensions for the Typical Mandibular Second Premolar Preparation

The mandibular second premolar, although better developed than the first premolar, resembles the latter fairly closely in dimensions. The bucco-lingual diameter is generally 1 mm greater and this tooth presents fewer problems when preparing these areas. In particular this tooth provides more potential length of preparation on the lingual and, because of its greater bulk, is not so subject to the risk of over-contouring by the ceramic technician. The suggested dimensions for a porcelain veneer crown are illustrated in Fig. 4-55.

The Molar Porcelain Veneer Crown

Since the introduction of metal-ceramic crowns there are few indications for using full veneer porcelain crowns on molar preparations. The cervico-occlusal length of molar crowns varies

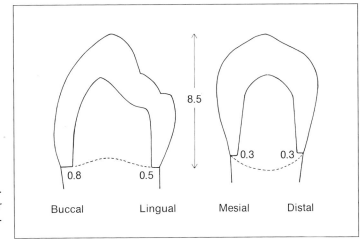

Fig. 4-54 Diagram of the recommended porcelain thickness for a mandibular first premolar preparation.

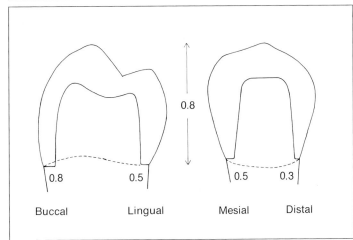

Fig. 4-55 Diagram of the recommended porcelain thickness for a mandibular second premolar preparation.

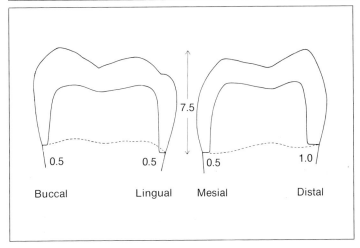

Fig. 4-56 Diagram of the recommended preparation for a mandibular first molar platinum bonded alumina crown. The bonded platinum should cover the full shoulder area and form a thin reinforcing collar (Fig. 3-43g and h).

between 7 mm for the first molars and 7.5 mm for the second molars (*Wheeler,* 1969), and these teeth can present problems with retention of the crowns if 1.5 mm of occlusal porcelain is provided. The strength of regular dental porcelain cannot be considered adequate if it is to withstand the more powerful occlusal forces present in the molar regions. However, if a molar tooth is prepared to receive a metal-ceramic crown, and a narrow lingual shoulder can be provided, then the new bonded alumina crown using 0.05 mm thick platinum foil as a strengthener can be used providing there is a 1 mm occlusal thickness (Fig. 4-56) (*McLean* et al., 1976). In cases where only a lingual chamfer can be provided then the cast metal-ceramic restoration is still preferred. The bonded alumina crown should not be used on molars where there has been gross destruction of tooth. Fracture will occur unless the metal is covered by an even thickness of porcelain. This principle also applies to the cast metal-ceramic crown; but in the latter case the casting can be designed to make up any deficiency in tooth structure.

The Atypical Preparation

Teeth that deviate from the anatomical average or have suffered from carious attack, erosion or traumatic injury, sufficient to destroy the outline form of a typical porcelain veneer crown preparation will be classified as atypical.
Atypical veneer crown preparations may be subdivided into the following categories:

Class 1: Crowns larger than anatomical average.

Class 2: Crowns smaller than anatomical average.

Class 3: Crowns which show marked anatomical deviation from normal.

Class 4: Crowns with loss of enamel and dentine on either the mesial or distal surfaces.

Class 5: Crowns with loss of enamel and dentine on both the mesial and distal surfaces.

Class 6: Crowns with loss of enamel and dentine at the incisal edge, e.g. traumatic injury or abrasion.

Class 7: Crowns with loss of enamel and dentine at the cervical margins.

Class 8: Crowns with generalised loss of surface enamel.

Class 9: Length of clinical crown greater than anatomical crown, i.e. loss of supporting gingival tissue.

The clinician is more frequently presented with an atypical tooth preparation than with a preparation conforming to the anatomical average. Methods of dealing with the atypical preparation are therefore of great importance to the student who is embarking on ceramic restorations. The atypical tooth will frequently present problems with regard to retention form and adequate dentinal support for the porcelain veneer crown. The designer of such a preparation must therefore take particular note of two important design factors, which have previously been discussed:

1. Retention form.
2. Achieving near uniform stress at all points in the surface of the crown.

Both these important design factors are exceedingly difficult to achieve with many atypical preparations since the loss of dentinal support can often be severe. In order to assess this loss it is wise to excavate all caries or fillings prior to commencing the preparation, since only then can the true loss of dentine be determined. A further preparatory step should be to measure the length of the anatomical crown and its width at the cervix, the cingulum, and the incisal third of the tooth. These measurements may be carried out quite rapidly with suitable crown and bridge calipers measuring to 0.1 mm. The anatomical dimensions of the tooth may then be determined and evaluated in relation to the anatomical average. It is of particular importance to note the measurement at the incisal one-third, since inadequate thickness in this area will either involve over-reducing the incisal edge of the preparation or providing inadequate thickness of porcelain for aesthetic purposes.

The recommended procedures for preparing teeth which are atypical in outline form are as follows:

Class 1: Crowns larger than the anatomical average

Teeth that exceed the average anatomical dimensions determined by *G. V. Black* and *Wheeler* (1969) will generally present fewer problems in veneer crown preparation than the typical tooth preparations already described. The design of the oversize preparation should conform to the typical preparation but it is often possible and desirable to increase the cross-sectional area of the porcelain veneer crown. For example, the anterior maxillary incisor may accommodate 1.5 mm of porcelain on the labial and lingual surfaces. Where the labio-lingual diameter of the cervix is 8.0 mm, the shoulder width may slightly exceed 1 mm. However, it should be noted that it is more desirable to increase the labial and lingual thickness of the porcelain rather than the mesial or distal shoulder width since maximum support should be given to the larger tooth where occlusal stresses can be more severe. At the same time the extra lingual thickness of porcelain will rein-

force the critical biting area. It is obvious that crowns larger than the anatomical average are the easiest to fit with metal-ceramic crowns.

Class 2: Crowns smaller than anatomical average

The undersize tooth crown will obviously present more problems in preparation than the typical crown. In the case of maxillary teeth, providing the tooth to be prepared has not suffered any loss of enamel and dentine, or exhibits any marked anatomical deviations such as a concave lingual surface with no cingulum or marked labio-lingual curvature of the incisal one-third, the fitting of porcelain veneer crowns can be very successful. Fortunately, few maxillary teeth will have a labio-lingual diameter at the cervix of less than 6.0 mm when compared with an average or typical tooth. The provision of a minimal thickness of 0.8 mm of porcelain is therefore possible without causing damage to the dental pulp. The shoulder thickness for these teeth should never exceed 0.8 mm on the labial and lingual surfaces and the mesial and distal shoulders should be restricted to under 0.5 mm in width. Maxillary teeth which present the greatest problems would be the undersize lateral incisor or premolar. In particular the latter may have a mesio-distal diameter at the cervix of only 4 mm, and minimal shoulder widths are obligatory. The smallest maxillary tooth is the lateral incisor and this tooth may also only have a mesio-distal diameter at the cervix of 4 mm. However, providing these teeth have normal anatomy, they can still be prepared for the construction of a porcelain veneer crown. These crowns may also be reinforced at the cervical one-third by using bonded platinum foil (*McLean* et al., 1976; *McLean,* 1977) (Fig. 4-57).

The mandibular incisors present greater problems since they are the smallest teeth in the mouth. The mesio-distal diameter at the cervix of some mandibular incisors may be as little as 2.5 mm but fortuantely the labio-lingual diame-

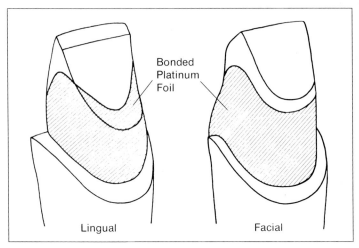

Fig. 4-57 Recommended design for a crown smaller than ana-tomical average. For very thin teeth or adolescent teeth, maxi-mum light transmission may be obtained by removing the bonded platinum foil from the incisal one-third. The cervical reinforcement is of particular value in the lower incisors.

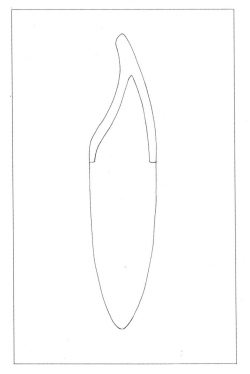

Fig. 4-58 Diagram illustrating the difficulty of provid-ing adequate dentine support to the porcelain veneer crown in very thin teeth. If a 0.8 mm thickness of porcelain is to be achieved then the preparation might become knife-edge or need to be shortened.

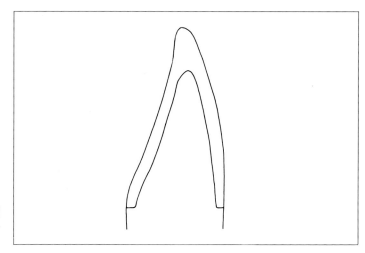

Fig. 4-59 Diagram of a typical preparation for a conical maxillary lateral incisor.

ter is much greater and is rarely less than 5.5 mm. Even in these cases, providing the tooth has a minimum labio-lingual thickness of 2.5 mm at the incisal one-third, it is still possible to fit a porcelain veneer crown, particularly of the bonded alumina type. The approximal shoulders of a small mandibular incisor preparation need only consist of a finishing line of sufficient thickness to provide a butt joint for the porcelain, since the approximal porcelain rapidly thickens as it flares out to the contact areas (Fig. 4-26a, b, c; Fig. 4-27 and 4-28).

In general, it may be stated that a markedly undersize tooth crown is not suitable for preparation for metal-ceramic crowns. Inevitably the ceramic technician will be forced to over-contour these restorations and a cervical stagnation area will be created with subsequent gingival irritation.

Class 3: Crowns which show marked anatomical deviations form normal

The most serious deviations from normal anatomy in a tooth crown which are likely to affect a porcelain veneer crown preparation would be the absence of a cingulum or very thin teeth. In the latter case this can present aesthetic problems in the incisal one-third of the preparation. If the labio-lingual diameter at the incisal third is less than 3 mm in the maxillary incisor teeth or 2.5 mm in the mandibular incisors, then it is almost impossible to provide 0.8 mm thickness of labial and lingual porcelain without thinning the incisal edge of the preparation to a dangerous level (Fig. 4-58). When this situation occurs it may be necessary to reduce the length of the preparation below the recommended two-thirds level, and in these cases it is essential to use platinum bonded alumina crowns. Incisor teeth with no cingulum are generally conical in shape. As previously described in this monograph, such a shape is highly deleterious to the retention of porcelain veneer crowns. When a conical maxillary incisor tooth is prepared for a veneer crown, the clinician will generally prepare the lingual surface so that it follows the original outline form of the tooth. This will inevitably produce a conical preparation when the tooth is viewed from the mesial or distal aspects (Fig. 4-59). The author prefers to use the cingulum step technique advocated for the typical maxillary canine preparation in these cases (see page 230). By creating an artifical cingulum, the labial and lingual axial walls can be brought nearer to parallelism, and the

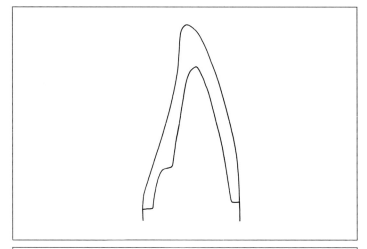

Fig. 4-60 Diagram of the modified cingulum step technique for improving retention in the conical maxillary incisor tooth preparation.

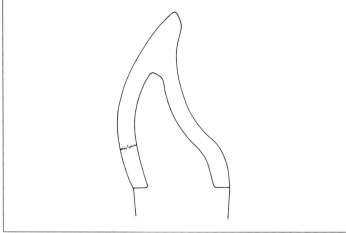

Fig. 4-61 Diagram illustrating the stress concentration and possible area of fracture in a preparation on a thin maxillary lateral incisor tooth with marked labial curvature.

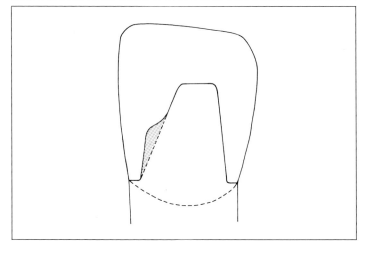

Fig. 4-62 Diagram illustrating incorrect removal of tooth structure when mesial dentine has been lost due to caries. Incorrect area of tooth removed is indicated by dotted line. Correct preparation is shown in shaded area.

porcelain veneer crown will only have one path of insertion (Fig. 4-60). In addition, by using aluminous core porcelain in this area the artificial cingulum strut will reinforce the crown against mid-line fracture. When the occlusion is unfavourable a bonded platinum foil lining will provide even further reinforcement and the author makes extensive use of this material in such cases (*McLean* et al., 1976).

If an absence of cingulum is combined with a very thin tooth labio-lingually, the problems become even more severe and unless such teeth are reinforced with bonded platinum foil, failure is almost certain to occur. The insertion of metal-ceramic crowns on these teeth is almost impossible unless the health of the pulp is endangered, and in addition the aesthetic problems can be formidable.

Other aesthetic and functional problems can also be encountered when the tooth crown curves sharply from labial to lingual at the incisal one-third. Frequently this anatomical abnormality is often associated with very thin teeth, and in these cases, although a porcelain jacket crown may be fitted, the patient should be warned that fracture of these crowns is very common. Generally the crown will develop a crescent-shaped fracture on the labial surface, since the curvature of the preparation on the labial is almost ideal for localising stress concentration at the cervical one-third (Fig. 4-61). Excessive curvature of the cervical line can also be associated with these teeth and may often involve the reduction of the crest of the line if a V-shaped notch is to be avoided. This will automatically reduce the width of the preparation which again is undesirable and at the same time there is great danger of damage to the epithelial attachment. In these cases the platinum bonded alumina crown will give better service.

Anatomical abnormalities in the posterior teeth generally present fewer problems, since it is often possible to correct the abnormality in the crown construction. By contrast the labial surface contour of the incisor teeth exercises a stern discipline on the ceramic technician, al-lowing him little leeway for error, if gingival health is to be preserved.

Class 4: Crowns with loss of enamel and dentine on either the mesial or distal surfaces

Approximal caries will normally commence at the contact areas of incisor teeth and the destruction of the enamel and dentine will generally occur at the middle third of the tooth. Unless the cavity is very large, the dentine will be intact at the cervical one-third of the tooth. The normal method of preparing these teeth for porcelain coverage is to excavate the remaining caries and to fill in the cavity with a lining cement. When a filling is already present, this too is removed and replaced with a lining cement. The tooth is then prepared for a typical veneer crown preparation, leaving the cement to fill in the area of dentine loss. During preparation there is a tendency for the clinician to taper the affected mesial or distal axial wall in order to provide a neat outline form. This may result in the loss of dentine at the cervical one-third and the mesial and distal axial walls will no longer be nearly parallel (Fig. 4-62). The retention form of the veneer crown will therefore be diminished.

It is preferable in these cases to replace the area destroyed by caries or fillings by aluminous core porcelain. Any undercut areas in the cavity are filled in with cement and the area of lost tooth tissue is rounded off at the incisal one-third of the preparation. This area will form a lingual step in the tooth and can provide an anti-rotational locking device when the aluminous core porcelain seats into the step (Fig. 4-63). At the same time maximum cervical support is provided for the crown by maintaining near parallelism of the preparation at the cervical one-third.

This principle should be applied to all atypical crown preparations involving destruction of dentine on either the mesial or distal surfaces of the tooth. Replacement of lost tooth tissue by

241

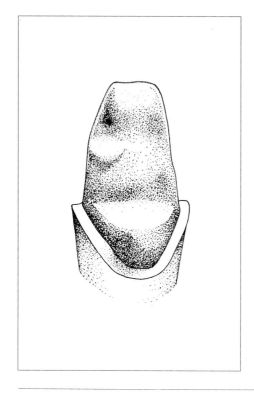

Fig. 4-63 Diagram illustrating a lingual step cut in a maxillary central incisor where the dentine has been destroyed by caries. This step provides an anti-rotational locking device when the crowns is fitted.

the stronger aluminous core porcelains combined with bonded platinum foil is preferable to filling in these areas with a weaker cement lining. As described earlier, if the tooth destruction is very severe, then a cast metal-ceramic crown should be used.

Class 5:
Crowns with loss of enamel and dentine on both the mesial and distal surfaces

Similar procedures should be adopted for a crown preparation, where loss of dentine occurs on both approximal surfaces. The mesial and distal cavities should be shaped to create twin lingual steps and the aluminous core porcelain can then fit accurately into these areas. If the remaining incisal spike of dentine is very

thin, and the removal of this spike would leave a preparation of only half the length of the clinicial crown, then other types of restoration should be used. For example, a high alumina backing sheet combined with bonded platinum foil could be used to reinforce the incisal dentine of the preparation or alternatively a metal-ceramic crown is indicated (Fig. 4-64). Other techniques which have been tried involve the use of thin gold copings to build up the destroyed dentine. However, the author has found this type of restoration to be rather difficult to construct due to lack of space. If the destruction of the dentine has involved over half the length of the anatomical crown it may be possible to provide retention by using TMS pins and core. However, where occlusal leverage is high, such a technique may fail due to shearing of the pins. In cases where tooth destruction is severe, devitalisation and insertion of a post crown is often preferred.

242

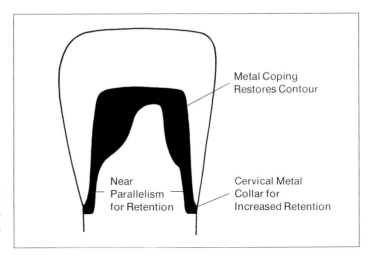

Fig. 4-64 Metal coping used to restore outline of preparation and give horizontal support to the porcelain. Metal collars may be used to improve retention.

Labels in figure: Metal Coping Restores Contour; Near Parallelism for Retention; Cervical Metal Collar for Increased Retention

Class 6: Crown with loss of enamel and dentine at the incisal edge

Loss of enamel and dentine at the incisal edges of tooth crowns is generally caused by abrasion or traumatic injury. Depending upon the amount of tissue loss, the restoration of these teeth with porcelain jacket crowns is often possible. It must be emphasised that if a deflective malocclusion exists and is causing the wearing down of anterior teeth, then this occlusion must be corrected prior to restoring these anterior teeth (see page 194). Porcelain jacket crowns inserted in such cases are otherwise doomed to failure. When the incisal edges of teeth are broken through traumatic injury, the clinician must assess the amount of supporting tooth structure left in relation to retention form and support for the crown. If two-thirds of the tooth crown remains intact then a typical veneer crown preparation can be easily prepared. It is in the marginal cases, where up to one-half of the original anatomical crown is destroyed, that shrewd clinical judgement is so necessary. Not only is it essential to study the pattern of occlusion but it is also vital that the inclination of the teeth be assessed. Proclination of the maxillary incisors is an unfavourable situation for the short jacket crown preparation, since the porcelain crown is easily dislodged during protrusive movements of the mandible.

Occasionally it is possible to construct a gold coping or small pinlay to extend the coronal portion of the preparation, but the greatest care must be exercised in the placement of the pins in relation to the dental pulp.

In cases of doubt, it is often better to insert a metal-ceramic crown on teeth where half the anatomical crown is missing. The added strength and retention of the gold casting will provide a more durable restoration, even though the aesthetic appeal of the crown may be reduced (Fig. 4-65).

Class 7: Crowns with loss of enamel and dentine at the cervical margins

The restoration of teeth with Class V cavities caused by caries or erosion does not present any great problem providing the cavity depth does not extend so far as to undermine the dentinal support of the preparation. The area of missing dentine may be filled in with cement prior to cutting the preparation, and standard procedures may be adopted for cutting the tooth. However, teeth may sometimes be so undermined by a deep labial cervical notch that

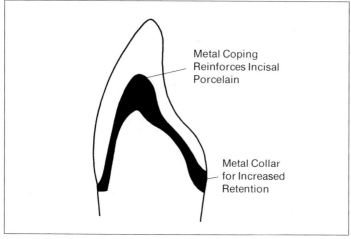

Metal Coping
Reinforces Incisal
Porcelain

Metal Collar
for Increased
Retention

Fig. 4-65 Metal coping restoring missing area of incisal dentine and giving support to the enamel porcelain.

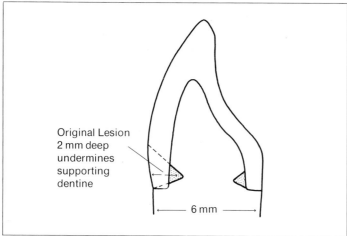

Original Lesion
2 mm deep
undermines
supporting
dentine

6 mm

Fig. 4-66 If cervical caries or erosion has undermined the tooth by more than 1 mm, the tooth preparation may be too weak to support a crown even when reinforcing gold collars are used.

the reduction of the lingual surface will only leave a thin supporting wall of dentine. It is therefore advisable to measure the labio-lingual diameter at the base of the notch prior to attempting any operative work. In most maxillary incisor teeth this notch should only encroach by up to 1 mm into the base of the preparation, if the dentine is to be left in a reasonably sound condition after a typical veneer crown preparation (Fig. 4-66).

In cases where cervical caries extends around the entire circumference of the tooth, considerable problems may arise. Firstly, it will be impossible to create a preparation with sufficient width to support a veneer crown due to heavy reduction of the mesial and distal shoulders, and secondly, the completed preparation may be so small that it could easily break off during function. It is sometimes possible to widen the preparation by inserting a thin gold coping, but this would still not solve the problem of strength. The strength of the dentine beneath these preparations is often low, since secondary dentine formation may have embrittled the stump area. In cases where cervical caries has encroached beyond 1.5 mm on the labial and lingual surfaces and 1 mm on the mesial and distal surfaces of maxillary incisors, it is often safer to devitalise the tooth and insert a post crown.

Class 8: Crowns with generalised loss of surface enamel

Incisor teeth which have suffered generalised loss of surface enamel can be some of the most difficult teeth to restore with porcelain veneer crowns. In cases where only a single tooth requires restoration, the problem becomes even more acute, since the clinician is restricted in both labial and lingual contour. These teeth may be so thin that it is impossible to reduce the surfaces by even 0.8 mm, if the dental pulp is not to be endangered. In these cases it is often impossible to restore a mandibular incisor without resorting to devitalisation. The maxillary incisors may not present such a problem but in the author's experience, it is far better to prepare all the incisor teeth, or at least the central incisors, for full porcelain coverage if good aesthetics are to be achieved. In this way it is possible to restore the original labial contour of the teeth by increasing the labial porcelain thickness. This small increase in cross-sectional area will not cause gingival irritation, providing the cervical area of the tooth is not over-contoured. When preparing these teeth it is important to reduce the lingual surface first since occlusal clearance must take first priority. A reversal of this procedure may leave such a thin lingual plate of porcelain that fracture is inevitable. Metal-ceramic crowns are seldom indicated in these cases.

Class 9:
Length of clinical crown greater than the anatomical crown

Recession of gingival tissue will expose the root surface and cervical line of the tooth crown. In order to cover this exposed surface and obtain an aesthetic result, the veneer crown preparation must be extended beyond the cervical line. If the approximal curvature at the cervical line is greater than normal, considerable problems in preparation will occur. The mesial and distal axial walls will require cutting back further than a typical preparation since the root diameter below the cervical line decreases as it moves apically. It is sometimes possible to deepen the labial shoulder by cutting into the root surface and then increasing the height of the approximal shoulders by maintaining their level above the gingiva. This will increase the width of the preparation but may also create a V-shaped notch in the approximal walls of the porcelain jacket crown. In order to cover the exposed labial root surface with porcelain the clinician must exercise careful judgement in deciding how deep the labial and lingual shoulders should be in relation to the approximal shoulders. The typical maxillary central incisor will have a curvature of cervical line at the mesial of 3.5 mm and this will be slightly less on the distal. In these cases it is sometimes possible to allow the labial shoulder to encroach by up to 1.0 mm into the root surface and still avoid the creation of V-shaped notches in the porcelain. However, when more than 1 mm of root surface is exposed, the deepening of the shoulder is not always practical since the diameter of the root at this level is often so narrow that the finished preparation would have insufficient width and dentinal support. In addition the pulp could also be exposed.

This situation can, to some extent, be predicted by using recording calipers to determine the difference in diameter between the anatomical crown cervix and the clinical crown diameter at the gingiva (see Fig. 4-73a). A difference of more than 0.5 mm in the average maxillary incisor tooth can be of great significance since differences of 1.0 mm would almost certainly involve removing so much dentine that the jacket crown would be without dentinal support and

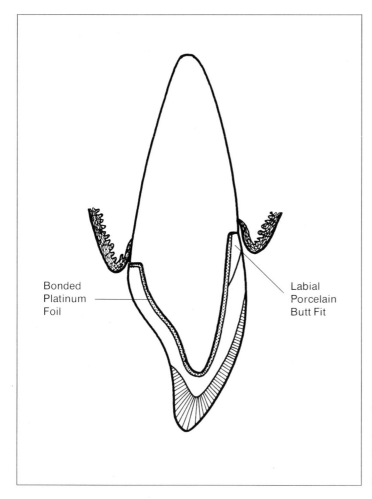

Bonded
Platinum
Foil

Labial
Porcelain
Butt Fit

Fig. 4-67 Platinum bonded alumina crown made with extended
labio-cervical shoulder, to prevent the labial margin from being
placed supra-gingival. Bonded
foil will prevent a crescent-
shaped fracture, as shown in the
clinical case illustrated in Figure
3-43 h and j.

the pulp endangered. In these cases it is far better to approach the preparation conservatively
and finish the porcelain jacket crown shoulder
at the anatomical crown's cervix. The patient
should be forewarned that the aesthetics of the
restoration will be less pleasing in order to
preserve the health of the tooth. If an existing
filling is already present in the labial root surface it may be advisable to prepare the tooth
with a deep chamfer at the shoulder and insert
a metal-ceramic crown with gold coller. Alternatively the platinum bonded alumina crown
can also be made to a restricted shoulder

width (Fig. 4-67) and be more pleasing aesthetically. (See clinical case in Fig. 3-43 h and j.)

Crown-Root ratio

Providing the length of a porcelain veneer
crown does not exceed the original length of the
anatomical tooth crown the typical preparation
will present no problem with regard to the alveolar bony support of the crown. Where bone
loss is extensive and the root is short, i.e. less
than 1:1 crown-root ratio, the mobility of the

tooth may increase the risk of fracture of a porcelain jacket crown. A stable occlusion will enable the operator to adjust the occlusal surface of the porcelain to a high degree of accuracy. Mobile teeth may often cause small discrepancies in occlusal registration and "high spots" can be easily left on the porcelain crown's surface. These high spots will inevitably act as stress concentrators from which microcracks can propagate. The degree of mobility of teeth is therefore often more important than the crown-root ratio since premature contacts on mobile teeth may cause severe damage to the periodontium if the porcelain remains intact, particulary where metal-ceramic crowns are fitted.

It will be noted that in the case of the anterior atypical preparation that the use of metal-ceramic crowns is limited and alternative systems should be used if the periodontium is to be preserved and a high standard of aesthetics maintained.

Summary of the requirements of the Atypical Preparation

1. Optimum retention form may be provided for the atypical preparation by preserving the maximum amount of dentine at the cervical one-third of the preparation. This area should be prepared so that near parallelism is obtained on both the approximal, lingual and labial axial walls, thereby ensuring that the crown only has one path of insertion.
2. Additional retention form and strength may be given to the porcelain veneer crown by providing an artificial cingulum step in cases where the tooth preparation would tend to be conical. This cingulum step will lessen the degree of taper of the lingual surface and bring it nearer to parallelism with the labial surface.
3. Approximal areas of missing tooth structure should not be entirely restored with cement but should be prepared to form small lingual steps in the preparation. These steps must be slightly rounded at all line or point angles and provide an anti-rotational locking mechanism for the porcelain veneer crown. It is recommended that high fusing aluminous core porcelain is used to restore these areas, thereby providing greater strength than a conventional cement lining. Alternatively the missing area can be built up with a cast metal coping when a metal-ceramic crown is fitted.
4. Additional anchorage for the porcelain veneer crown may be provided by constructing thin gold copings or pinlays which will restore the missing areas of incisal dentine. The use of accessory gold anchorage in porcelain veneer crown work is limited by the amount of space available, and should only be used as a last resort if a strong and aesthetic result is to be obtained. The metal-ceramic crown or platinum bonded alumina crown will often provide more suitable alternatives. The use of pins with a composite resin core is not satisfactory on front teeth due to the risk of shearing of the pins or micro-leakage at the resin tooth interface due to the low modulus of elasticity and low shear strength of the composite fillings.

The factors affecting the treatment planning for porcelain veneer crown preparation have been previously discussed on pages 213 and 215.

A healthy periodontium and dental pulp are prerequisites. The clinician must then assess his proposed design of preparation for the tooth in relation to the following anatomical features:

1. The relationship of the anatomical tooth crown to the gingiva.
2. The amount of remaining tooth structure left to support the crown.
3. The crown-root ratio and remaining bony support for the crown.

4. The occlusal pattern and any deviation from normal in the tooth anatomy.
5. Relationship of the tooth pulp to the crown surfaces.

A clinical and radiographic examination should be made to assess any pathological changes or abnormalities in the tooth and its supporting structures. Diagnostic study casts will also aid the clinician in his planning. The tooth dimensions should also be determined with crown and bridge calipers and the tightness of the approximal contact areas and occlusal contacts assessed with thin plastic shims.

occlusion but they lack the texture of human enamel, as described in Monograph III. The use of an Epimine resin (Espe Scutan*) will produce more life-like detail of the surface characteristics of a tooth. This resin may be injected into an alginate or silicone impression of the teeth, and due to its very low shrinkage, will reproduce the surface anatomy of the teeth to a high degree of accuracy. In order to reduce the cost of preparing these dies, the "Scutan" resin is only injected into the tooth to be prepared and its adjoining neighbours or the contralateral tooth. Old burs or small pieces of roughened wire may be embedded in the resin and provide a key for securing it in the stone cast which is subsequently poured into the full mouth impression. The fine reproduction obtained with the Scutan resin will enable the ceramic technician to copy the original tooth anatomy in great detail and this can often eliminate a try-in of the finished porcelain crown at the high bisque stage.

The Typical Maxillary Central Incisor Preparation

Complete Porcelain or Platinum Bonded Veneer Crown Operative Procedures

Registration of surface characterisations of tooth

Before any operative work is started it is essential to furnish the ceramic technician with details of the surface anatomy of the tooth to be prepared. Alginate or elastomeric impressions of the complete arch should have been taken at the time of treatment planning and these diagnostic stone casts would normally be used by the technician to duplicate the tooth anatomy during the porcelain crown construction. Stone casts can be very satisfactory for studying

Shade Determination

A detailed procedure for determining the shade of the tooth to be reproduced has been given in Monograph III. The reader is advised to study this in depth before commencing any operative procedures.

Elimination of gingival trauma

The design of the preparation should have already been determined during the planning stage and an estimate of the required thicknesses of porcelain made. Efficient cutting of a tooth for placement of a porcelain veneer crown depends upon definite but restricted cutting action. The sequence of these cutting

* ESPE, Seefeld, West Germany.

operations should be clearly determined by the operator if he is to exercise maximum control over his operative procedures. The protection of the dental pulp and gingival tissue must be paramount in his mind and every effort should be made to leave the gingival tissue intact after the preparation. The term "bloodless cutting" has been used to describe this desirable goal and graphically depicts the alternative state in which the gingiva may be left.

The gingival crevice in a healthy tooth will vary in depth between 1.5 to 3 mm. If a shoulder preparation is carried to the maximum depth of the crevice, the epithelial attachment is almost certain to be damaged and no matter how accurately the crown fits the tooth, a violent intrusion into the crevice will have been made. This often results in the development of a chronic marginal gingivitis which can only be relieved by removal of bone and alteration of the gingival line and contour. Microscopic examination of the margins of porcelain crowns has revealed that no crown can fit within an accuracy of much less than 20 microns (*McLean,* and *von Fraunhofer,* 1970). This discrepancy will not be easily tolerated by gingival tissue and the deeper the shoulder extends into the gingiva the greater the risk of plaque accumulation. Extension of crowns under the gingiva to depths of over 1 mm has been taught in the past in order to avoid subsequent "gum shrinkage". However, in the light of modern periodontal thinking, such extension is more likely to cause detachment of the epithelial attachment and gingival inflammation, and hasten the process of tissue loss.

a major problem. A healthy periodontium will be maintained for many years and the gingival tissue will remain static (Fig. 4-68a and b). By contrast, a crown that extends too closely to the epithelial attachment, even though it is accurate in fit, may often produce an inflammatory response from the tissue (Fig. 4-69).

Additional advantages may be gained by avoiding deep intrusion into the gingival crevice. Impression-taking is made easier since there is much less chance of the tissue folding in over the shoulder preparation, and the fitting of temporary crowns can be made with less trauma.

It should be a basic rule that porcelain veneer crown shoulders should only extend subgingivally by 1.0 to 1.5 mm on the buccal and labial surfaces and where possible be placed at the level of the mesial, distal and lingual surfaces. The latter recommendation should be qualified where additional retention of the crown must be provided or where weakened enamel margins might be left. The student should be advised that he may enter the gingival crevice but not trespass upon its hospitality.

Depth of Shoulder

If a porcelain veneer crown shoulder only enters the gingival crevice to a maximum depth of 1.0 to 1.5 mm, or not more than half the depth of the crevice, then gingival recession will not become

The Preparation

Theoretical Considerations

The introduction of high-speed cutting has greatly facilitated the rapid removal of dental enamel. However, the speed of this cutting action demands efficient control by the operator, if accurate preparations are to be obtained. The sequence of enamel removal in a veneer crown preparation must be very definite and planned with great care. Over-cutting of a preparation can never be corrected and this would apply particularly to the incisal and approximal areas of the tooth. Once these areas are over-reduced, support for the porcelain veneer crown will be diminished very rapidly.

Removal of an even layer of enamel from a tooth surface may be made by approaching the preparation either from the cervical area of the tooth or from the incisal edge. Alternatively a combination of these two approaches may be made.

Cervical approach

Tylman (1970) advocates a combined incisal and cervical approach in which he starts by reducing the incisal edge by 1.5 to 2 mm and then cuts the approximal surfaces with a safe-sided diamond disc. Removal of the labial and lingual enamel is then commenced by cutting a narrow groove from the mesial to distal approximal cuts; this groove is cut parallel to the gingival curvature of the soft tissue and is placed level with the crest of the gingiva. A small knife-edged stone is recommended for this operation. Once these cervical depth cuts have been made the remaining labial and lingual enamel is removed by successive grooving and stripping of the enamel with knife-edged diamond discs and chisels.

Fraser (1969) has described an elegant technique for reducing the enamel via the cervical approach, and designed special diamond instruments for this operation. His method resembles that described by *Tylman* but deviates in one important aspect. *Fraser* advocated the reduction of the lingual surface before any labial enamel is removed since, quite rightly, he wished to concentrate on the most critical area of tooth preparation first. Inadequate removal of lingual enamel often occurs if the labial reduction has been too severe.

Both *Tylman* and *Fraser* recommended that the shoulder should be extended sub-gingivally as the final operation in their preparation. This may sometimes involve further reduction of the axial walls of the preparation since, as the shoulder extends sub-gingivally, the tooth diameter may decrease. If the axial walls are not further reduced, the shoulder could be too narrow or disappear completely (Fig. 4-70). This situation is made even worse when the shoulder has to be extended beyond the cervical line in cases of gingival recession.

In order to avoid further cutting of the axial walls after the completion of the shoulder, the author prefers to use an incisal approach to cutting a porcelain veneer crown preparation. This technique establishes shoulder depth at an early stage in the preparation. This method combined with cutting one half of the tooth at a time so that the other half acts as a depth guide as advocated by *Johnston* et al. (1967) provides a very simple method for the beginner.

Fig. 4-68 a and b (a) Four maxillary incisor complete porcelain veneer crowns (Vitadur) which only entered the gingival crevice to half its depth shown five years later. (b) Diagram showing ideal placement of a veneer crown shoulder in relation to the gingival crevice. Shoulder preparation indicated by dotted line.

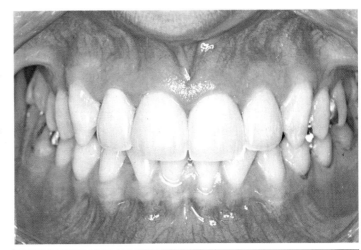

Figure 4-68 a

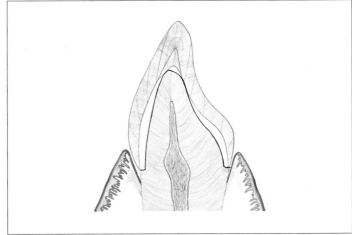

Figure 4-68 b

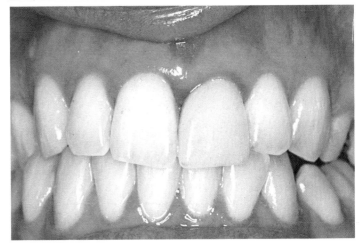

Fig. 4-69 Photograph of a central incisor crown on 21 which has been extended too near the epithelial attachment. Patient suffers from a permanent chronic gingivitis.

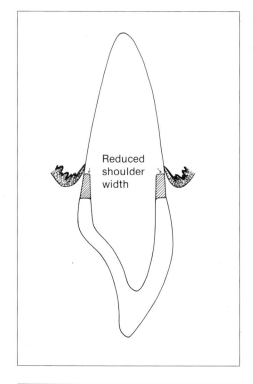

Reduced
shoulder
width

Fig. 4-70   Diagram illustrating the effect of deepening the crown shoulder after completion of the preparation. If the root diameter is decreasing as the cut is made then the shoulder width could be inadequate.

Preparation for the Porcelain Veneer Crown using the Incisal Approach

The basic steps described below will also apply to the preparation of teeth for metal-ceramic crowns

Measurements required for establishing the design of preparation

1. Measure the labio-lingual diameter of the tooth at the cervix, the cingulum and incisal one-third (Fig.4-73a).

Design factor: These measurements will determine the amount of tooth structure that can be removed on the labial and lingual surfaces for optimum aesthetics without causing damage to the dental pulp or leaving a knife-edged incisal preparation.

2. Measure the length and width of the clinical crown.

Design factor: The ultimate dentine support for the porcelain veneer crown will depend upon these measurements. The preparation must have adequate width and length. (See page 228 and the optimum dimensions for porcelain veneer crowns.)

3. Mark the centre-line of the tooth by slightly scoring the enamel with a knife-edged diamond stone (Fig. 4-73b).

Design factor: The centre-line of the tooth will act as a guide when the labial and lingual depth cuts are made in the enamel.

Design factor: This level should be the proposed length of the preparation but may require modification if the measurement of the labio-lingual section is less than 3 mm for the maxillary central incisor (see page 228).

The stages in preparations are as follows:

1. Labial and lingual depth cuts made from the incisal to gingival margin. These cuts should enter the labial gingival crevice by 1.0 mm and be level with the gingiva on the lingual.

2. Reduction of half the lingual surface. The other half is reduced at the second stage of the preparation. Removal of the lingual surface enamel should be level with the lingual depth cut, i.e. at the same level as the gingiva. The lingual shoulder may be prepared at the same time.

3. Reduction of the labial surface, one half at a time. Removal of the labial surface enamel should not extend sub-gingivally but the midline sub-gingival depth cut will still control the amount and depth of enamel removed, and allow final shoulder preparation to be carried out without further reduction of the labial surface.

4. Reduction of the mesial axial wall and creation of a shoulder at level of gingiva.

5. Creation of labial sub-gingival shoulder.

6. Removal of other half of tooth using same procedure as above and relating the cutting process to the prepared half of the tooth.

7. Reduction of incisal edge.

8. Construction of epimine resin temporary crown to determine correct thickness for the porcelain restoration.

9. Refinement of shoulders and rounding of all line angles and point angles except those at the external cervical margins.

Operative technique

The cutting of a porcelain veneer crown preparation should employ both high and low speed instrumentation. High speed cutting (>100,000 r.p.m.) should be employed for gross removal of enamel and low speed cutting (<40,000 r.p.m.) for the refinement of shoulders and rounding of line and point angles. A copious supply of water is required during all cutting procedures in order to avoid over-heating the tooth, or causing aspiration of odontoblasts by excessive dehydration.

Instrumentation

Every operator will develop his own system of instrumentation and the following recommendations are only intended as a guide and largely reflect the personal preferences of the author.

High speed cutting

Recommended handpieces (Fig. 4-71):
Adem 350 – ball-bearing turbine*
Kavo Super-torque turbine handpiece**
with Vario-air coupling

Advantages:

1. When running at top speed, there is no alteration of speed of the bur or diamond resulting from slight variations in cutting pressure.

2. Increased torque allows the use of large diamonds, up to 5 millimetres or more in diameter.

3. Improved visibility of bur tip.

* Micro Turbines Ltd., Blackpool, England.
** Kavo – 7950 Biberach/Riss, West Germany.

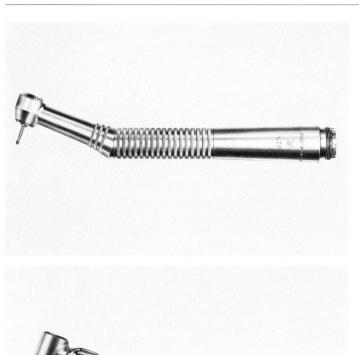

Fig. 4-71   Kavo Super-torque turbine handpiece and Vario-air coupling.

Fig. 4-72a and b Ash electric motor with Kavo handpiece for slow speed cutting.

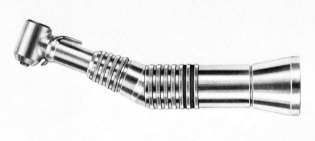

Figure 4-72a

Figure 4-72b

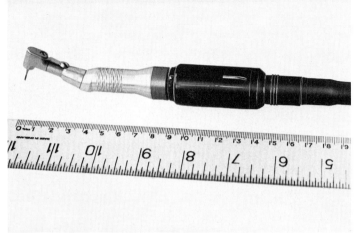

Courtesy of Kavo Dental Manufacturing

Courtesy of AD. International Ltd.

Vario-air coupling (Kavo Super-torque)

The coupling comprises a precision air-flow control valve attached to the rear end of the Super-torque handpiece. Speed alteration is effected very simply by twisting the black sleeve which locates into one of the three speed settings. There is no need for the dentist to alter his grasp of the handpiece in his right hand, even with the handpiece head still held in the patient's mouth, the speed change sleeve being easily rotated by the forefinger and thumb of his left hand. The higher the speed setting the more a red indicator strip is exposed, so that it is obvious at a glance not only at which speed the handpiece is set, but also which way the sleeve should be rotated to select a different speed.

Basic speed settings of the Super-torque/Vario-air assembly are:

Setting	r.p.m.	Appropriate speed and torque for cutting or grinding of:
Top speed	325,000	Enamel
Medium speed	230,000	Dentine
Low speed	160,000	Carious dentine and fine finishing

Low-speed cutting

Recommended handpieces:
Kavo intra contra angle 23 (Fig. 4-72a)
Micro-Mega intra contra angle 120 E
Motors – ADEM electric (Fig. 4-72b)
Siemens Sirona

The Kavo or Micro-Mega handpiece used in an electric motor provides the ideal instruments for fine finishing of line and point angles. Both these handpieces use friction grip burs which ensure even and smooth cutting. It should be noted that the Kavo Super-torque handpiece set at LOW SPEED may also be used for the finishing of the preparation.

Labial and Lingual Depth Cuts

The purpose of a depth cut is to control the amount of enamel removed from the tooth surface. A depth cut therefore assists the clinician in developing restricted but efficient cutting. Depth cuts are usually made in the enamel with small knife-edged diamond stones as described by *Tylman* (1970). The author prefers to use tapered cylindrical diamond stones and to restrict the depth cuts in the enamel to the midline of the tooth. This centre line cut may then be easily continued into approximal areas of the tooth if one half of the tooth has been left intact as a depth guide.

A small tapered cylindrical diamond stone measuring 1.5 mm at the shank and tapering to 1 mm at the tip (HiDi 554 or 555)* is used at high speed to deepen the score mark in the mid-line of the labial enamel (Fig. 4-73). The tip of the stone may then be directed sub-gingivally to a depth of 1.0 mm to establish the shoulder. This depth cut should then extend from the shoulder to the incisal edge of the tooth (Fig. 4-74). In the typical maxillary central incisor tooth the shoulder should be 0.8 to 1 mm wide and the reduction of labial enamel in the groove may be as much as 1.3 mm. Controlling the depth of this cut may be done by viewing the diamond stone laterally and making sure that it is just visible above the level of the labial enamel. The final refinement of the depth cuts should preferably be made at low speed using the Kavo Super-torque/Vario air handpiece or Adem electric motor with geared handpiece. Never use a latch type bur due to the danger of eccentricity, and damage to the gingiva.

The labial depth cut should now establish the exact amount of labial enamel that will require

* A.D. International Ltd. London. W.I.

255

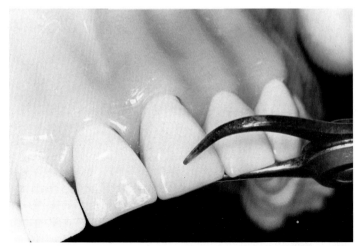

Fig. 4-73 a to c   (a) Measuring labio-lingual diameter at incisal one-third with recording calipers. (b) Marking centre line of tooth. (c) Labial depth cut extended 0.5 mm sub-gingivally.

Figure 4-73 a

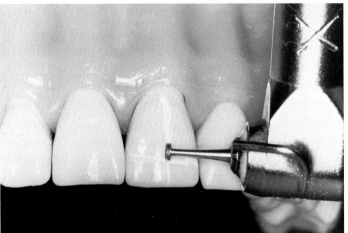

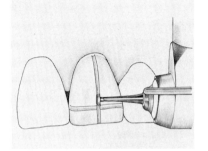

Figure 4-73 b

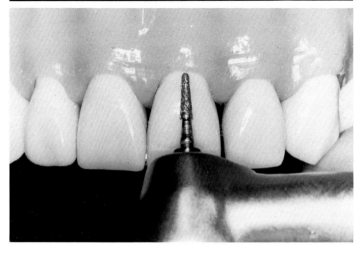

Figure 4-73 c

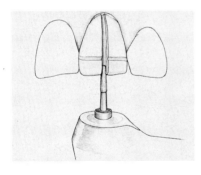

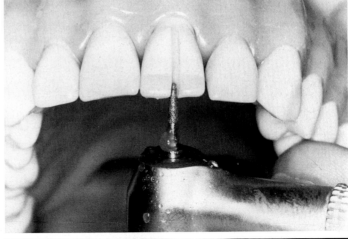

Fig. 4-74 Completed labial depth cut extending along centre line score mark and through the incisal enamel at two-thirds the height of the anatomical crown.

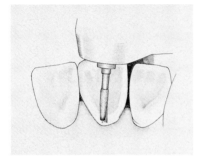

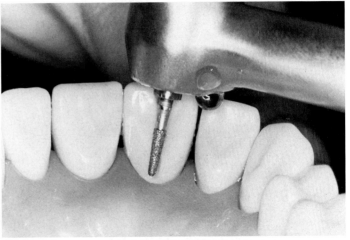

Fig. 4-75 a and b (a) Depth cut prepared in lingual surface with a small tapered diamond stone. (b) Lingual surface grooved with small wheel stone.

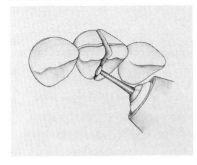

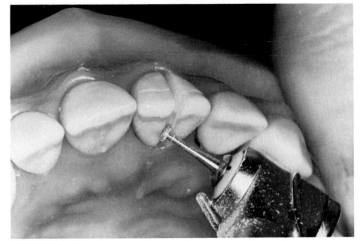

Figure 4-75 b

removal, and this will include the shoulder area.

The lingual depth cut is made in a similar fashion except that the shoulder cut is maintained level with the gingiva. The same tapered diamond stone may be used for creating the shoulder cut and, if necessary, the remaining lingual surface can be grooved with a small knife-edged diamond stone which has a 1 mm deep cutting edge (Fig. 4-75a and b).

The labial and lingual depth cuts are then joined at the incisal edge by making a groove through the incisal enamel and dentine at the score-mark placed at the two-thirds level of the anatomical crown (see Fig. 4-75). Because the incisal edge has not been reduced prematurely, it is now possible to view the tip of the preparation and relate it to the labial and lingual enamel which is silhouetted either side of the incisal groove. This silhouette will exactly depict the outline form of the completed porcelain veneer crown. At this stage it is comparatively easy to determine whether a preparation cut to two-thirds the length of the original anatomical crown will allow sufficient depth of porcelain and also leave sufficient dentine support at the incisal edge of the final preparation.

The reasons for using a tapered diamond stone to establish the dept cuts may now become clearer since the wider depth cut allows the clinician to view the lateral walls of the groove more easily (Fig. 4-76).

The accuracy of the depth cuts may be checked by the beginner with crown and bridge calipers. If the labio-lingual width of the intact enamel is determined, it is a simple procedure to calculate the difference between this measurement and the dimensions at the bottom of the grooved depth cuts.

Reduction of the Lingual Surface

The lingual surface of a porcelain veneer crown is the most critical area during tooth prepara-

tion. Sudden changes of thickness from the lingual plate of porcelain to the approximal axial walls is a common site for fracture (see page 222). The reduction of the lingual tooth surface should always be done before cutting the labial surface, in order to avoid creating thin lingual plates of porcelain.

Nuttall (1961) has suggested leaving the enamel in the cingulum area intact at the start of the lingual preparation since this prevents the extension of the preparation in an axial direction, and ensures a shoulder of uniform width. By contrast, if the entire lingual enamel is removed too soon, the softer dentine does not resist the axial penetration of rotary instruments, resulting in a lingual shoulder that may be too wide.

Lingual surface removal should therefore be commenced by extending the lingual depth cut at the shoulder so that it connects with the approximal enamel. This may be easily achieved with the tapered cylindrical diamond stone running supragingivally and at high speed. A lingual shoulder of 0.8 to 1 mm wide may now be rapidly created and the intact cingulum will act as a guide for determining a near degree of parallelism with the mesial axial wall at the cervical one-third (Fig. 4-77).

The remaining half of the lingual enamel is now removed, with a small diamond wheelstone (Fig. 4-78). The occlusal clearance on a typical maxillary central incisor should be at least 1 mm and in many cases this may be increased to 1.3 mm. The final accuracy of this clearance will be determined by measuring the lingual thickness of a temporary Epimine crown which will duplicate the ultimate thickness of porcelain. The technique for constructing this crown will be described later.

Reduction of the Labial Surface

The mesio-labial enamel is now removed, using the same tapered cylindrical diamond stone as employed for the depth cuts. The enamel is removed at high speed with the diamond stone

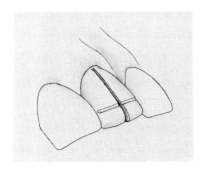
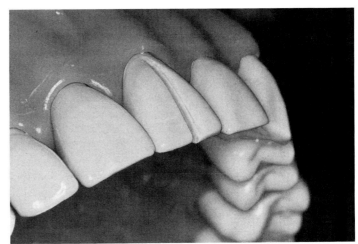

Fig. 4-76 Lateral view of incisal depth cut showing tooth profile.

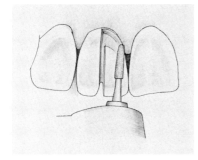
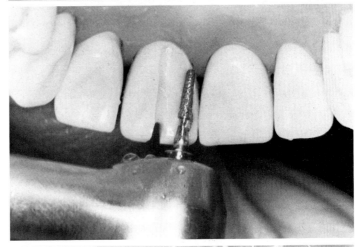

Fig. 4-77 Lingual shoulder prepared on one half of the tooth.

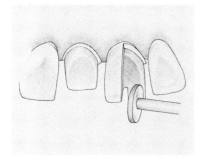
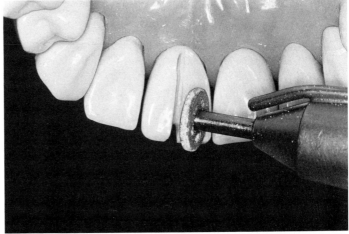

Fig. 4-78 Removal of one half of lingual enamel.

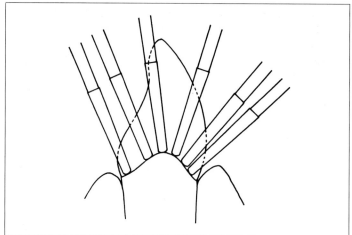

Fig. 4-79a to c (a) Diagram showing the correct placement of the approximal shoulder in relation to the interdental papilla. (b) Removal of approximal enamel using protective steel matrix band to protect adjacent tooth. (c) Final removal of labial enamel.

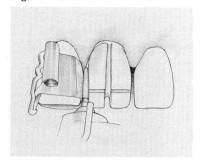

Figure 4-79a

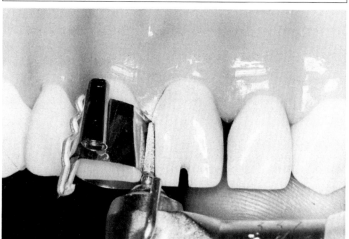

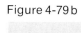

Figure 4-79b

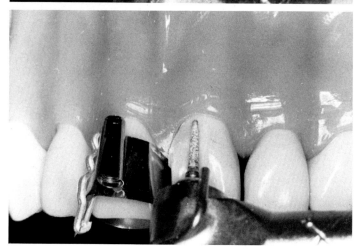

Figure 4-79c

placed just level with the gingiva. At this stage, no attempt should be made to enter the sub-gingival labial depth cut, but the enamel removal should be level with the depth of the axial wall created by this depth cut. As the diamond tool is directed towards the approximal enamel, it will follow the tooth curvature and resultantly the shoulder width should be narrowed as it approaches the approximal enamel. For example, in the typical maxillary central incisor, the labial shoulder should decrease in width from 1 mm to 0.5 mm at the maximum mesio-distal diameter.

Relationship of the shoulder to the interdental papilla

The cutting of the approximal shoulders is a very critical procedure. Under no circumstances should the preparation encroach into the epithelial attachment. Although this may appear obvious to the clinician, it is a simple matter to level the shoulder with the labial and lingual shoulder cuts without realising that the cervical line of the tooth has risen sharply in the approximal areas. It is therefore essential to watch carefully the contour of the gingival crest and the approximal cut must rise in harmony with the anatomy of the tooth (Fig. 4-79 a to c).

Creation of the Labial Sub-Gingival Shoulder

All sub-gingival cutting operations must be done at slow speed if the gingival tissue is to remain undamaged. The forming of the sub-gingival labial shoulder requires meticulous attention during the cutting operation, since it is very easy to encroach into the gingival crevice too far. Equally a shoulder which only remains at the level of the gingiva may cause a porcelain crown edge to become rapidly visible to the patient. The tapered cylindrical diamond stone, of 1 mm diameter at the tip, should be used in a friction grip handpiece at a speed of 20,000 to 40,000 r.p.m. in order to provide the minimum degree of eccentricity and maximum amount of control. The clinician is also advised to use the index finger of his left hand placed over the head of the handpiece as an additional control guide. The tip of the diamond stone is now inserted at the base of the labial depth cut and gently moved sideways until it rises clear of the gingiva at the approximal shoulder. Gentle pressure will assure that the sub-gingival depth of 1.0 mm is maintained and visibility will be improved if the cutting is done under water-spray. The spray will slightly displace the gingiva and expose the enamel at the cervical line.

At this stage some of the sub-gingival enamel may be left intact at the cervical line if the shoulder depth is only 1.0 mm under the gingiva. Providing this enamel is not too thin it may be left in situ. However, in the author's experience the shoulder will generally terminate at the cervical line or just below it in adult teeth so that problems of weakened enamel edges do not often occur.

The original sub-gingival mid-line depth cut will have controlled the amount of labial enamel removed and the necessity for further removal of labial dentine and enamel to provide adequate shoulder width is avoided.

At this stage the outline form of the preparation should be completed on one half of the tooth. A careful inspection of the profile of the uncut half will allow the student to see in three dimensions his future porcelain crown in silhouette. If he is in any doubt, the cut walls of the tooth can be marked with a pencil to highlight the surfaces (Fig. 4-80a). Once the depth and form of the preparation have been established, it is a simple matter to repeat all the procedures for the removal of the other half of the tooth (Fig. 4-80b).

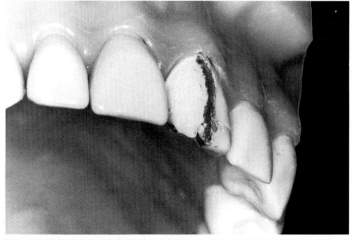

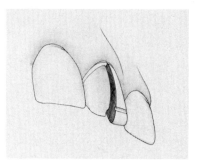

Figure 4-80 a

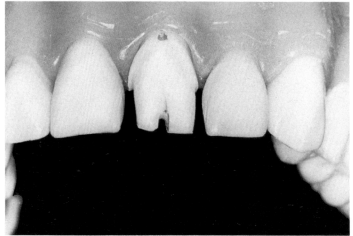

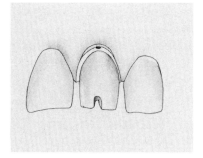

Figure 4-80 b

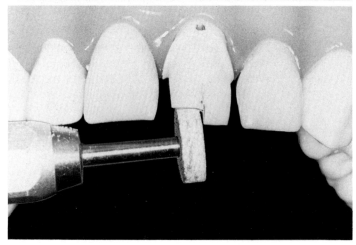

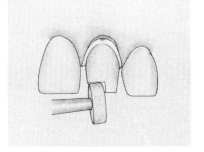

Figure 4-80 c

Reduction of Incisal Edge

The removal of both the labial and lingual enamel and the mid-line incisal depth cut will have already reduced the incisal length of the preparation. It is now a simple procedure to refine the bevel at the incisal edge of the preparation with a small diamond wheelstone. Generally this bevel should be cut at a 45 degree angle to the lingual surface. However, the ultimate rounding of the incisal edge is the more important operation and should be carried out when all line and point angles are rounded off.

The length of the preparation will have been determined by the incisal depth cut but if the tip of the incisal edge is too thin, then modifications may have to be made. In the average or typical incisor tooth, the preparation will nearly always accommodate a length of two-thirds of the original anatomical crown (Fig. 4-80c). In the case of atypical teeth, slight reductions in length may be required.

The importance of leaving the incisal edge reduction until last is self-evident, since the tooth structure in this area is so easily destroyed by premature cutting, and support for the porcelain crown is reduced. The outline form of the preparation should now have been completed and it is at this stage that a temporary crown can be made to assess the accuracy of preparation. Providing a low-shrinking resin is used, it is possible to monitor the future thickness of the crown by using the temporary restoration as a master template.

Monitoring the Depth of the Preparation by Using a Temporary Crown as a Master Template

A temporary crown should fulfill the following function:

1. Possess sufficient mechanical strength to maintain occlusal stability during construction of the porcelain veneer crown.
2. Preserve the vitality of the dental pulp.
3. Maintain the health and stability of the surrounding periodontium.
4. Serve as a master template for determining the ultimate thickness of the porcelain veneer crown.
5. Provide reasonable aesthetics which will satisfy the patient.

The maintenance of occlusal stability and a healthy periodontium will depend upon the marginal fit of the temporary crown and the accuracy with which it duplicates the original tooth contour. In addition, any damage to the dental pulp or gingival tissue will be influenced by the biological compatibility of the temporary crown material.

The cold-curing acrylic resins will never reach a high degree of polymerisation and will inevitably continue to leach free acrylic monomer after setting. These materials will always produce some irritation at the gingival margin and may induce a degree of gingival recession. Free monomer may also cause pulpal inflammation but this can be mitigated by protection of the dentine stump with vaseline during setting of the acrylic and cementing it with temporary zinc oxide cements. Cold-curing acrylic resins also have a high polymerisation shrinkage and do not produce a good marginal fit. This is further exacerbated by an undue tightness of fit, particularly on the axial walls of the preparation.

The use of cold-curing acrylic resin in temporary crown forms made from polycarbonate, methyl methacrylate, cellulose acetate or metals is

263

therefore always prone to the above disadvantages. In addition it is extremely difficult to reproduce original tooth contour with preformed crown forms. Inevitably some occlusal adjustment is required, and incorrect labial or cervical contour can cause some reaction from the gingiva. This will become even more apparend when the crown is left in position for long periods.

The Epimine Resin Temporary Crown

A new polymeric material has recently been introduced for temporary crown work in dentistry. This material uses ethylene imine side groups which enable the material to be cross-linked with aromatic sulphonates or related compounds (*Braden* et al., 1972). The material (ESPE Scutan*) is dispensed from a syringe as a base paste containing a methacrylate filler, and a bottle containing the sulphonate cross-linking agent. The setting reaction is only very slightly exothermic and there is no free monomer. Gingival reaction to this material is therefore much less than that experienced with the cold-curing acrylics. In addition, these epimine resins have a very low shrinkage during polymerisation and will provide a remarkably accurate fit when polymerised in situ on a tooth. Their withdrawal from tooth preparations is also facilitated by their slow rise in modulus of elasticity (rigidity) after initial set. When compared with cold-curing acrylic resins they are therefore considerably more flexible, but after approximately 15 minutes, will cross-link to a degree where they become extremely rigid.

The Epimine resins possess several advantages over cold-curing acrylics, both in their low toxicity, good fit and low shrinkage. However, their mechanical properties are definitely inferior (*Braden,* and *Causton,* 1970). The impact strength, tensile strength and extension to

* ESPE, Seefeld, West Germany.

break are markedly inferior to polymethacrylate, and considerable care is necessary in the handling of any intricate or thin-walled appliances made from this new material.

Despite these defects in mechanical properties, the author considers that this type of material represents a major advance in the chemistry and concepts of temporary crown and bridge materials. Not only do these materials preserve the health of the pulp and periodontium during crown construction but the clinician is offered the opportunity of rapidly making restorations that can exactly reproducd the original tooth contour. Further development of stronger and more colour-stable resins of this type can usher in a new era in temporary crown and bridge construction.

Construction of an Epimine Resin Temporary Crown

An alginate or elastomeric impression should be taken of the teeth to be prepared for veneer crown construction prior to any operative work. Any missing areas of tooth structure may be restored with wax or a cold-curing resin prior to taking the impression (Fig. 4-81a and b).

The preparation of the tooth should now be finished up to the stage of its final outline form. Final finishing of the preparation should be delayed until after the fabrication of the Epimine temporary crown. This crown will serve as a master template for assessing the ultimate thickness of the porcelain veneer crown. If the Epimine master template is measured with calipers and examined visually, it will reveal any faults in preparation which can be corrected prior to finishing the dentine surfaces.

Fig. 4-81 a to e   (a) Teeth prior to crowning. (b) Alginate impression taken of teeth prior to crown preparation. (c) Scutan resin injected into areas of alginate impression where teeth have been prepared for veneer crowns. (d) Scutan resin temporary crowns in position on teeth after removal of the alginate master impression. (e) Removal of flash on crowns with sandpaper discs. Note the accuracy of the epimine resin in duplicating the surface anatomy of the alginate impression.

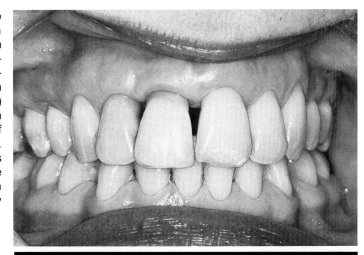

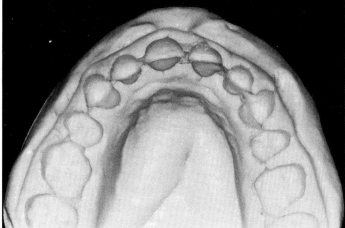

Figure 4-81 b

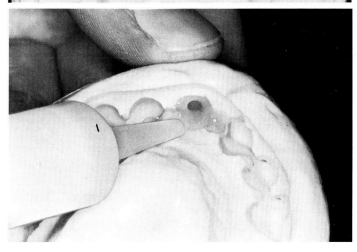

Figure 4-81 c

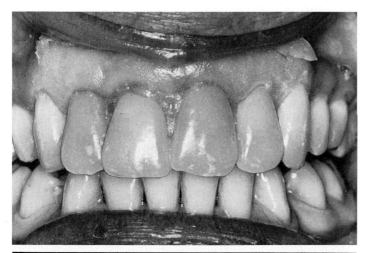

Figure 4-81 d

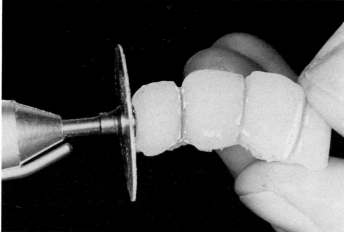

Figure 4-81 e

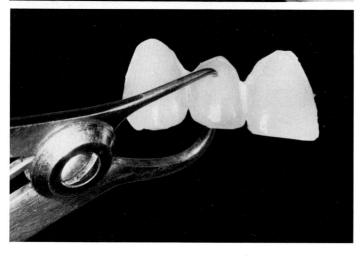

Fig. 4-82 Measuring the thickness of the epimine resin crown to determine any areas of inadequate thickness.

The liquid Epimine resin is dispensed from the syringe onto a special mixing pad calibrated in centimetres. One drop of liquid catalyst is added for each centimetre of paste and mixing of the liquid resin may be carried out very rapidly. The resin is then injected into the tooth area of the impression which is to be restored (Fig. 4-81c). Great care must be taken to avoid trapping air in the resin and this is one of the disadvantages of the current material. Special syringes are supplied to inject the resin but disposable syringes are equally satisfactory.

The tooth preparation is wiped dry with cotton-wool and the impression seated in the mouth. The resin will flow and adapt itself very accurately to the preparation and when set (ca. 3 to 4 minutes) the impression is removed from the mouth. Completion of set may be checked by testing the hardness of the Epimine resin which is left on the mixing pad. On removal of the impression the Epimine crown may be removed cleanly in the impression or it may be left intact on the tooth (Fig. 4-81d). At this stage it will be seen that a very detailed replica of the original anatomical crown of the tooth has been produced. If the crown has remained on the tooth preparation, it can be gently teased off, and the resin's flexibility will prevent any locking in the approximal spaces. Alternatively the resin crown may now be removed from the impression. Due to the very low viscosity of the resin, an extremely thin flash will be present, and this can be rapidly removed with a sandpaper disc and polished with a rubber wheel (Fig. 4-81e). The crown should be tried on the preparation and checked for fit which should be very accurate and free-sliding.

Multiple crowns may be made quite easily by this technique and the author has constructed up to eight crowns at a time. When multiple crowns are made, it is important to allow a longer setting time since the resin can be easily broken if removed too quickly, i.e. cross-linking of the resin will increase the strength. This extra strength will be more necessary when crowns are removed from elastomeric impressions.

Where distinct changes of colour are desired, the basic dentine colour of the Epimine resins can be modified at the time of mixing with colour modifiers. Alternatively the addition of a little silicate cement powder will increase the opacity and often give more life-like colours.

The completed crown may now be measured with crown and bridge calipers to determine the thickness of the labial and lingual surfaces (Fig. 4-82).Visual examination will also reveal any sharp internal line angles. The clinican is strongly advised to check any marked changes in thickness at the axial wall line angles. Sudden changes in thickness at the lingual surface line angles is probably the most serious fault that occurs in veneer crown preparation, since it is here that cleavage planes may be set up in the porcelain veneer crown (see page 222). The Epimine crown may also serve as a good indication of retention form. If it is easily placed in position on the tooth preparation via more than one path of insertion, then the taper of axial walls may be too great.

The low shrinkage of the Epimine resins will provide a very close approximation to the original tooth dimensions and if thin areas are observed on either the labial or lingual surfaces, it is a simple operation to return to the tooth preparation and remove more dentine to eliminate these deficiencies. The student could then reline the Epimine crown with a little more resin to check his accuracy. The very low viscosity of the resin is ideal for this purpose.

The importance of using liquid resins to form a master template for checking accuracy may now be apparent since alternative methods of using various thicknesses of articulating paper can never provide the same accuracy.

In many cases it can be a great advantage to construct duplicate crowns, one of which is sent to the technician. This will furnish him with an anatomical picture of the tooth in relation to the gingiva and indicate the cervical contour which he must seek to achieve. A duplicate crown could also be used as an alternative to the diagnostic cast technique described previously in which the surface characterisation of the tooth may be clearly seen. A duplicate crown is of particular value in obtaining accurate contour of the posterior teeth and in many cases it can serve as a guide to functional occlusion, where it is not planned to alter the tooth anatomy. The use of liquid resins as master templates is advocated by the author as a basic concept in temporary crown construction. The current resins possess inadequate mechanical properties for long-term temporary restorations and lack the toughness of methylmethacrylates or polycarbonates. However, even the present Epimine resins can function satisfactorily for several weeks and it is hoped that future research in this area will produce materials that will offer both clinicians and technicians the opportunity of creating restorations that are in complete harmony with the periodontium and surrounding teeth.

Finishing the Typical Maxillary Central Incisor Preparation

It will be obvious that the final finishing of the jacket crown preparation should be delayed until after the calibration of the preparation with the Epimine temporary crown. If modifications have to be made to the preparation, then fine surface finishes would be destroyed.

Once the correct outline form of the preparation has been established then it is essential to refine the surface detail to provide as smooth a surface as possible for impression taking. In addition, a smooth surface is more easily wetted by the new hydrophilic polycarboxylate and glass-ionomer cements.

Conventional instrumentation will rely on the use of fine sandpaper discs, finishing burs, abrasive stones, files or chisels. There is little doubt that fine sandpaper discs can produce extremely smooth surfaces to dentine (*Street*, 1953). However these discs cannot reach all surfaces of the preparation and may cause some gingival damage. Twelve-bladed finishing burs are reasonably satisfactory but tend to lose their cutting efficiency and also may cause stepping of the shoulder preparation. Chisels are not very useful instruments for full crown preparation, except for refining the shoulder area, since sharp internal line angles are nothing more than stress concentrators (see page 226). The chisel is much better used for planing external cavo-surface angles. Fine abrasive stones of the carborundum type can be made to produce a very smooth finish but they are bulky and soon loose their original shape, due to rapid wear of the bonding matrices.

The electroplated diamond stone is available in a variety of sizes and may be made to very small dimensions. It is a durable instrument and difficult to break; however, due to the nature of its construction, it does not easily fulfill the requirement of a finishing tool. Firstly, it is extremely difficult to electroplate very fine diamonds onto the end of a bur shaft and, secondly, once these diamond chips become dislodged from the plated bur surface, the cutting action diminishes rapidly. Indeed, examination of some of these tools will reveal actual loss of diamond chips at the time of manufacture, the diamond particles becoming dislodged during the electroplating process. Recent improvements in the diamond tool industry have resulted in finer diamond plated stones being produced and these tools are becoming more acceptable for finishing procedures.

Sintered Diamonds Finishing Stones

Studies on this problem revealed that modern industrial techniques of producing sintered diamond tools might be applied to dentistry. In this case it is possible to produce cutting tools which contain much finer diamond particles, the metal powder and fine diamonds being intimately mixed and then compressed and sintered onto the end of a steel shank.

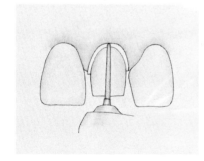

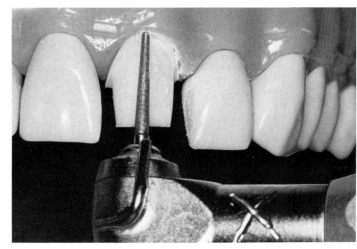

Fig. 4-83 Finishing of preparation with micro-diamond plated stone or sintered diamond stone.

These finishing stones have a uniform continuous distribution of diamond particles within the shank itself. Consequently, the metal and the diamond wear at the same rate to continously expose a fresh cutting surface during operation which ensures the maintenance of cutting efficiency and bur shape.* This is but one approach to the production of a dental finishing tool but the important aspect is the concept of obtaining smooth surfaces to dentine. Basically all finishing techniques rely on a cutting or milling action and it is a matter of selecting the most efficient abrasive to produce a "micro-finish" rather than a "macro-finish" to dentine. The abrasive must be held in a matrix material which will wear slightly faster than the abrasive used; on the other hand, the matrix must not wear away so fast that the tool quickly loses its geometric form. The cutting tool must also show no signs of glazing if the fine abrasive is to perform satisfactorily and it must be free from clogging by tooth debris.

* Sintered diamond finishing stones. A.D. International Ltd. London W.J.

Micro-diamond finishing

Cutting speeds for micro-diamond finishing stones, whether of the sintered or plated type, should lie within the range of 5,000 to 40,000 r.p.m. for all finishing operations on full crown preparations. Initial finishing operations on teeth should be done under water-spray. Final inspection under an air-spray will allow the operator to observe the precision of his work. Shoulder preparations are best finished with a sintered tapered cylindrical stone of 1.5 mm shank and 1 mm tip, using light pressure (Fig. 4-83). The slight rounding at the edge of this stone will then produce an equal rounding of the internal axial wall line angle, which avoids stress concentration (see page 226). This rounding of the internal line angle should not produce a chamfer (see page 226), and the main object should be to smooth off the cervical margins at the shoulder and eliminate any overhanging or weak enamel prisms. Because of the very smooth surfaces of sintered diamond tools, they are ideal for the finishing of shoulders placed sub-gingivally. Damage to tissue will be minimised and the tool cannot overcut and create undercuts on the axial walls.

Micro-diamond tools may also be used to smooth off all internal surfaces and line and

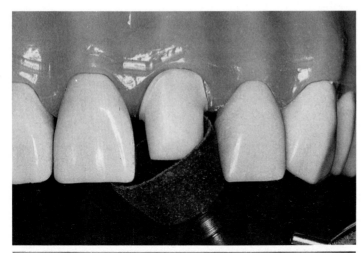

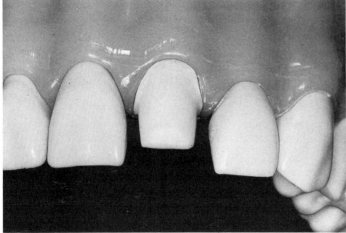

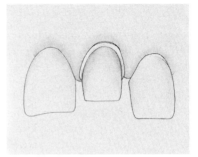

Fig. 4-84 Polishing of preparation with rubber cups under water spray.

Fig. 4-85 Completed porcelain jacket crown preparation for maxillary central incisor.

point angles. Alternatively fine sandpaper discs may perform equally well providing access to all areas is possible.

Tungsten-Carbide Finishing "Stones"

An interesting approach to the finishing of cavo-surface margins has been made by *Boyde* (1973). He observed that the degree of chipping out of embrasure or cervical margins depended upon the designed cutting angle of the tungsten bur blades and their actual sharpness. He sur-

mised that a bur with very low blades or a stone with a very fine grit could be used to finish the exit margins when used in clockwise rotation at very high speeds in the air turbine handpiece. A bur was produced and deliberately ground longitudinally but with a finite number of blades, to produce a 40-bladed bur.

Subsequently *Boyde* demonstrated that a smooth bladeless tungsten-carbide bur in an air turbine handpiece produced a high quality finish on enamel margins. *Barnes* (1974) assessed cervical margins finished with one of these new "tungsten carbide stones" and found the quality of margin achieved was superior to that achieved with newly-sharpened gingival margin trimmers and comparable with the best finish achieved by other methods. *Baker* and *Curson* (1974) designed three finishing burs based on the tungsten carbide stone for finishing the margins for both amalgam and cast gold restorations. These new stones are now available commercially and can be useful in finishing the shoulder preparation.*

Polishing the Preparation

As explained previously, if the new hydrophilic polyacrylic acid bonded cements are to be used, then better wetting and adhesion is obtained on well-finished dentine surfaces.

The highest possible finish that may be given to the surfaces of a porcelain veneer crown preparation would be by use of rubber bonded carbide abrasive cups** (Fig. 4-84). Polishing of the preparation must be done under continuous water-spry when abrasive wheels are used, since this procedure can quickly produce over-heating of the pulp. A preparation which has been polished should exhibit an ivory-like surface and no scratch marks should be visible. The completed porcelain veneer crown preparation is illustrated in Fig. 4-85. The ideal preparation should have the following features:

1. Adequate height and width to support the porcelain crown.
2. Sharp external line angles at the cervical margin.
3. Flat shoulder at just over 90° to the axial walls.
4. No sharp internal line or point angles.
5. Maximum parallelism at the cervical axial walls, allowing only one path of insertion.

* Baker-Curson finishing stones. A.D. International Ltd., London, W.1.
** Aaba rubber cups. Identoflex A.G. Buchs/SG Switzerland.

Pre-packing of the gingiva

It is sometimes found that the relationship of the porcelain veneer crown shoulder with the gingiva alters slightly after the use of sub-gingival packing cord. Pre-packing of the gingiva has been recommended as a means of overcoming this problem and the shoulder is cut in relation to the displaced gingiva.

The author does not recommend this procedure since it may result in the gingival packing cord being left in position for too long a period. Permanent damage to the tissue may then ensue.

If it is found that the shoulder preparation is not deep enough then it is better to increase its depth at the time of the impression taking. Sintered diamond stones have been found particularly useful for this operation since they will not entagle with the cord or damage the gingiva.

Common Causes of Fracture in Porcelain Jacket Crowns

Fractures in porcelain jacket crowns may be attributed to the following causes:

1. Insufficient tooth support for the porcelain restoration.
2. Sudden changes in thickness of the porcelain creating planes of weakness (cleavage planes).
3. Incorrect condensation and firing of the porcelain causing mechanical weakness in critical sections, e.g. large air bubbles present at the linguo-axial line angles (cleavage planes) or micro-cracks produced by thermal shock.
4. Deflective malocclusions which have not been corrected prior to placement of the restoration.

5. Parafunctional movements of the mandible producing excessive stress, e.g. bruxism, clenching, etc.
6. Traumatic injury.

The types of preparations most likely to cause fracture have already been described and may be summarised as follows:

1. Conical preparations

A conical preparation will not provide sufficient retention form and the crown may become dislodged and crushed between the jaws. Alternatively the stress concentration may become too high due to inadequate supporting dentine and a longitudinal fracture may occur. Conical preparations will allow several paths of insertion for the crown.

2. Preparations with insufficient lingual reduction

A thin lingual plate of porcelain will cause a sudden change in thickness of the porcelain at the linguo-axial walls. These areas create planes of cleavage and result in crescent-shaped fractures of the porcelain.

3. Short preparations

If the coronal support for the jacket crown is reduced, crescent-shaped fractures may occur on either the labial or lingual surfaces. Short preparations increase the stress created by leverage, i.e. protrusive movements of the mandible (Fig. 4-37).

4. Undercut preparations

Undercuts, when present at the cervical one-third, will increase the stress concentration due to inadequate support for the porcelain. Although the ceramic technician may succeed in building a crown on such a preparation, he too might over-stress the crown during removal from the die. This type of preparation is also very likely to cause a tensile fracture of the crown during cementation.

An understanding of the stresses applied to a porcelain jacket crown during function and the designing of preparations to resist these stresses should enable the student to diagnose his failures. If a porcelain jacket crown breaks soon after insertion then the clinician is strongly advised not to replace it without giving further consideration to the stress analysis of his restoration.

The Metal-Ceramic Veneer Crown

Successful bonding of porcelain to metal alloys is not only dependent upon the handling of materials in the dental laboratory, but also upon the design of the preparation and the metal coping. It has been shown in Monograph II, page 61 that the bonding of porcelain to metal largely eliminates any flaws in the porcelain with a result that this brittle material takes on a new character. Because of the absence of flaws on the fit surface, the glassy porcelain can more nearly achieve its theoretical strength which can be of a very high order.

Unfortunately when porcelain is fired onto the metal surface it is a common experience to find that the metal coping never fits as well after completion of the baking.

The cause of this is:

1. Metal creep due to the close approximation of melting temperatures of the gold alloys and porcelain (ca. $150\,°C - 200\,°C$).

2. Differences in thermal expansion and rate of cooling between gold alloys and porcelain.

3. Sintering shrinkage of the porcelain.

The labial or buccal margins, where the thickness of metal is limited by aesthetics, is the region most often subject to distortion. The design of the preparation must therefore take into account all the above factors and the following objectives should always be paramount in the operator's mind:

1. Reduction of stress on the porcelain.

2. Minimising creep of the metal coping, particularly at the fit surface.

3. Optimising the aesthetics of the labial or buccal porcelain.

4. Maintenance of marginal fit.

5. Providing adequate retention form.

Reduction of stress and creep in the metal porcelain combination

The principles of stress analysis and the design factors described for the complete porcelain veneer crown on pages 218 to 228 must be observed when preparing teeth for metal-ceramic crowns. However, because of the improved strength of these crowns, many clinicians are tempted to prepare teeth without giving due' consideration to stress factors. Such an attitude has led to the cult of the shoulderless preparation which, as will be shown, hardly fulfills any of the objectives set out above. It is also imperative to establish what effect full or partial coverage of metal by porcelain has on the strength of the restoration and the effect such procedures have on the residual stresses left in the porcelain after cooling.

The firing of porcelain onto a rigid body has always presented problems to the ceramist. The success of this operation is dependent upon the control of the firing or sintering shrinkage, matching of the thermal expansion of the porcelain, and the stability of the body during firing. The shape of the rigid body will have a great effect on the ease of this operation and one of the simplest shapes to coat with a glaze porcelain (veneer porcelain) would be a rod, in which the porcelain will sinter and shrink evenly. This situation is very similar to that of a thermally-induced shrink fitted collar where the tensile stresses are balanced by reciprocal compressive stresses in the porcelain.

The most difficult shapes to coat with porcelain would be ones with sharp re-entrant angles, and these are to be avoided under all circumstances (Fig. 4-86). Even when porcelain is applied to a convex surface, if only one surface is coated, the sintering shrinkage will drag the porcelain towards the area of greatest bulk. This is illustrated in Fig. 4-87 where an aluminous porcelain of matched expansion to high alumina has been applied to a dove-tail high alumina profile. On sintering, the edges have lifted and shrunk away from the alumina profile as indicated by the

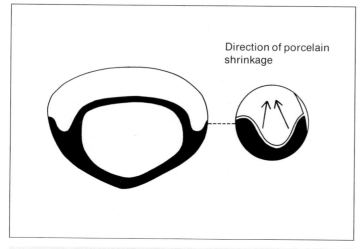

Direction of porcelain
shrinkage

Fig. 4-86 Diagram illustrating unfavourable design of metal coping with re-entrant angles.

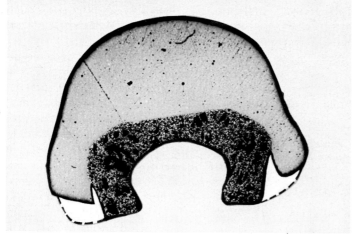

Fig. 4-87 Polished section of an
aluminous porcelain/high alumina bridge pontic showing areas
of sintering shrinkage.

dotted line in Fig. 4-87. The effect of surface tension during sintering of the porcelain is well demonstrated here and illustrates the difficulty of firing dental porcelain accurately to a fine edge. On cooling, it was also observed that in some cases the tensile stress which developed around the middle of the high alumina backing was sufficient to crack it (*McLean,* 1966). This is a dramatic demonstration of the forces exerted by the sintering shrinkage and thermal contraction of porcelain and one that is sometimes overlooked by the dental ceramist. If the alumina profile was replaced with metal in such a design, then, on cooling from the glaze temperature the metal would creep and distort if it was too thin.

From a study of Fig. 4-87 it will be seen that the application of porcelain to only one surface of a metal crown is the least favourable procedure. If the sintering shrinkage and thermal contraction of the porcelain are to be harnessed with advantage to produce good bonding, then the optimum design must be one in which the entire coping is covered with porcelain and all the tensile stresses developing in the metal on cooling are equally

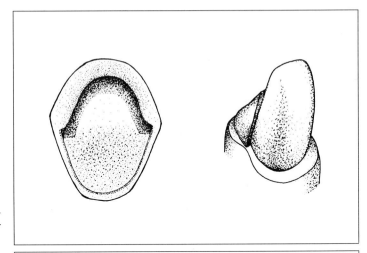

Fig. 4-88 Diagram of a metal-ceramic preparation designed for lingual metal coverage.

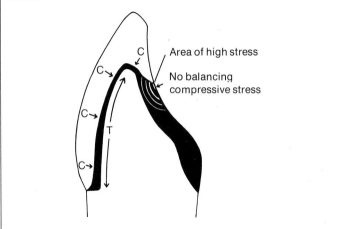

Fig. 4-89 Diagram of a preparation designed for full metal coverage on lingual. Tensile stresses in lingual metal are not balanced by compressive stresses in porcelain thereby creating high stress at porcelain/metal interface. C = Compression; T = Tension.

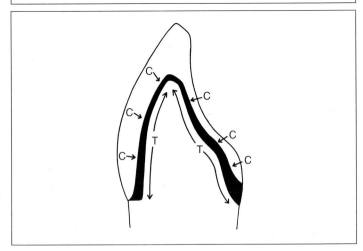

Fig. 4-90 Preparation designed for full porcelain coverage of metal. Compressive stresses set up in the porcelain on cooling are balanced by the tensile stresses developing in the higher thermal expansion metal. C = Compressive stresses; T = Tensile stresses.

balanced by compressive stresses in the porcelain. A preparation design (Fig. 4-88) which deliberately sets out to create full gold backings on the lingual surface is therefore undesirable since the stresses at the metal/ceramic interface will be unevenly balanced (Fig. 4-89). By contrast, when full porcelain coverage is used these stresses are markedly reduced (Fig. 4-90).

The Labial Shoulder

Optimising the aesthetics and maintaining the marginal fit of the labial and buccal porcelain

It has already been illustrated on page 224 (Fig. 4-44), that the optimum type of shoulder preparation which will cause the least stress on a restoration is one in which the shoulder is very slightly rounded at the angle between the axial wall and the gingival floor. The only sharp line angles should be those at the external cervical margin (Fig. 4-44, Model 1).

The preparations which have been advocated by many clinicians for the metal-ceramic crown are the chamfer Model 2, Fig. 4-44, the flat shoulder Model 4, the shoulder with bevel as in Model 6, and the modified flat shoulder illustrated in Model 1, Fig. 4-44.

Since all four types of shoulder preparation are used, it is important to consider the effect upon the design of the metal coping, the latter's effect upon the aesthetics of the porcelain and, finally, the fit of the restoration. The four types

of shoulder preparation are illustrated in Fig. 4-95 and the metal copings are shown in black. A further modification where the angle between the axial wall and the shoulder is increased to 135° is shown in Fig. 4-95e, page 279.

The shoulder versus the bevel

It is important to establish the role of the bevel in improving the fit of the metal-ceramic crown. *McLean* and *Wilson* (1978) have examined the effect of angle of bevel on rate of diffusion at the margins of a crown, the latter controlling the rate of solubility and disintegration of the cement. They showed that moderate angles of bevel below 45° (Fig. 4-95a) are not effective in reducing diffusion and that diffusion was only reduced to a major degree at angles greater than 70° Fig. 4-91.

Unfortunately, extending the angle of bevel from 45° to 70° also increases the risk of damage to the epithelial attachment since if the metal collar is to be hidden sub-gingivally, the gold bevel must be extended even further into the crevice (Fig. 4-92).

An additional problem with thin and long gold bevels is one of finishing. Not only is there a risk of metal distortion during firing of the porcelain (Fig. 4-93) but finishing and polishing of these fine edges presents major problems.

Effect of burnishing

Rosensteil (1957) considered that if the angle of the gold margin was less than 30° to 45° then the edge will be too thick to allow spinning of the gold. Unfortunately these ideal bevels are the ones that cannot provide any improvement in diffusion rate of the cement unless the gap is closed by burnishing as in a cast gold inlay. A metal bevel can only be burnished if the operator can overcome the inherent yield strength in

Fig. 4-91 Graph showing that the rate of diffusion of cement decreases as the angle of bevel α increases. Diffusion is only reduced to a significant clinical degree when bevels of 70° or more are used Calculations based on an average crown with a diameter at cervix of 8 mm, shoulder width of 1.0 mm and bevel width of 0.5 mm. (From *McLean, J. W.,* and *Wilson, A. D.* The butt joint versus bevelled gold margin in metal-ceramic crowns. Unpublished data 1978.)

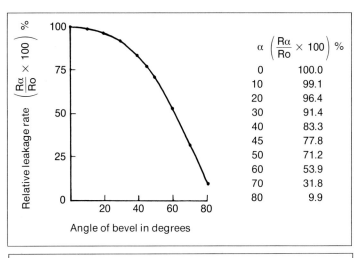

α	$\left(\dfrac{R\alpha}{Ro} \times 100\right)$ %
0	100.0
10	99.1
20	96.4
30	91.4
40	83.3
45	77.8
50	71.2
60	53.9
70	31.8
80	9.9

Relative leakage rate $\left(\dfrac{R\alpha}{Ro} \times 100\right)$ %

Angle of bevel in degrees

Fig. 4-92 (a) 45° bevel with a gold collar 1 mm thick can only just be accomodated in a gingival crevice of 3 mm depth. (b) 70° bevel (the long bevel) extends too far and would damage the epithelial attachment.

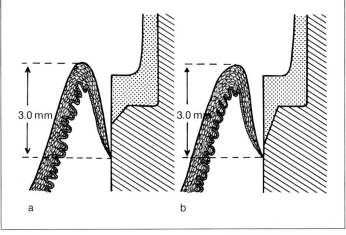

Fig. 4-93 Long gold bevels (70°) cannot be easily finished to a fine edge and may distort on firing the porcelain.

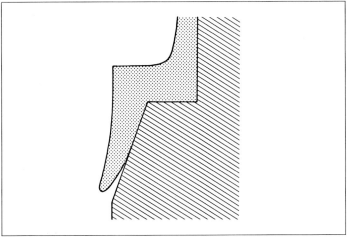

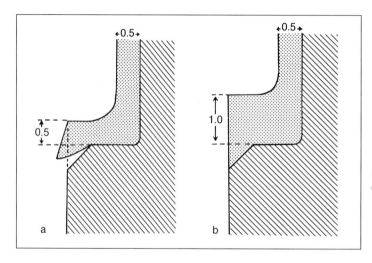

Fig. 4-94 (a) 45° gold bevel may distort during firing of the porcelain if the gold collar is too thin. (b) Gold collars of 1 mm depth will buttress the gold bevel and resist distortion.

the metal, and the metal also has a reasonably high elongation percent. It was shown by *McLean* and *Wilson* (1978) that the burnishing of ceramic bonding alloys is extremely difficult since the relationship between hardness values and percent elongation gave a burnishability number too high on the scale developed by *Moon* and *Modjeski* (1976).

In practice the ceramic bonding alloys are not as easily burnished as the Type III gold alloys and it is highly doubtful whether burnishing can close the gap at a bevelled margin, unless bevels of around 70° are used.

The gold collar and bevel

Confusion over the merits of using gold collars still exists since, in some clinicians' minds, the gold collar is associated with a gold bevel and has been accepted as improving fit and resistance to microleakage. However, as described previously, unless the bevel is at an angle of at least 70° then little resistance to microleakage can be expected. It must be clearly understood that if a gold collar is used with or without a bevel, then the fit of the metal-ceramic crown will generally be better than firing porcelain to a butt joint. The benefits of using a gold collar

are therefore related to a direct porcelain versus gold fit, not an improvement in the fit of a straight gold casting. For this reason the important factor when designing a gold collar is one of thickness, since the cross-sectional area of the collar will determine its resistance to creep during firing of the porcelain. Long gold bevels will creep and even a 45° bevel may lift if the gold collar is not thick enough (Fig. 4-94). The design of a gold collar should be one of a strong reinforcing ring of at least 1 mm thickness, independent of whether a bevel is used or not.

Unfortunately, placing a thick gold collar subgingivally will result in a dark shadow at the gum margin which is unacceptable to the more discerning patient.

In view of the fact that only bevels greater than 70° are capable of making a major reduction in microleakage, a strong case can be made for eliminating them from the metal-ceramic crown preparation. For this reason the preparation using either a shoulder or deep chamfer should be considered.

Fig. 4-95 Coping designs for various types of shoulder preparation illustrated in Fig. 4-44. (a) Model 6. Shoulder with bevel. (b) Model 4. Standard type, flat shoulder, (c) Model 2. Deep chamfer. Dotted line indicates area of tooth which would be cut in a full shoulder preparation. (d) Model I. Flat shoulder, internal line angles rounded. (e) 135° angle shoulder with internal line angles rounded. In this case a slip joint is provided which improves fit and the axiogingival floor line angle is not placed too deeply so as to endanger the pulp.

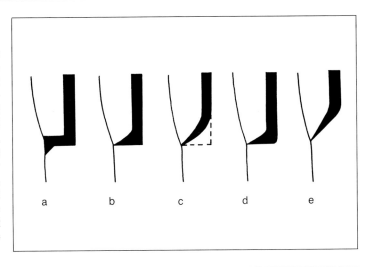

a   b   c   d   e

The Shoulder and Chamfer Preparation

In the case of the 90° shoulder illustrated in Fig. 4-95 b (standard type flat shoulder), the gold coping is accommodated comparatively easily on the axial wall and can be thinned down to almost a knife-edge at the external cervical margin. The fused porcelain may therefore be kept in correct contour and the opaque porcelain is more easily concealed by a reasonable depth of gingival dentine porcelain. The axiogingival area can be heavily reinforced with gold and the chances of metal creep affecting fit are lessened. By contrast, when the chamfer preparation (Fig. 4-95c) is used, the thickness remaining for the porcelain is reduced by exactly the amount of tooth structure retained at the axiogingival floor line angle. This area is outlined by the dotted line in Fig. 4-95c. The deep chamfer, although producing a low stress concentration factor does increase the problems of obtaining good aesthetics. In addition, the lack of bulk metal at the axiogingival floor also increases the risk of metal creep and poor fit, unless as will be shown a gold collar is used.

When Model 1 (flat shoulder internal line angles rounded) is considered (Fig. 4-95 d) it would appear to have all the advantages of Model 4 (standard type flat shoulder) without the higher stress concentration factor (Fig. 4-95b). In addition, the flat shoulder also allows the maximum amount of room for porcelain (Fig. 4-95 d). It will be seen that the shoulder provides an overall improvement in properties when compared with any other type of preparation. The metal coping is of sufficient thickness to resist much of the metal creep and it can be masked by a good depth of porcelain. Where the preparation has to be extended into the root face, it is advantageous to increase the angle at the shoulder with the axial wall by up to 135° (Fig. 4-95e).

Influence of shoulder design on Metal Creep

The influence of shoulder geometry on the creep of the metal coping has been studied by *Shillingburg* et al. (1973). A master die was made in wax and then cast in a chromium-cobalt alloy to provide a reference that would not be easily damaged. It represented a preparation for a metal-ceramic restoration on a maxillary central incisor, similar to that described by

Johnson et al. (1967). The labial margin was prepared to assess what effect four labial finishing lines would have on the stability of the labial margins of metal-ceramic crowns during the stages of porcelain firing. The distance between the labial finishing line of each coping and a reference mark on the die was measured with a filar eyepiece and recorded at six stages:

1. before any firing procedures;
2. following degassing;
3. after the addition of the opaque porcelain;
4. after the first addition of body porcelain;
5. after the second body bake;
6. following the final glazing.

The results of these tests were recorded on the following types of finishing lines:

1. the chamfer,
2. the heavy chamfer with bevel,
3. the shoulder with bevel,
4. the shoulder.

The types of shoulder finish and the results of the measurements are recorded in Fig. 4-96. All four finishing lines exhibited successively greater increases in labial opening during the first firing of body porcelain, and these changes continued during all stages when porcelain was added. All restorations continued to open with the second bake of porcelain with the exception of the shoulder with bevel. *Shillingburg* and associates concluded that the amount of opening exhibited by the chamfer (47.1 μm) and the heavy chamfer with bevel (29.3 μm) was large enough to be of clinical significance. If shrinkage of porcelain during firing and cooling is the primary reason for marginal distortion, increasing the bulk of metal seems to be a sound means of minimising distortion. Aesthetic considerations prohibit the overall thickening of the coping, so reinforcement of the coping must be limited to an inconspicuous area. They therefore recommended that some variation of the shoulder on the labial surface should be made

in order to provide space for an extra bulk of metal without encroaching on the space required for the porcelain veneer.

This study, and the evidence previously given in this monograph, confirm the importance of rethinking the current approach to the preparation of teeth for metal-ceramic crowns. Although a shoulderless or chisel edge preparation is easy to do and makes impression-taking less tedious, this should be no excuse for continuing with a preparation that falls short of our clinical requirements. It is for the above reasons that the shoulder will be the main type of finishing line advocated for metal-ceramic crowns in the monograph. The deep chamfer should only be used where space is limited and aesthetics of prime importance, otherwise it must be buttressed with a strong reinforcing gold collar to prevent distortion during firing.

The Approximal and Lingual Shoulders

In the case of the lingual aspect of the tooth where aesthetics is of no importance, then the design of the shoulder preparation should only be concerned with minimising the stress concentration at the margins of a restoration and maintaining the fit of the metal casting. A study of Fig. 4-44 will show that either Model 1 (flat shoulder, internal line angles rounded) or Model 2 (deep chamfer) are ideal in this respect. The common practice of using a deep chamfer preparation on the lingual surface can therefore be well supported on scientific grounds. Providing the preparation allows sufficient thickness of metal (>1.0 mm) then there is little risk of lifting of the margins during baking of the porcelain. However, when the deep chamfer preparation is extended to the approximal regions, then problems can arise. If the reduction of the approximal margins is minimal (<0.5 mm), there is a risk of the metal having an

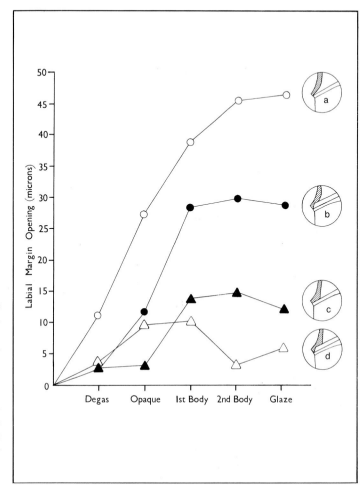

Fig. 4-96 Types of finishing line in relation to the amount of marginal distortion caused during five stages of baking the porcelain veneer. (a) Chamfer. (b) Chamfer with bevel. (c) Shoulder. (d) Shoulder with bevel. Adapted from *Shillingburg, H. T., Hobo, S.,* and *Fisher, D. W.* Preparation design and margin distortion in porcelain-fused-to-metal restorations. J. Pros. Dent. 29, 276−284. 1973.

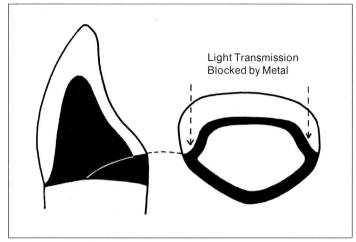

Fig. 4-97 Standard coping design for a restricted chamfer preparation in the approximal zones. Light transmission is restricted by the metal collar.

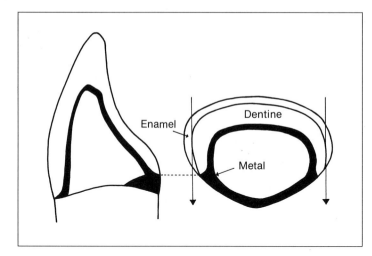

Fig. 4-98 Coping design for a widened approximal shoulder area. There is ample space for enamel porcelain in the approximal areas and a natural tooth effect is more easily achieved. Light transmission through the porcelain highlights the enamel as indicated by the arrows.

undesirable influence on colour. A typical preparation and coping (reduced approximal and lingual shoulder) is illustrated in Fig. 4-97. Transmission of light at the cervical one-third is restricted and the opportunity for providing a natural approximal enamel effect is reduced (see page 132, Monograph III). It is clear, therefore, that the preparation of the approximal regions of the tooth deserves as much attention as the labial if the crown is to achieve its maximum cosmetic effect. Even when a deep chamfer preparation is used, it is essential that the shoulder area should have a depth of at least 0.5 mm. This widened approximal shoulder allows the coping design to be restricted to the axial walls with no metal showing at the external cervical margins. Enamel porcelain can then be baked around the approximal zone to give the classical approximal translucency of the natural tooth (Fig. 4-98).

Recommended Designs for the Preparation and Metal Coping in Metal-Ceramic Crowns

The ideal types of preparation involving a butt joint are:

1. the flat shoulder,
2. the 135° shoulder,
3. the deep chamfer.

The recommended designs are as follows:

Facial Shoulder

1. Flat shoulder (90°) with all internal line angles rounded (Fig. 4-99 a).

1. Distinct labial shoulder with axiogingival line angles rounded. No external cervical margin bevel. (Thin gold margins are lifted during the firing of the porcelain.)
2. Lingual surface to be finished to a deep chamfer with a depth of at least 1.0 mm.
3. Approximal region to be finished to a flat shoulder or long chamfer. Depth of cut must be at least 0.5 mm.

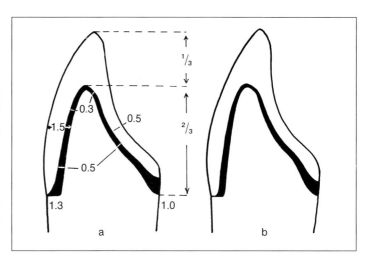

Fig. 4-99 (a) Flat shoulder (90°) with all internal line angles rounded. Recommended design for gold coping finished to a knife edge where preparation does not extend up root face and aesthetics is of primary importance. (b) Flat shoulder (90°) showing porcelain fired directly to the labial margin and gold coping cut back to the axiogingival line angle.

4. Metal coping should be strongly reinforced at the cervical collar (0.5 mm) but may be reduced to 0.3 mm at the labio-incisal one-third, where aesthetics is of prime importance.
5. All internal line and point angles should be slightly rounded.
6. Metal coping should exhibit smooth convex surfaces for the application of porcelain and where possible allow an even thickness of porcelain veneer.
7. Full porcelain coverage of the coping is recommended wherever possible in order to create a balanced stress system at the metal/porcelain interface.

Advantages. Preparation will produce the least stress in the cervical area. Maximum room for porcelain and metal. Porcelain can be fired to the metal edge and provides good aesthetics. Alternatively porcelain may be fired directly to the labial margin (Fig. 4-99 b).

Disadvantages. Labial porcelain butt fit more difficult to achieve than using a gold collar.

2. **Deep Chamfer** (Fig. 4-99 c)

Advantages. The deep chamfer is an excellent preparation to use where gold collars can be employed without interfering with aesthetics.
Provides a slip joint.
The chamfer produces low stress concentration.
The chamfer can easily enter the gingival crevice.

Disadvantages. Unless used with a gold collar there is greater risk of metal creep at the thin chamfer edge.
The deep chamfer does not provide as much space at the shoulder for porcelain veneering (Fig. 4-99 c).

Chamfer with bevel

This preparation is not recommended since the bevel can easily lift during firing of the porcelain unless very thick gold collars are used.

3. **135° Shoulder with all internal line angles rounded** (Fig. 4-99 d)

This preparation is a modification of the flat shoulder.

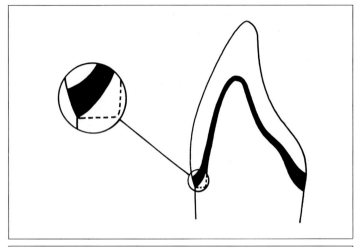

Fig. 4-99c Deep chamfer showing design of gold coping with collar. Recommended for teeth where aesthetics is not of primary importance. Area outlined by dotted line shows the loss of buttressing metal when a flat shoulder (90°) is compared with the chamfer.

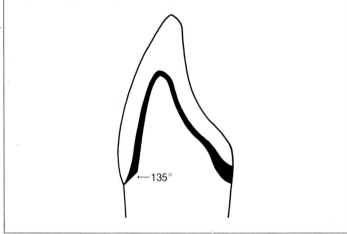

←135°

Fig. 4-99d 135° shoulder with all internal line angles rounded. Recommended preparation for labial shoulder which extends into the root face, and aesthetics is of primary importance.

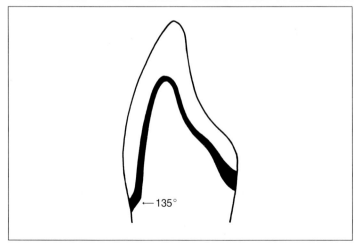

←135°

Fig. 4-99e 135° shoulder showing design of gold coping with collar. Recommended for teeth with marked loss of facial supporting tissue and where aesthetics is not of primary importance.

Advantages. Very useful preparation to use where the labial shoulder is extending well into the root face, e.g. canines with marked gingival recession. The finishing line can be placed sub-gingivally and the axio-gingival floor line angle left at a higher level.
Low stress concentration.
Provides a slip joint.
Easy to enter gingival crevice.

Disadvantages. Same as the flat shoulder if porcelain is fired to a butt fit.

Lingual Shoulder

Since the lingual shoulder can be finished in metal it is obvious that a low stress concentration preparation may be used without regard to its effect on aesthetics. Most operators are agreed that the deep chamfer preparation meets all the requirements for general usage.

Recommended designs for the preparations and metal coping

Standard metal-ceramic crown involving only the anatomical crown and where aesthetics is of primary importance (Fig. 4-99 a or b).
Labial – Flat shoulder (90°)
Lingual – Deep chamfer with gold collar

Standard metal-ceramic crown involving only the anatomical crown and where aesthetics is not of primary importance (Fig. 4-99 c).
Labial – Deep chamfer with 1 mm gold collar
Lingual – Deep chamfer with gold collar

Metal-ceramic crown where there is marked loss of labial supporting tissue and aesthetics is of primary importance (Fig. 4-99 d).
Labial – 135° shoulder or deep chamfer
Lingual – Deep chamfer with gold collar

Metal-ceramic crown where there is marked loss of labial supporting tissue and aesthetics is not of primary importance (Fig. 4-99 e).
Labial – 135° shoulder or deep chamfer with 1 mm gold collar
Lingual – Deep chamfer with gold collar

The Metal-Ceramic Crown Preparation

Typical Maxillary Central Incisor Preparation Operative Procedures

The basic operative procedures for the full porcelain veneer crown described on page 252 of this monograph will still apply when cutting teeth for metal-ceramic restorations . All stages of the porcelain veneer crown preparation should be followed with the exception of the provision of a deep chamfer preparation on the lingual surface, and an increase in labial shoulder width. The stages are as follows:

1. *Labial and lingual depth cuts*

   Instruments – HiDi tapered diamond stones 554 (1.5 shank 1 mm tip) and 555 (1.3 shank 0.8 mm tip). Handpiece – highspeed Kavo super-torque or Adem 350 ball bearing turbine.
   Make a labial depth cut of just over 1.0 mm from the incisal to gingival margin. This cut should enter the labial gingival crevice by 1.0 mm. Extend the depth cut through the incisal edge (one-third height of anatomical crown) and make a lingual depth cut at shoulder area of 0.5 mm (Fig. 4-100).

2. *Preparation of half the lingual shoulder*

   Extend the lingual depth cut at the shoulder so that it connects with the mesial approximal enamel. The approximal enamel should be removed at the same time as a 0.5 mm shoulder is created. The smaller diamond stone (HiDi 555) should be used to open up the approximal space. Protect the adjoining tooth enamel with a steel matrix band during cutting (Fig. 4-101). Make sure that the approximal cut is not more than 10° out of parallel (see page 223) and that the lingual shoulder is not

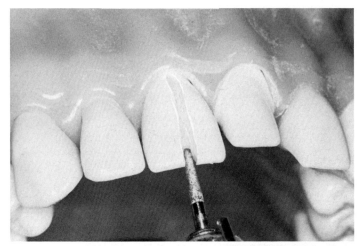

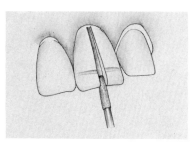

Fig. 4-100 Preparation of a typical maxillary central incisor for a metal-ceramic crown. Labial and lingual depth cuts made with HiDi diamond stone 554 or 555.

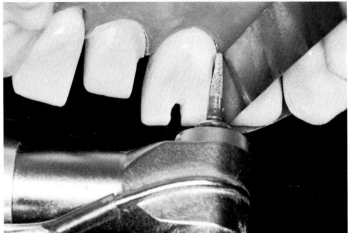

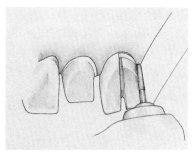

Fig. 4-101 Preparation of a typical maxillary central incisor for a metal-ceramic crown. Lingual shoulder prepared and mesial approximal enamel removed.

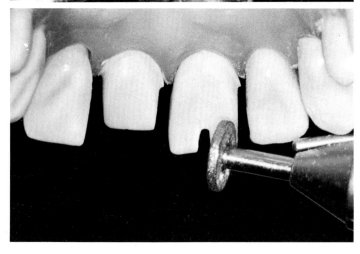

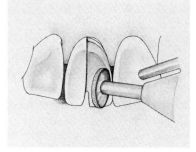

Fig. 4-102 Preparation of a typical maxillary central incisor for a metal-ceramic crown. Reduction of half the lingual surface.

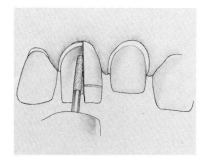

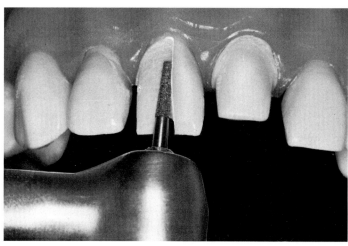

Fig. 4-103 Preparation of a typical maxillary central incisor for a metal-ceramic crown. Reduction of half the labial surface and establishment of shoulder.

deeper than 0.5 mm since this area is to be refined at a later stage with a torpedo-shaped diamond stone.

3. Reduction of half the lingual surface

Remove the remaining half of the lingual enamel with a small diamond wheelstone (HiDi 514 [Fig. 4-102]). The occlusal clearance for a metal-ceramic crown should be at least 1.3 mm if full porcelain coverage is to be achieved. The final accuracy of this clearance may be determined by measuring the lingual thickness of a temporary Epimine resin crown which has already been described on page 263.

4. Reduction of half the labial surface

Remove the mesio-labial enamel using the HiDi 554 or 555 diamond stones at high speed. The shoulder is prepared to the full extent of the original depth cut and should be 1.0 – 1.3 mm deep. The labial shoulder may then be connected with the approximal cut but when doing this it is essential to avoid widening the approximal shoulder which must remain at 0.5 mm (Fig. 4-103).

5. Preparation of labial sub-gingival shoulder

Final deepening of the labial shoulder should be carried out at slow speed in order to avoid damage to the tissues. This may conveniently be done using the Kavo super-torque handpiece running at slow speed (160,000 r.p.m.) or with the Adem electric motor and Kavo intra contra angle handpiece running at 20,000 – 40,000 r.p.m. The average depth of the shoulder should be 1.0 to 1.5 mm below the gingival crest or half the depth of the gingival crevice. Do not deepen the approximal shoulder which should be just level with gingival crest. Where a deep chamfer is required on the labial shoulder, a torpedo-shaped sintered diamond stone should be used at slow speed.

6. Preparation of distal half of tooth

After completion of the mesial half of the tooth preparation, inspect the cut half (Fig. 4-104) and check that the silhouette of the uncut half clearly outlines the ideal section illustrated in Fig. 4-99 (the typical maxillary central incisor prep-

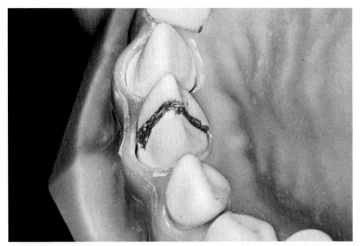

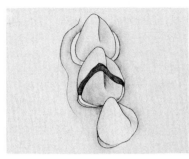

Fig. 4-104 Preparation of a typical maxillary central incisor for a metal-ceramic crown. Silhouette of uncut half of tooth clearly outlined with graphite.

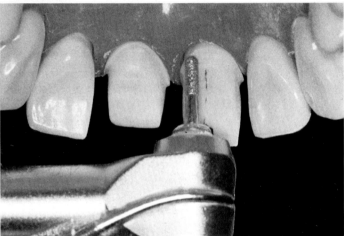

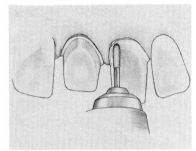

Fig. 4-105 Preparation of a typical maxillary central incisor for a metal-ceramic crown. Preparation of lingual chamfer with torpedo shaped sintered diamond stone or HiDi stone No. 544.

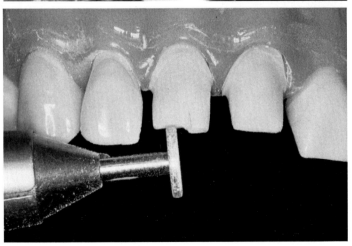

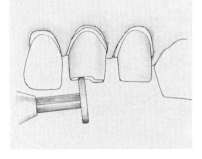

Fig. 4-106 Preparation of a typical maxillary central incisor for a metal-ceramic crown. Reduction of incisal edge.

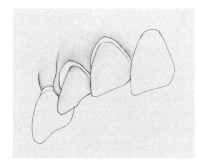

Fig. 4-107a and b Completed preparation of a typical maxillary
central incisor on 11 for metal-
ceramic crowning. (a) Labial
view; (b) Lingual view. Note the
extra width of shoulder on 11
compared with the reduced
shoulder width for the complete
porcelain veneer crown on upper
left central incisor.

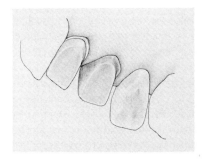

Fig. 4-107c HiDi sintered diamond stone of 1.5 mm diameter
used incorrectly. When directed
towards the preparation or beyond half its depth it will create
a lip on the preparation and
weaken the shoulder margin (a).
When used correctly it will create
a chamfer, providing the diameter
of the stone is at least twice as
great as the depth of the chamfer
(b). The stone should be gently
stroked downwards and out-
wards to ensure that the chamfer
is correctly finished to provide a
slip joint (c).

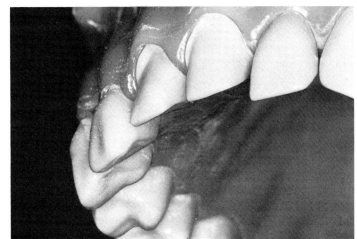

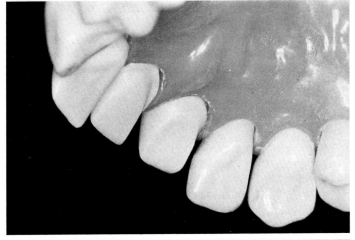

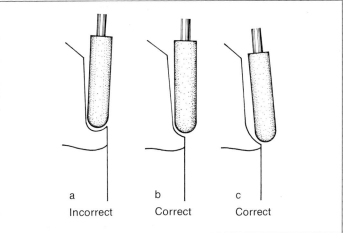

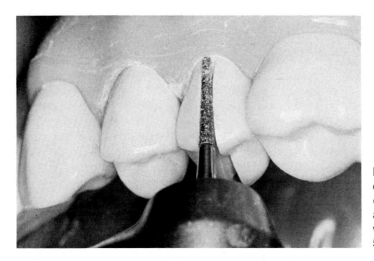

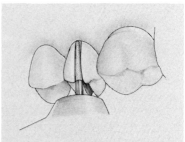

Fig. 4-108 Preparation of a typical maxillary premolar for a metal-ceramic crown. Buccal, lingual and occlusal depth cuts made with tapered HiDi diamond stone 555 as in Fig. 4-75.

aration). If this profile is correct it is a simple matter to repeat all the stages outlined in 1 to 5 above and remove the other half of the tooth.

7. *Preparing lingual long chamfer*

On completing of the outline form of the preparation, a torpedo-shaped sintered diamond stone should be used to create the lingual chamfer. This chamfer is easily superimposed on the original shoulder made at the time of the initial depth cuts (Fig. 4-105).

8. *Reduction of incisal edge*

Refine the bevel at the incisal edge of the preparation with a diamond wheelstone: Cut the bevel at approximately 45 degrees to the lingual surface. Ideally the final length of the preparation should be two-thirds that of the original anatomical crown (Fig. 4-106).

9. *Monitor the depth of the preparation by using a temporary crown as a Master Template*
(see page 263).

10. *Finishing the preparation*

Once the correct outline form of the preparation has been established the surface of the tooth should be smoothed with fine abrasives. The most suitable tools have been discussed on page 268 and each operator must make his own choice of finishing instruments. The completed preparation is illustrated in Fig. 4-107a and b. When a deep chamfer is selected for the labial shoulder finish, the torpedo-shaped sintered diamond tool (A.D. International Ltd.) is an ideal instrument for refining the shoulder Fig. 4-107c.

Typical Maxillary Premolar Preparation for Metal-Ceramic Crown for Full Porcelain Veneer Coverage

1. *Buccal and Lingual Depth Cuts*

Make a buccal depth cut of just over 1.0 mm from the incisal to gingival margin using a tapered diamond stone (HiDi 554 or 555). Repeat this operation on the lingual surface but restrict the gingival cut to a depth of 0.5 mm

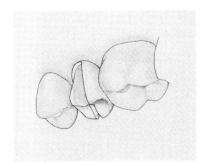

Figure 4-109a

Fig. 4-109a to c   Preparation of a typical maxillary premolar for a metal-ceramic crown. (a) Buccal enamel removed on mesial half. (b) Removal of mesial approximal enamel and creation of a chamfered shoulder. (c) Removal of mesial half of the lingual enamel.

Figure 4-109b

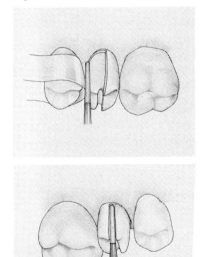

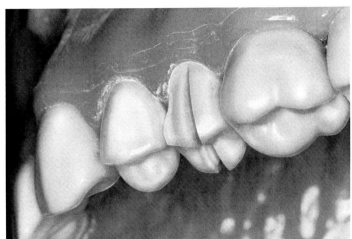

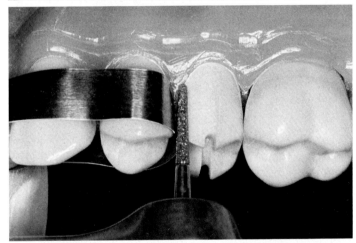

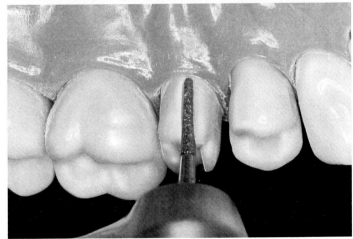

Figure 4-109c

(Fig. 4-108). Connect the two depth cuts by joining them across the occlusal surface. The same diamond stone or a torpedo-shaped stone may be used from two angles and when placed in the cut should be level with the occlusal surface, i.e. the shank of the stone is 1.0 to 1.3 mm in diameter and corresponds to the depth of the cut. The occlusal depth cuts are illustrated in Fig. 4-109 a.

2. *Reduction of mesial half of tooth*

Starting from the buccal depth cut, insert the stone in the base of the cut and reduce the buccal enamel at high speed (Fig. 4-109 a). Continue through the mesial aspect of the tooth so that the approximal enamel is removed to leave a very slight chamfer finish at the margin. Protect the opposing tooth with a steel matrix band (Fig. 4-109 b). Extend the cut lingually and remove the mesial half of the lingual enamel up to the line of the depth cut (Fig. 4-109 c). The lingual shoulder should be just under 0.5 mm deep.

3. *Removal of mesio-occlusal enamel*

Using the same tapered diamond stone, remove the occlusal enamel to a depth of 1.3 – 1.5 mm, taking great care to follow exactly the contour of the occlusal surface (Fig. 4-110). Do not deepen the central fossa unnecessarily and round off the buccal and lingual cusps. In particular, failure to provide room at the cusp tips for metal and porcelain is a common fault often resulting in the technician widening the occlusal table to provide room for porcelain (see page 194).

4. *Removal of distal half of enamel*

On completion of the removal of enamel from the mesial half of the tooth the distal half should now be silhouetted quite clearly (Fig. 4-111 a and b). If the silhouette is correct, it is now a simple matter to repeat all the above steps and remove the distal half of the enamel (Fig. 4-112).

5. *Preparing mesial, distal and lingual chamfer*

On completion of the outline form of the preparation, use a torpedo-shaped sintered diamond stone to create a fine chamfer at the mesial, distal and lingual margins. This chamfer preparation should be not more than 0.3 mm wide on the mesial and distal aspects and not more than 0.5 mm on the lingual aspect. However, it is important that sufficient tooth is removed lingually, otherwise there is again a risk of the technician widening the occlusal table. It is the author's experience that failure to remove sufficient lingual enamel is the commonest cause of over-contoured posterior teeth where full porcelain coverage is desired.

6. Monitor the depth of the preparation by using the Epimine resin crown technique described on page 263.

7. Finishing of the preparation should follow the steps previously described on page 268.

Preparation of the Typical Maxillary Premolar for Partial Porcelain Veneer Coverage

It has already been shown that if the stresses at the metal-ceramic interface in porcelain veneer crowns are to remain minimal then full porcelain coverage of the metal is essential. However, there are occasions where, for occlusal reasons, tooth conservation or provision of adequate retention form, partial coverage of porcelain is desirable. For example, at the beginning of this monograph the problems of developing occlusion in porcelain have been discussed, and many operators still prefer to use gold occlusal

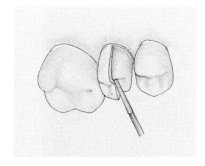

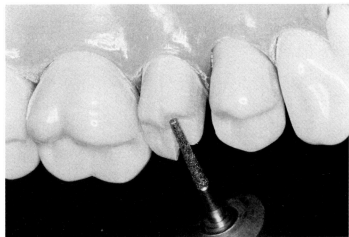

Fig. 4-110 Preparation of a typical maxillary premolar for a metal-ceramic crown. Removal of mesio-occlusal enamel.

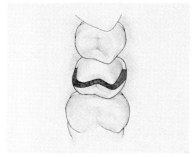

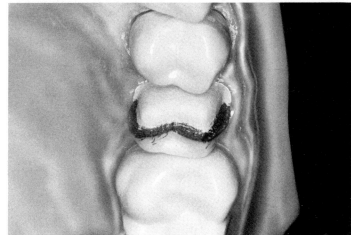

Figure 4-111 a

Fig. 4-111 a and b Preparation of a typical maxillary premolar for a metal-ceramic crown. (a) Completion of occlusal enamel removal from mesial surface revealing silhouette of distal half. (b) Diagram of the silhouette of the distal half of the enamel showing correct contour and ideal shoulder depths. The buccal shoulder may be modified to a 135° angle or deep chamfer where required.

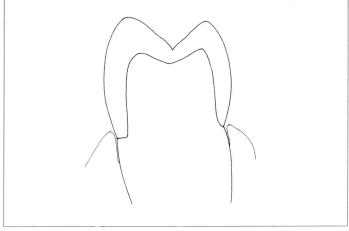

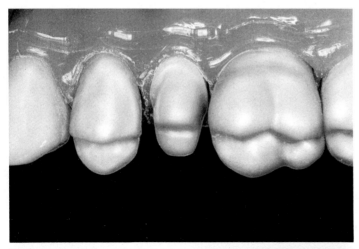

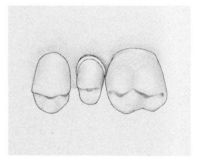

Fig. 4-112a and b   Preparation of a typical maxillary premolar for a metal-ceramic crown. Removal of distal half of enamel completed and preparation finished with sintered diamond stones and polishing cups; (a) buccal view; (b) occlusal view.

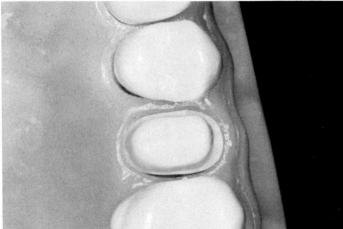

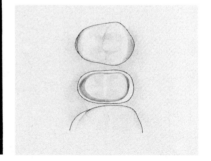

surfaces. There are also some occasions where the clinical crown is too short or the whole tooth is too small to accommodate both metal and porcelain. For these reasons a more conservative preparation is desirable and can be achieved when only porcelain coverage is used on the buccal or labial surfaces.

The preparation of a tooth for partial veneer coverage should follow all the principles laid down for full porcelain coverage except for reduction of the amount of space available on the occlusal, mesial, distal and lingual surfaces since only metal will be used here. The width of

the mesial, distal and lingual shoulders may be reduced to 0.3 mm to provide only a chamfered finishing line. The metal occlusal surface may also be reduced to 0.5 to 0.8 mm. However it is essential that enough space is provided for porcelain on the buccal shoulder which should be cut to its full width (ca. 1.3 mm). In addition, the metal should never be thinned out at the bucco-occlusal margins to accommodate the porcelain (Fig. 4-113a). The reverse should be aimed for and a definite chamfer made in the tooth at the bucco-occlusal table area to accomodate the metal and porcelain (Fig. 4-113b). The de-

Fig. 4-113a and b Diagram of an (a) incorrect preparation of the bucco-occlusal table for porcelain veneer coverage; (b) correct preparation of the bucco-occlusal table for porcelain coverage. A distinct bevel should be made in the buccal cusp so that the porcelain may be finished to a thick metal edge.

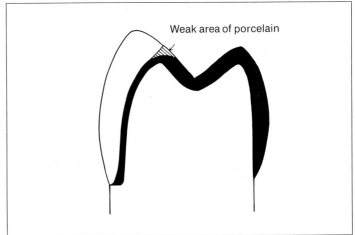

Figure 4-113a

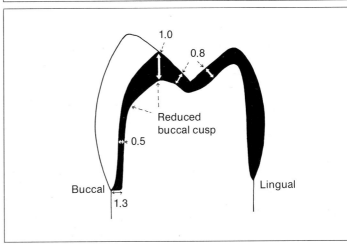

Figure 4-113b

sign of the metal coping may then follow this slope and the metal can be chamfered to provide a butt joint for the porcelain. Under no circumstances should the metal coping exhibit any re-entrant angles or concavities since these are very detrimental to the retention of porcelain. Providing the porcelain covers the outer buccal cusps of the tooth then it has a good chance of resisting fracture.

The doubtful quality of the bond between base metal alloys and dental porcelain does not make them suitable for partial veneer coverage. In addition, the development of occlusion in nickel-chromium alloys is extremely difficult and can be even more of a problem than a pure porcelain surface. For these reasons the author strongly advises only the use of high-fusing gold alloys where metal occlusal surfaces are contemplated. Even where gold alloys are used it is essential to avoid any occlusal contacts at the junction between porcelain and metal if fracture of the porcelain veneer is to be avoided. For this reason the buccal shearing cusps must not be in contact once the patient moves out of centric relationship.

Improving Retention of Metal-Ceramic Crowns

In cases where there is doubt about the retention of metal-ceramic crowns such as in short teeth or heavily destroyed cusp areas two main methods are open to the operator for improving this retention.

1. *Teeth with cusps missing*

   a) Accessory pin anchorage using cast pins in the metal-ceramic crown.

   b) Accessory pins either threaded or friction grip with amalgam or glass ionomer cement cores. Composite resin cores may also be used if carefully lined with cement.

2. *Short teeth*

   Preparation of mesial and distal rails in the tooth with, if necessary, additional rails in the buccal and lingual. Occlusal pin anchorage may also be used as a last resort.

Advantages of Partial Veneer Coverage of Porcelain over Full Veneer Coverage

1. Tooth preparation may be more conservative.
2. Gold occlusal surfaces are more easily built to accurate occlusion.

Disadvantages of Partial Veneer Coverage of Porcelain over Full Veneer Coverage

1. Less aesthetic, particularly in the lower jaw.
2. Increased retention of plaque because of the large volume of metal surface.
3. Increased risk of porcelain fracture because of higher stresses at the metal-ceramic interface.
4. Increased risk of metal creep at the margins after fitting since the metal is not reinforced

by the porcelain. (The non-ductile porcelain prevents any movement of the metal when full coverage is used unless the porcelain fractures.)

Preparation for the periodontally involved tooth

Metal-ceramic crowns are frequently used to splint periodontally involved teeth. The gingival margins around these teeth can be situated well below the original anatomical crown and resultantly the preparation, particularly on the front teeth, must involve the root area. It has already been shown on page 252 that as a preparation extends cervically it enters an area of decreasing circumference of tooth root (see Fig. 4-70). It is therefore impossible to create an adequate shoulder on the labial to accommodate a metal-ceramic crown. A compromise must be made and the following procedures can be adopted.

1. Terminate the preparation supra-gingivally (Fig. 4-114a).
2. Prepare a labial deep chamfer or 135° shoulder terminating just at the gingival margin (Fig. 4-114b).
3. Prepare a deep chamfer with extended bevel Fig. 4-114c). This preparation is not recommended unless a 1 mm thick gold collar is used. The angle of the bevel at the shoulder should be around 70° if an improvement in seal is to be obtained (see page 276).

Aesthetically the extended bevel in Fig. 4-105c will only be acceptable providing the gold collar remains sub-gingivally. However, if the gold collar becomes visible due to gum recession, then the supragingival preparation in Fig. 4-114a can often be a better choice.

In the author's experience the preparation in Fig. 4-114b – the deep chamfer – has proved the best all-around compromise. However, once again, this must be dependent on the length of root exposed since if more than 2−3 mm is in-

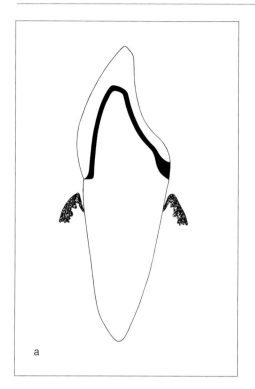

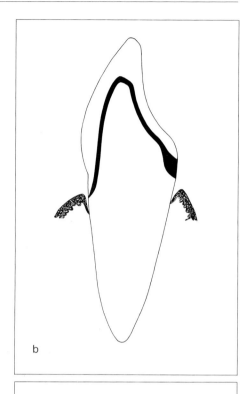

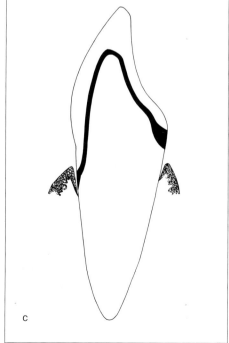

Fig. 4-114a to c (a) Diagram illustrating the preparation of a periodontally-involved tooth in which the shoulder is terminated supra-gingivally. (b) Diagram illustrating the deep chamfer preparation for a periodontally-involved tooth. (c) Diagram illustrating the deep chamfer preparation with gold collar and bevel for a periodontally-involved tooth.

volved, it is far better to decide on a supragingival preparation. It is vital to make this decision prior to commencing the preparation and warn the patient of the technical and biological problems involved. In addition, no matter how expert the ceramist, when he is faced with a decreasing diameter of tooth and reduced thickness for porcelain and metal, inevitably the necks of the teeth prove very difficult to build aesthetically. If the tooth is to remain in correct contour, then there is generally room for only a thin coat of opaque and enamel glaze. This can present great problems due to the high reflectivity and resultant brightness from the opaque porcelain. In order to mitigate this effect it is useful to use a heavily colour-saturated neck dentine powder which will effectively mask the opaque but still provide some depth of translucency (see Figs. 4-29 and 4-30). Alternatively a direct porcelain butt fit might be attempted.

Where aesthetics is not of great importance then a deep chamfer may be used with a 1 mm thick gold collar as advocated on page 283.

Common Faults in Preparation

1. Insufficient removal of buccal or labial enamel particularly at the labio-incisal one-third of the preparation (Fig. 4-115).
2. Insufficient removal of occlusal enamel in posterior teeth particularly at the cusp tips (see Fig. 4-11).
3. Insufficient removal of lingual enamel which may force the ceramist to widen his occlusal table or reduce the gold coping thickness which can increase the risk of metal deformation.
4. Increasing the taper of the preparation beyond 10° and reducing retention of the casting particularly on short posterior teeth.
5. Failure to round off all internal line and point angles, thereby creating stress concentration areas which may cause "pop-off" of the porcelain veneer.

6. Flattening occlusal tables in the preparation instead of following the line of the cusp angles.
7. Inadequate removal of approximal enamel, particularly on the front teeth, leaving insufficient space for metal and porcelain at the cervical third of the tooth.

Biological Considerations

1. Never allow teeth to dry out during preparation. Use a copious supply of water coolant. (Dehydration of teeth will cause aspiration of odontoblasts and an inflammatory response from the pulp which may not be reversible).
2. Avoid injury to gingival tissue by using slower speeds when cutting sub-gingivally.
3. Do not cut into the epithelial attachment. A one-millimetre sub-gingival shoulder depth should be adequate in many clinical situations.
4. Immediately on completion of each preparation, coat the tooth with a polymerisable silicone polyester varnish.* Sealing of the dentine surfaces will prevent accidental dehydration during any subsequent operative procedures. Renew this varnish at each sitting if temporary crowns are removed at "try-in" stages. Clean off the varnish prior to cementation when polyacrylic-based cements are used if good adhesion is to be obtained.
5. Check the sub-gingival margins for any deposits of calculus. These must be removed prior to taking the impression. In particular, calculus in the approximal regions is much more easily removed at the time of crown preparation and often can be present despite careful pre-operative prophylaxis.

---

* Tresiolan varnish. ESPE, Seefeld, West Germany.

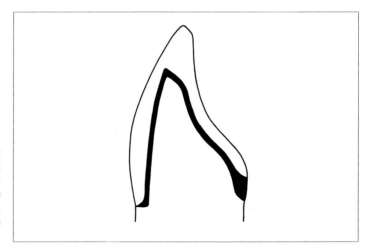

Fig. 4-115 Diagram illustrating the effect of removing insufficient tooth at the labio-incisal one-third. The metal is too near the surface if the tooth is to remain within the original contour of the labial face.

The Impression

The selection of impression materials and the viability of their various clinical techniques will continue to arouse controversy amongst clinicians. To a large extent this has been brought about by the tremendous increase in the number of impression materials available and the development of new elastomers for dental use. The clinician has therefore been tempted into believing that one particular material or technique will ultimately solve all his problems.

In order to appreciate the problems in securing accurate impressions of tooth preparations it is better for the student to understand the biological problems involved and relate them to the properties of the impression material.

The main factors involved in impression taking are the condition and position of the gingival tissue, the surface smoothness of the prepared tooth and the working properties of the impression material. The latter properties will be directly related to the viscosity and rate of set of the impression materials, and its visco-elastic behaviour when applied to the tooth.

If all tooth preparations could be finished supra-gingivally there would be few problems in impression taking. The control of gingival tissue

and the formulation of materials and techniques to displace gingival tissue have been necessitated mainly by aesthetic considerations. In these instances impressions of the full crown preparation can often present the greatest problem since we are concerned with reproducing to a high degree of accuracy an uninterrupted sub-gingival margin. By contrast the intra-coronal preparation can often be an easier proposition since control of the gingival tissue is more easily achieved over a limited area and approximal margins lend themselves very well to the retention of gingival retraction cords.

However, the intra-coronal preparation makes severe demands on the impression material. For example, in some class II cavities when the impression material is withdrawn from the tooth, it may have to survive undercuts which can exert a tensile extension of 30 percent or more (McLean, 1962). Materials that will reproduce accurately these types of intra-coronal preparations must have excellent elastic recovery. In technical terms they must have a low tension and compression set and high resistance to shear.

In the case of the porcelain veneer crown preparation, which is the subject of this monograph, the physical demands on the impression materi-

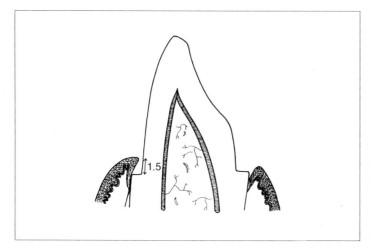

Fig. 4-116 Diagram illustrating the difficulty of taking impressions when shoulder depths of more than 1.5 mm are used. The gingival tissue may easily fold in over the shoulder when the retraction cords are removed.

al are less severe. Although the impression material may have to be withdrawn from undercuts sub-gingival to the shoulder, the amount of strain induced in the material is comparatively small.

When considering the full crown impression material, good dimensional stability, high tear resistance and adequate working properties are more essential than low tension set properties. Although for multiple preparations a high degree of elastic recovery may still be desirable, since non-parallel preparation may be necessary in cases where precision attachments have to be used to overcome badly tilted teeth.

A full crown impression material must also have sufficient initial viscosity to resist displacement by gingival tissue, saliva, tissue fluid or even blood. It must also easily wet the tooth surface but not stick to the tooth on removal.

Relationship of the gingival tissue to the crown or margin

The ease with which an impression of a full crown preparation may be taken is largely determined by the condition and position of the supporting gingival tissue. Shoulder prepara-

tions on full crowns which enter the gingival crevice by more than 1.5 mm will generally prove more difficult to record accurately in any material.

A crown shoulder which has been placed more than 1.5 mm sub-gingivally can present great problems. Even assuming that the gingival condition is healthy, it is apparent that the shoulder is very close to or has already encroached upon the epithelial attachment. Two difficulties will immediately arise during impression taking; the gingival cuff may fold in over the shoulder and the gingival crevice may be obliterated (Fig. 4-116). Either condition will make impression taking very difficult since the gingival retraction cord will not easily displace the collapsed tissue and, because of the absence of a gingival crevice, there may be no room for the retention cord. A false crevice could be created by electrosurgery but this can advance the onset of periodontal disease by damaging the epithelial attachment and forcing a new attachment level too near the alveolar bone (Fig. 4-69).

Even in cases where the epithelial attachment is well below the shoulder, the risk of the gingiva collapsing over the shoulder is still there. It is therefore desirable that after the shoulder preparation is completed that all the margins of the preparation should be completely visible. This type of preparation will only enter the gingival crevice to a depth of just over 1.0 mm. The relationship of the gingival tissue to the shoulder should allow easy access for the impression material and the final restoration may be kept clean at the margins because of this relationship. Once this correct relationship has been established the decision as to what type of impression material or technique to use is not so critical. Access for a copper ring or alternatively an elastomeric material is made easier and the operator's visibility is improved.

Selection of Impression Materials and Techniques

There are two basic techniques for taking impressions of full crown preparations. The copper tube contoured and cut to fit the preparation and the elastic impression taken in a custom-built full or sectional tray.

The Copper Tube Impression

The use of close-fitting and accurately contoured copper tubes containing impression compound is a well tried and widely-taught technique for registering impressions of full crown preparations. The very high viscosity of the impression compound confined in a copper tube is capable of displacing gingival tissue, saliva or blood and, providing the tissue is not trapped under the edges of the band, very accurate impressions of crown shoulders can be recorded. Unfortunately, a copper tube is equally capable of displacing the epithelial attachment and when used carelessly can produce quite severe gingival damage.

For impressions of one or two crown preparations the copper tube technique is a viable system, but when multiple preparations are contemplated, the technique can become time-consuming and tedious. In addition, the problem of locating all the dies made in the copper tube impressions in a full arch impression is a formidable task. Even when only one or two preparations are involved, location of the dies is still a problem. Various techniques have been adopted; for example, early techniques used a wax impression of the tooth stump surrounded by a master plaster impression. The die prepared from the copper tube impression was then located in the wax impression. More recent methods use high viscosity silicone or polysulphide elastomers in a full tray. However, in these cases it is difficult to locate a die in an elastomeric impression of the tooth preparation due to the springiness of the rubber. Alternatively an elastomeric impression may be taken of the copper tube impression in situ. Once again, removal of these impressions may introduce distortion and some inaccuracy.

The Transfer Coping

The most sophisticated approach to locating the individual die prepared from a copper tube impression is by the use of transfer copings. In this case a metal coping is cast to fit the die and the coping is then tried on the tooth preparation in the mouth. An overall arch impression in an elastomeric impression material may then be taken of the transfer coping and the master die located in the coping which is removed in the impression. Again, this system is very adequate for one or two crowns but can introduce inaccuracies when multiple preparations are involved. Unfortunately most copings only fit the master dies with an accuracy of about 40 to 160 μm and resultantly errors can be compounded when several transfer copings are involved. The use of transfer copings will also involve both patient and dentist in an additional visit for the location with all the attendant discomfort of crown removal. However, transfer copings have certain advantages in that they allow the clinician to try the copings in the mouth and establish the accuracy of his master dies. It is therefore desirable when using a copper tube technique to adopt the transfer coping system if maximum accuracy is to be obtained.

The transfer coping can also be used as an aid to registering centric relationship. In this case the copings can be used as a foundation onto which the acrylic occlusal rims can be attached to form a platform for the occlusal registration wax or paste. Alternatively the copings can be used to control the interocclusal space in cases of full mouth reconstruction. For example, a cuspid disclusion could be evaluated by constructing a coping with an anatomically correct lingual surface and any minor correction can then be made by grinding in the mouth.

Although the copper tube technique is still widely used and strongly advocated by some clinicians, the author never uses this technique in ceramic crown and bridgework. The accurate lacation of dies, even where transfer copings are used, remains the main problem. The stone cast made from a full arch elastomeric impression or its equivalent in metal or plastic supported silver plated dies cannot be surpassed in accuracy when multiple restorations are involved.

The following procedures are therefore recommended:

1. Use α-hemihydrate stone models for all intracoronal preparations. (The setting expansion of the stone will improve the fit of MOD castings.)
2. Use silver plated dies for all full crown restorations where porcelain veneers are to be used.

The Elastic Impression

It is important for the clinician to have a good working knowledge of the physical properties of elastic impression materials. Equally an understanding of the basic clinical requirements of an elastic impression material will enable him to select his materials judiciously.

As stated previously, we are concerned with reproducing an uninterrupted sub-gingival margin in the full crown preparation. The control of the gingival tissue is therefore our greatest obstacle. In order to reproduce the shoulder area of a full crown preparation, any elastic impression must be of sufficient viscosity and under sufficient pressure to resist displacement by the gingival tissue. Equally the material, in its fluid state, should not be displaced by seepage of tissue fluid or even blood during setting. Here, then, is the key to the formulation of all elastic impression materials; they must have a limiting viscosity.

If we consider the problem of maintaining intimate contact between the elastic impression material and the tooth preparation during setting, there are several possible ways of doing this.

A low viscosity mix could be used to wet the tooth preparation and this is then adapted under pressure and confined in a high viscosity mix. Alternatively a high viscosity mix could be used to register an impression of the tooth preparation and then re-based with a low viscosity mix which is pressurised and brought into intimate contact with all surfaces of the tooth on reseating the impression.

Other methods that could be used might involve the spraying or brush application of a low viscosity rubber varnish which would act as a primer to wet all the tooth surfaces. The thin elastic film could then be withdrawn attached to a standard elastomeric impression.

However, at the present time the two current approaches to elastic impression taking involve the use of low viscosity syringe mixes. The main methods are as follows:

1. A low viscosity syringe mix is used to "wet" the tooth preparation and is then confined in a high viscosity mix which forms the main bulk of the impression.
2. A high viscosity elastomeric impression of the tooth taken prior to preparation is re-based with a very low viscosity syringe mix.

Both of the above methods rely on the use of high viscosity materials to force the syringe mix material to place and hold it there during setting. Unfortunately, theory does not always work in practice. If the syringe mix material has too low a viscosity, it may still be displaced by tissue fluid, blood or gingival tissue. An elastic gingival tissue can still displace a low viscosity material despite its more viscous backing material. It is for this reason that the relationship of the gingival crevice to the crown shoulder is so important and why the condition of the gingiva has such a marked influence on the accuracy of the impression. Equally the preparation of the gingival crevice to receive the impression material requires careful attention.

The limitations imposed by the oral conditions can now be related to the clinical requirements of an elastic impression material. In the author's opinion the following list of requirements and properties are desirable:

1. *Visco-elastic behavior*

The unset material should be hydrophilic and "wet" the tooth structure. It should not tend to rebound from internal line angles or exhibit any "springiness". Syringe mixes should be capable of being injected through fine bore nozzles and yet have a limiting viscosity which will prevent displacement by gingival tissue or serumal seepage. The set material must not stick to the tooth on removal.

2. *General properties and dispensing techniques*

An elastic impression material should mix easily and have a pleasant taste and smell. The dispensing technique should not involve any elaborate preparation of the material and must give a high degree of repeatable values for quantity of material dispensed.

Impression powders or pastes should not undergo any deterioration during storage periods of at least 2 years at any temperature experienced throughout the world where operative dentistry is feasible.

The mixed material should not cause any inflammatory response from human tissue.

3. *Working time*

The working time of an elastic impression material is the interval between start of mix and the onset of the initial set. This interval is required for insertion of the material into a tray and the seating of the tray in the mouth. An ideal clinical working time for one or two crown impressions would be $1^1/_2$ to 2 minutes and for multiple preparation the working time should not be less than 3 minutes.

4. *Setting time*

The setting time of an elastic impression material at mouth temperature should not be more than 5 minutes for a single crown impression and not more than 8 minutes for multiple preparations. Longer periods than this are irritating for the patient and the clinician.

Surface Reproduction

A dental impression material should reproduce the tooth surface accurately. Generally, it is recognised that if a material will reproduce a 10μm line it is satisfactory (*Hosoda*, and *Fusayama*,

1959). Surface reproduction will depend to some extent on the degree of wetting of the tooth surface and, as described previously, is closely connected to visco-elastic behaviour. Good surface reproduction is also related to the material's resistance to deterioration in the presence of blood or moisture.

Compatibility with Model Materials

An elastic impression can only be considered versatile if it is compatible with all our current model materials. The impression should be easily electroplated and compatible with stone, resin or cement dies. The material should also be capable of having more than one stone cast poured into it without suffering any dimensional change.

Dimensional Stability

An elastic impression material, after its final set period, should undergo the minimal dimensional change. A linear shrinkage of not more than 0.05 to 0.1 percent can be tolerated during the first hour but shrinkages in excess of 0.2 percent must be regarded as undesirable (*McLean,* 1962). In particular, once these higher figures are reached, electroplating of dies becomes increasingly hazardous due to the longer period required for this procedure.

Coefficient of Thermal Expansion

The dimensional changes occurring in an impression material on cooling from mouth to room temperature may be of significance if the coefficient of thermal expansion is high. If a material contracts by more than 0.2 percent on cooling from 37 °C to 22 °C, then errors in model fabrication can occur. However, in cases where the elastic impression has a high coefficient of expansion, the use of an incubator to store the impression during pouring of the cast at 37 °C can solve the problem.

Elasticity

The elastic recovery of a set impression material determines to a large extent the permanent distortion that occurs when the impression is withdrawn from undercuts in the mouth. This elasticity should be maximal up to 30 percent strain in the material since, as previously explained, strain levels above this figure are not likely to occur in the mouth. The elastic recovery of a deformed elastomer is time dependent and will vary with different materials.

In the case of the full crown impression, strains of 30 percent are seldom incurred. However, a good elastic recovery is still a most desirable property in an impression material and ideally materials should be developed that will not distort permanently at 30 percent strain. The failure of recovery in an elastic impression material is generally measured in terms of "Tension or Compression set". The rubber would be stretched or compressed and any permanent distortion measured after release of the force producing the strain. This failure in recovery could then be expressed in centimetres per centimetre. For example, if a length of polysulphide rubber was stretched by 20 percent, this induces a 20 percent strain. A polysulphide rubber at this level of strain would generally have a "Tension set" of around 0.002 to 0.003 cm per cm, i.e. for every one centimetre of length of rubber the permanent distortion would be 0.002 to 0.003 centimetres (20−30 μm). The permanent distortion in an elastic impression could therefore be expressed in terms of percentage, either for compression or tension set.

In the case of the British Standard 4269 Pt I for Elastomeric impression materials, the tension set for silicone and polysulphide elastomers at 50 % strain is required to be 1.0 and 2.5 percent respectively: materials that meet these requirements have been found to be very accurate under clinical conditions.

Tearing Energy

When an elastic impression material is withdrawn from an undercut it should not tear easily. This applies particularly to material present in the sub-gingival crevice. Thin sections of rubber entrapped in the crevice may easily be torn on withdrawal of the impression, and sometimes might even be left inadvertently in the crevice. The tearing energy of an elastic impression material is therefore of great importance, and may be defined as the energy per unit area of new surface formed in the tearing process. When taking impressions of multiple full crown preparations it is therefore very important that syringe type rubbers should have a high tearing energy. The general order of tearing energies for the elastic impression materials is as follows:

Polysulphide > polyether > silicone > alginate > reversible hydrocolloid

Cost

The cost of any impression material plays some part in a clinician's decision as to whether it should be used. However, if one relates the cost of current impression materials to the total overhead on any type of full crown construction, the impression material represents only a small fraction of the total. Inaccuracy leading to the remake of a crown is the most expensive item in any crown and bridge practice and one re-make far outweighs differences in cost between impression materials. Other factors such as the necessity for employing auxiliary help in mixing, or the need for custom-built trays may influence the cost of full crown construction a little more. However, if an impression material is consistent in its performance and its clinical technique is not over-elaborate, then cost should be a small factor in considering its use. Versatility should be the key-word for any impression material since every clinician or technician has his own ideas on impression taking or model preparation. In particular with laboratory work sharing an even greater part in crown and bridge practice, an impression material's ability to remain dimensionally stable during storage and also its compatibility with all types of die materials is becoming increasingly important.

As yet, there is no material that fulfills all the above requirements but manufacturers are constantly striving to make the all-purpose material.

Types of Elastic Impression Material

There are four main types of elastic impression material:

Reversible Hydrocolloid

Polysulphide Rubber

Silicone Rubber

Polyether Rubber

Details of the various physical properties of these materials have been well documented by *Phillips* (1973) and *Braden* (1975). However, it is useful to consider briefly the chemistry and properties of the newer elastomeric impression materials. These may be classified as follows:

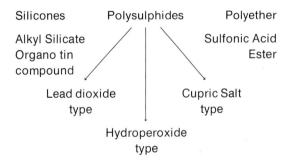

Silicone rubbers used for dental impressions are mainly of the α-w hydroxy terminated type, using organo tin compound activated alkyl silicate setting reagents (*Braden,* and *Elliot,* 1966). They are usually dispensed as a paste, containing the polymer and filler, and a catalyst liquid containing the setting reagents. Unfortunately, during setting the current silicones liberate alcohol during their condensation polymerisation which results in high shrinkage of the material when stored for long periods.

More recently a new type of silicone rubber has been introduced using a chloroplatinic acid catalyst. This new type of silicone is of great interest since during setting the cross-linking reaction is one of addition (not condensation), so that no by-products are formed. These materials exhibit almost zero shrinkage and are very easily dispensed as a two-paste system.

Dental Polysulphides are based on Thiokol LP-2, a standard industrial polymer and consist of a two-paste system. The base paste consists of Thiokol LP-2, a filler such as titanium dioxide, lithopone or zinc sulphide, and a plasticiser (e.g. a chlorinated paraffin). The activator or catalyst paste contains the setting reagent, some filler and a plasticiser as in the base (*Braden,* 1974).

Lead dioxide (PbO_2) is the most common setting reagent, and is responsible for the dark brown colour of the catalyst pastes. Typical of these materials are Permlastic, Coe-flex and Neo-Galt. Alternative catalysts are based on organic hydroperoxides such as t-butyl hydroperoxide and typical examples are products such as MIM and Rubber-Jel.

A newer material, Omniflex, contains a copper salt as a setting reagent which gives the material a blue colour.

A recently-developed polysulphide developed by *Braden* at the London Hospital utilizes a zinc oxide catalyst.

Polyether Rubbers were developed at ESPE in West Germany and the base paste consists of an imine terminated polyether polymer, a silicate filler and a glycol ester plasticiser. The catalyst paste contains a benzene sulphonate ester as a setting reagent together with filler and plasticiser as in the base paste. Setting results from reaction of the sulphonate and the terminal imine groups.

It is now essential to consider how these materials satisfy the requirements listed previously for an ideal elastic impression material and to compare their advantages and disadvantages.

Reversible Hydrocolloid

Advantages

Simple dispensing technique with the material always available if kept in a storage bath. May be used in stock trays, easily wets the tooth surface and has excellent flow.

Not affected by increased temperature or humidity.

Good shelf life.

Adequate working time but with rapid setting (gelation) time on cooling.

Low cost and all equipment is easily cleaned and maintained.

Disadvantages

Viscosity too low and may be displaced by gingival tissue.

Poor tension set by comparison with the elastomeric materials. The material is easily torn. Sensitive to blood or saliva.

Not dimensionally stable if two casts are poured.

Cannot be electroplated. Should not be stored due to high shrinkage on dehydration.

Polysulphide Rubber

Advantages

May be prepared in varying degrees of viscosity and is not easily displaced by gingival tissue.
Compatible with all types of die material and can be silver plated.
Remains dimensionally stable when more than one cast is poured.
Good working time.
Good shelf life.
Better elastic proportions than the reversible hydrocolloids.
High tearing energy.

Disadvantages

Sensitive to temperature and humidity.
Material is hydrophobic and does not easily wet the tooth surface. Air bubbles may be entrapped which can cause collapse of small surface areas.
Unpleasant taste and odour.
Stains clothing and is messy to use.
Long setting time for individual restorations.
Requires accurate dispensing since reduction of catalyst concentration (brown paste) will markedly slow the set and prevent the development of good elastic properties.
High coefficient of thermal expansion.

Silicone Rubber (Organo-tin catalysts)

Advantages

May be prepared in varying degrees of viscosity to resist displacement of gingival tissue.
Remains dimensionally stable over short periods when more than one cast is poured.
Simple dispensing and mixing technique. Pleasant taste, odour, and clean to handle.
Excellent elastic properties giving a very low tension or compression set.

Disadvantages

Sensitive to high temperatures.
Material is hydrophobic and does not easily wet the tooth.
Short working time for multiple crown impressions.
Higher shrinkage than polysulphide rubbers.
Cannot be electroplated very easily.
Poor shelf life.
Small variations in catalyst concentration can markedly affect the working and setting time.
May exhibit high shrinkage during storage.

Silicone Rubber (Chloroplatinic acid catalyst)

Advantages

May be prepared in varying degrees of viscosity to resist displacement by gingival tissue.
Best dimensional stability of all the elastomeric materials.
Simple dispensing and mixing technique.
Pleasant taste, odour, and very clean to handle.
Excellent elastic properties giving a very low tension or compression set.
Can be electroplated.

Disadvantages

Material is hydrophobic and does not easily wet the tooth surface.
High cost due to platinum catalyst.
Lower tearing energy.

Polyether Rubber

Advantages

May be prepared in varying degrees of viscosity to resist displacement by gingival tissue.
Excellent dimensional stability when stored dry.
Compatible with all types of die material and can be silver plated.

Remains dimensionally stable when more than one cast is poured.

May be prepared to give various working times to suit all types of impression taking.

Good shelf life.

Pleasant taste, odour, and clean to handle.

Disadvantages

Difficult to remove from the mouth due to its hardness. It tears more easily than the polysulphides.

May stick to the teeth during removal due to hydrophilic nature of material.

Fine margins or thin preparations may be broken from stone casts during removal of the impression, due to hardness of rubber.

High absorption of water.

Insufficient catalyst results in long set and sticky surfaces.

Prolonged immersion in electroplating solutions may cause swelling of the impression.

Evaluation of Elastic Impression Materials

The reversible Hydrocolloids will continue to set a high standard for all impression materials. When used in every type of restoration they provide impressions of exceptional accuracy. However, their main disadvantage in ceramic crown and bridgework is their inability to accept metal plating or remain dimensionally stable during the pouring of two or more casts. It is possible to use a master cast from a reversible hydrocolloid and duplicate it in a material that will accept electroplating but this does tend to compound any errors in dimensional stability. It is the author's opinion that extensive ceramic work should be made on metal dies and this applies particularly to the student in ceramics where dies are very easily damaged. Stone casts involving several teeth can also be easily broken when metal splints or bridgework are being made.

Silicones (organo-tin compounds) have some attraction, particularly with regard to their ease of handling and general cleanliness. However, their major fault is shrinkage due to the use of volatile liquid catalysts. In addition, where extensive preparations are involved, the short working time of the silicone is a disadvantage.

The use of heavy body (high viscosity) silicone rubbers for use as preliminary impressions of the tooth preparation and to act as a tray is receiving increasing attention. The rebasing of these impressions with a low viscosity silicone mix has great appeal for many dentists who find the polysulphide elastomers rather messy to handle. However, as previously stated, the organo-tin catalysed silicone elastomers have a higher shrinkage than the polysulphide rubbers and this will occur even in the heavy body materials. It should also be noted that even when a heavy body silicone impression is employed, the rebase technique using the low viscosity mix will not easily displace gingival tissue. Some form of gingival retraction is usually necessary. The author considers that the only main advantage with this type of material lies in its ease of handling for multiple crown preparations. However, this can easily be outweighed by problems of dimensional stability, and the author has never experienced consistent clinical results with any form of rebase technique using silicone elastomers based on organo-tin compounds.

Silicones (chloroplatinic acid catalysts) represent a major step forward in the chemistry of the silicone elastomers. Because they set by an addition reaction, their shrinkage is minimal. Secondly, they can be manufactured as a two-paste system which greatly facilitates the dispensing and mixing technique, since both pastes can have the same viscosity. They are also not particularly sensitive to humidity or temperature so that their setting time is very consistent. In addition, these new silicones can be electroplated. The development of the chloroplatinic acid catalysed silicones has very nearly achieved all that is required in an impression material, with one major exception. Like all silicone materials, they are hydrophobic and do not easily wet the tooth surface. In addition they still have low tearing energy. This means that in multiple full crown impression the recording of the sub-gingival crevice can be more difficult than with the polysulphides. The high cost of these new silicones must also be taken into account but, as explained previously, this represents a minor part of the overall cost of crown and bridgework.

The polyether elastomers must now be considered close rivals to the polysulphides with regard to their dimensional stability and working properties. By using a two-paste system the manufacturer has overcome the problem of shrinkage caused by volatile liquid catalysts. However, a reduction in the hardness of the polyether rubbers is very desirable if they are to rival the polysulphides. A lesser disadvantage is their high water absorption but this is only of clinical significance during prolonged immersion in water. The polyether impression materials tend to stick to teeth and particularly in the case of the intra-coronal preparation, inaccuracies may occur due to distortion on removal. Another aspect which deserves attention is their failure to penetrate the gingival crevice quite as easily as the polysulphide rubbers, with the result that sub-gingival registration is a little less sharp although the margins of the preparation can be unaffected. One of their great advantages is the ease with which they accept electroplating.

The polysulphides still offer a great number of advantages, but the new chloroplatinic acid catalysed silicones must rival them for many usages. The high tearing energy and wettability of the polysulphides still make them the materials of choice in complex crown and bridgework. A criticism levelled at them of their long setting time may be easily corrected for the single tooth impression by the incorporation of one or two drops of water which hasten cross-linking of the rubber.

Their main disadvantage is that they are messy materials to handle and can easily stain clothing. However, never types of catalyst are improving this aspect and materials such as Omniflex (cupric salt), or the newer zinc oxide or carbonate type are cleaner to handle and can be made faster setting. The hydroperoxide types are also cleaner to handle but due to their volatile catalyst will shrink more than the other types. In addition, the hydroperoxides have a rather pungent smell and unpleasant taste. Of the three types of polysulphides on the market, the lead dioxide and cupric salt types are generally most satisfactory.

Clinical Recommendations

1. For registering multiple full crown impressions, polysulphide materials should be used in the syringe. Newer types of cupric salt or zinc carbonate catalysed polysulphides are cleaner to handle in the syringe. Heavy body polysulphides should then be used for the tray mix.
2. For individual or limited numbers of full crown preparations, the new chloroplatinic acid catalysed silicones possess the best dimensional stability, working qualities and cleanliness. However, care must be taken with these materials to secure a dry field if the sub-gingival crevice area is to be recorded accurately.
3. Intra-coronal preparations involving deep undercuts may be recorded most accurately with the chloroplatinic acid catalysed silicones.
4. If rebase techniques are employed in which an elastomeric impression is taken of the teeth prior to preparation, then systems using polysulphide rubber in the syringe are preferable when rebasing the impression. Current systems such as Kerr's "Accralastic" or Coe's "Speed Tray" are suitable. The use

of a polysulphide system reduces shrinkage of the impression. However, it must be noted that with all rebase techniques, the set tray mix has minimal elasticity and will not easily withdraw from undercuts. The tray mix should therefore allow plenty of room for the rebase syringe mix so as to use the latter's elastic recovery properties to the maximum. It is for the above reasons that the system outlined in 1 above is to be preferred, since an elastomeric material with excellent tension or compression set properties may be used in the tray.

Procedures for taking Polysulphide or Polyether Elastomeric Impressions

A full arch impression is necessary for most cases involving ceramic crown and bridgework. Such an impression allows both dentist and technician to evaluate any occlusal abnormalities and ensure that his restoration is in harmony with the adjoining teeth. A custom-built tray is an essential part of this technique if the polysulphide or polyether rubbers are to be used to their best advantage.

Custom-built trays may be made either by hand-forming a cold-curing acrylic resin or by vacuum-forming ready-made acrylic sheeting onto a diagnostic stone cast. Instructions for using these materials are supplied by the manufacturers.

Requirements for a Custom-Built Tray

1. The tray must be close-fitting and not extend further than 3.0 mm beyond the gingival margins of the teeth.

2. The correct spacing for the elastomeric impression material should not exceed 3.0 mm and be not less than 2.0 mm. Wax covered with tin-foil or asbestos liners will provide this space during moulding of the tray.

3. At least three occlusal stops should be provided on the tray, centred over the incisor and molar regions. Such a tripod will stabilize the tray and maintain correct thickness of impression material during seating. Occlusal stops may be easily provided by removing the wax or asbestos spacers over the fossae of the first or second molars and the incisal edges of the centrals (Fig. 4-117).

4. The tray must have sufficient thickness to resist distortion during removal. It must also be provided with strong handles. The importance of controlling the thickness of the elastomeric impression cannot be over-emphasized. It has been shown by a number of workers (*Phillips,* 1973; *McLean,* 1958) that a large bulk of elastomeric material is liable to greater distortion or shrinkage than an even layer of material. A 3.0 mm layer of elastomer will show very little linear shrinkage when restrained in a tray and linear contraction figures of less than 0.1 percent can be maintained even after 24 hours.

Preparation of the Gingival Tissue

In order to obtain accurate impressions of a full crown preparation, certain requirements must be fulfilled.

1. There must be sufficient space between the crown shoulder and tissue to provide access and ensure adequate bulk of impression material.

2. The gingival tissue should suffer the minimum of trauma commensurate with the prevention of serumal seepage or haemorrhage.

The importance of starting with healthy gingival tissue has already been emphasized. Equally

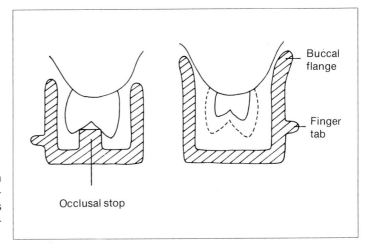

Fig. 4-117 Diagram of section through a custom-built tray showing placement of occlusal stops and ideal thickness for impression material.

the correct relationship between the crown shoulder and the gingival crevice has been defined. The shoulder should never enter the crevice by more than half the depth of the gingival crevice. In the average case this will give a shoulder depth of not more than 1.5 mm.

If these requirements have been fulfilled it may then be stated that the use of strong chemicals or electro-surgery to expose the cervical margins of a preparation are both unnecessary and can be positively injurious.

Methods of retracting gingival tissue may be classified into three groups (*Brown,* 1967; *Tay,* 1974):

1. Mechanical

2. Mechanical-chemical

3. Surgical

The mechanical and mechanical-chemical methods obtain adequate retraction by displacing tissue laterally and are conservative in nature.

The surgical methods remove interfering or pathologically-involved tissue and should be regarded as a radical approach to impression taking.

Mechanical Retraction

Mechanical retraction of the gingival tissue may be undertaken with the use of heavy gauge rubber dam or untreated cotton cord placed in the gingival crevice. The author does not use rubber dam either in the preparation of the full crown or in impression taking. The reasons for this are that the rubber dam must obscure the relationship between the crown shoulder and the gingival tissue. Secondly, an impression taken with the rubber dam in place prevents the operator from obtaining an accurate recording of the position and topographical anatomy of the surrounding gingiva. A failure to record this relationship places the ceramic technician at a serious disadvantage if he is to do full justice to the contour of the cervical region of the crown. The rubber dam has many vital uses in operative dentistry but its routine use in porcelain or metal-ceramic work can result in incorrect relationship between restoration and tissue.

By contrast the use of chemically untreated cotton cord placed in the gingival crevice is to be strongly advocated. If the gingival crevice can be exposed by such means without resort to astringents, then a healthy gingiva is even more certain to be secured. Unfortunately, the control of serumal seepage or haemorrhage is not always achieved by this method and the use of chemicals is forced upon the operator.

Mechanical-chemical Retraction

The use of chemically impregnated cord is the most common method to retract gingival tissue. The decision as to which chemical or chemicals to use in the cord is more controversial.

The use of several strands of adrenaline cords can be highly dangerous, particularly when applied to lacerated tissue. Increase in heart rate and a rise in blood pressure may· occur. Adrenaline cords should never be used on persons suffering from cardiovascular disease, diabetes or hyperthyroidism. The British National Formulary recommends that the maximum parenteral dose of adrenaline 1:1000 is 0.5 ml. This dose may easily be exceeded even by the use of 5 cm lengths of 8:100 solution adrenaline hydrochloride impregnated cords.

Cords saturated with escharotic or caustic drugs such a zinc chloride and trichloracetic acid will also cause severe tissue reaction and even necrosis.

For this reason the author never makes use of these chemicals.

A useful gingival retraction cord used in the author's practice is "Racestyptine".* Each cord consists of four thin strands which may be separated to give various thicknesses of cord. Each centimetre of cord is impregnated with:

Aluminium trichloride	500 mcg
Lignocaine	325 mcg
Oxyquinol	2 mcg

Whatever the choice of retraction cord, it cannot be emphasized too often that if impression

* Racestyptine, Specialites Septodont, 29 Rue les Petites, Eurics, 75010, Paris.

taking is to be made easy, then the gingival tissue must be healthy. If tissues are ulcerated or lacerated, the operator will be fighting for time against pinpoint areas of bleeding and serumal seepage. The chances of securing an accurate impression of multiple preparations will be minimal.

Technical considerations

On completion of the crown preparation, it is generally far better to place accurately fitting temporary restorations and have the patient return for impression taking in a week to ten days. Not only does this enable the tissues to recover but any slight recession of the gingiva can be compensated for by deepening of the crown shoulder. In particular, this period of "tissue resting" is often invaluable when multiple crown preparations are undertaken. Under no circumstances should overextended temporary crowns be used to retract tissue. The damage that can be caused by this technique can seldom be corrected.

The interval prior to impression taking can also be a useful period to encourage the patient to be even more vigourous in his oral hygiene technique. Often well-made temporary crowns can eliminate the defects of badly-fitting restorations and a rapid improvement in the gingival condition may occur in periods even as short as one week.

The following procedures should now be adopted:

1. Cleanse all the preparations with atomised water and a 3 % solution of hydrogen peroxide.
2. Isolate the preparation with cotton-wool rolls and pack fluffed-out cotton-wool around the margins. This can prove a far more effective way of drying the gingival crevice than using a warm-air spray.

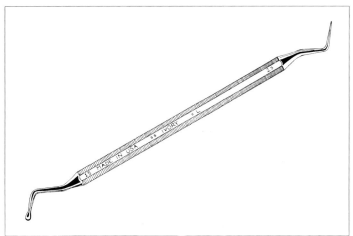

Fig. 4-118 Gingival packing instrument.

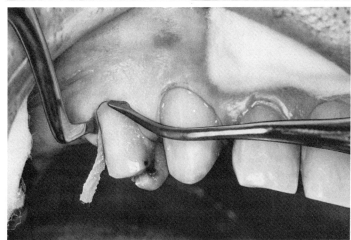

Fig. 4-119 Insertion of primary gingival packing cord using two instruments, one to hold the free end and one to pack the cord.

3. After 2 or 3 minutes, remove the cotton-wool around the preparation and pack one strand of gingival retraction cord into the crevice where the tooth undercut is greatest.

Gingival packing instrument

In order to avoid damaging tissue, it is preferable to use a blunt edged instrument. However, if the blade of this instrument is too thick, it cannot easily enter the gingival crevice. The author has designed a suitable instrument for this purpose and the blade is thin, blunt and oval in shape, making it easy to insert sub-gingivally (Fig. 4-118).

4. Hold one end of the cord in position and, using a second gingival packer, gently push the next section of cord to position (Fig. 4-119). Always make sure that the cord is being packed in the direction of the "warp". Generally the cord is coiled anticlockwise so that it should be packed with the warp in a clockwise direction.

5. The excess length of cord is cut so that the

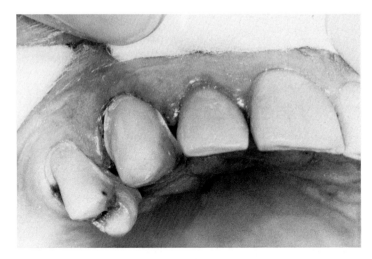

Figure 4-120a

Figure 4-120b

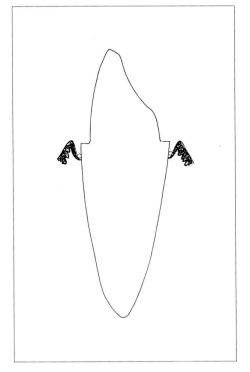

Fig. 4-120a and b   (a) Primary cord in position on 14, 13 showing all the shoulder areas of the preparation clearly visible. (b) Diagram showing placement on a maxillary central incisor.

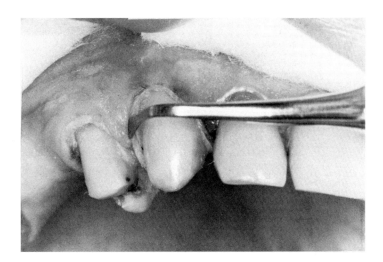

Figure 4-121a

Figure 4-121b

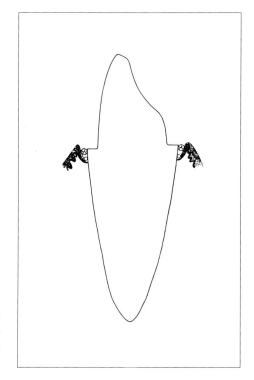

Fig. 4-121a and b (a) Secondary gingival retraction cord in position with free end left for removal. (b) Diagram showing placement, on a maxillary central incisor.

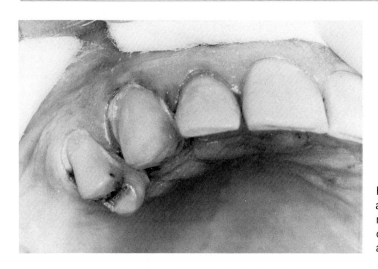

Fig. 4-122 Removal of secondary cord prior to injecting syringe mix. Gingival crevice should be clearly outlined and free of blood and debris.

free end can be tucked into the gingival crevice. At this stage the cord should completely encircle the tooth and the shoulder of the crown preparation be completely visible (Fig. 4-120). This cord, termed the "primary cord" is often left in situ during impression taking.

6. A double strand of gingival retraction cord is now packed over the primary cord and will provide lateral displacement of the gingiva (Fig. 4-121). This cord must not be forced to position, otherwise the circular fibres of the epithelial attachment could be damaged and a false pocket created in which the impression material could lodge.

7. The cords should not be left in position for more than ten minutes and generally it is advantageous to leave them only during the dispensing and preparation of the impression material. This should not occupy more than five minutes.

During the preparation of the tooth for impression taking, it is vital not to allow the dentine to dry out. The use of silicone polyester varnish has already been advocated and the author also uses loose cotton-wool to cover each tooth during the packing of gingival cords. This is particularly advantageous when multiple preparations are being treated. The clinician has only to see the pain produced by dehydration of multiple crown preparations without local anaesthetic to realise how severe the effects of dehydration are on large exposed tracts of dentine. When a local anaesthetic is administered, it is easy to forget that a pulp is being exposed to severe trauma even when no instruments are being used.

8. If the tissues are in a healthy condition and the cord correctly placed, once the retaining cotton-wool and the secondary cord is removed the margins of the preparation should be clearly visible (Fig. 4-122). In addition, there should be no haemorrhage or saliva present which might cause failure of wetting of the tooth surface by the impression material.

If these conditions do not exist then it is generally a waste of time to proceed with the impression. A good idea of the tissue's condition can often be obtained when the temporary restorations are removed. Oedematous or bleeding tissue will be immediately apparent and steps must be taken to correct this. Firstly, the temporary restorations must be checked for fit or else a longer period of healing and meticulous hygiene must be instituted. Failing this, periodontal surgery and a further review should be considered.

Preparation of Shoulder areas

If, after removal of the secondary packing cord, the shoulder preparation is almost level with the gingival margin, it may be advisable to deepen the shoulder very slightly with a slow-running sintered diamond stone or chisel. In particular, the student is advised to take careful note of any gingival creep in the canine areas since these teeth are particularly susceptible to post-operative gingival recession.

Surgical Retraction

The most widely-used surgical method of creating space for impression materials in the gingival crevice is by the use of electro-surgery. A high-frequency current emitted from the electrode will cut the tissue and widen the crevice. There should be no associated haemorrhage and minimal tissue damage with a resultant short period of healing.

Electro-sectioning using fine wire J-loop electrodes produces the least amount of tissue coagulation whereas electro-coagulation requires a deeper penetration and necessitates the use of conical solid electrodes or flexible silver cylindrical electrodes. If the current is too high, excessive sparking and coagulation of tissue occurs whilst too low a current causes the tissue to cling to the electrode. For this reason current setting is often done by trial and error on a piece of raw meat.

The author makes very limited use of electro-surgery during impression taking but prefers to use this instrument for preparatory work on the tissue prior to cutting teeth. Removal of hyperplastic tissue, recontouring gingival "cuffs" or treating pathologically-involved tissue may all be done at the time of tooth preparation. A temporary restoration must then be placed to allow the tissues to heal and assume their new position in relation to the tooth margins. If the tissues are allowed to heal and the gingival margins are pink and healthy, then the use of electro-surgery to widen the crevice is unnecessary and may result in exposure of the labial margins of the tooth preparation. The routine use of electro-surgery is not recommended for gingival retraction.

The so-called "tooling" of the gingiva with flame-shaped diamond stones is equally deprecated except for removal of pathologically involved tissue. If gingival tissue is to remain near to its original level after impression taking, then the cardinal point for any student to bear in mind is that "he may enter the gingival crevice but not trespass upon its hospitality." More damage is done in the name of gingival retraction than any other procedure and phrases such as "management of gingival tissue" are used often because the tissues have been made unmanageable during tooth preparation and construction of temporary restorations.

Steel scalpel and electrosurgical cutting on gingival tissues and alveolar bone*

Oringer (1976) has given an excellent summary on the merits of electrosurgical cutting. It is impossible for any clinician, because of superior expertise, to improve the effects of electrosurgical cutting on gingival tissues and underlying alveolar bone. Conversely, the lack of optimal expertise in the use ot this method can degrade its cutting efficiency with accompanying destructive effects on the gingiva and alveolar bone.

Second, different factors influence the quality and effects of steel scalpel and electrosurgical cutting. Tissue is cut with a scalpel by forcing the blade into the tissue with manual pressure. The sharpness of the blade and the amount of pressure used are the only factors that the clinician controls that directly influence the cutting. The former determines the quality and the latter the depth of the cutting. (Sterility is an indirect factor; its influence is limited to the post-operative effects on the wound healing).

Electrosurgical cutting results from conversion of the radiofrequency (RF or CWRF) current into heat energy by the resistance of the tissues to passage of the current. The heat disintegrates and volatilizes the tissue cells in the path of the activated electrode, causing them to split apart without manual pressure. If the RF current is applied to the tissues properly and the correct amount of current is used, there is virtually no destructive effect on the immediately adjacent and subjacent tissues. However, if the current is improperly applied or the improper amount of current is used, the cutting efficiency is greatly impaired, causing a destructive increase in the lateral heat penetration into the adjacent and subjacent tissues. If the heat energy is permitted to accumulate, the destruction is greatly increased and more widespread. The destructive effect on underlying alveolar bone is particularly devastating when this occurs.

Thus, although efficient scalpel cutting requires special knowledge of anatomy and physiology, it does not require the same degree of expertise in the manipulation of the instrument as does electrosurgical cutting.

Factors governing optimal electrosurgical cutting

Optimal electrosurgical cutting involves more than substituting an activated electrode for a steel scalpel, since experience in the use of electrosurgery is no insurance of its optimal use. Experience is predicated on time and familiarity; expertise is predicated on skill, and the two are not necessarily equal. Use of elec-

trosurgery with indifferent skill for a long time may qualify the user as experienced, but not as an expert.

When using electrosurgical cutting the following factors should be adhered to rigidly.

– The electrosurgical cutting should be performed with either fully rectified or continous wave current.
– The optimal cutting power of the electrosurgical device used should be predetermined before cutting is begun.
– Activated electrode contact with the tissues should not be maintained for more than a brief fraction of a second per application.
– The electrode should be kept in rapid motion while in contact with the tissues.
– The electrode should be used with the maximum speed compatible with efficient, "surgically pure" cutting.
– The cutting should be performed with the predetermined optimal cutting power output.
– At least five to ten seconds should be permitted to elapse after each application of the activated electrode, to prevent destructive retention of heat in the tissues.
– The electronic cutting should be performed biterminally (simultaneous, combined use of the surgical electrode and the patient indifferent electrode).
– During instrumentation, the normal surface tension of the tissues should be maintained.

* by *Maurice J. Oringer,* DDS. Abstracted with permission, J. Am. Dent. Assoc. 92:850, May 1976.

Impression Technique

The following technique may be applied either for polysulphide or polyether impression materials.

1. Coat the tray thinly with the adhesive supplied by the manufacturer. The adhesive must be allowed to dry thoroughly, otherwise the impression material can pull away on the sticky adhesive. A minimum period of ten minutes should be allowed.
2. Equal lengths of the heavy body base and catalyst pastes are extruded onto the mixing pad in sufficient quantity for the tray mix. A well-fitting tray will require nearly twice its length in material.
3. Dispense 2−3 cm of the lighter body base and catalyst onto a separate pad for the syringe mix (Fig. 4-123). Many of the syringe mixes are too low in viscosity to resist displacement by serumal seepage or even blood with the result that the unset material is displaced before it is set and this will occur even after the operator has achieved what he thinks is perfect wetting of the tooth. Elastomeric impression materials should have a "limiting viscosity", i.e. the viscosity of the unset mix must be high enough to resist displacement by fluid seepage. For these reasons it is preferable to use a regular body material in the syringe if the light body materials is too low in viscosity. This can become apparent when moving from one quadrant to the other in the upper jaw. The syringe mix will tend to drip off the tooth.
4. Mix the heavy body pastes with a stirring motion and the spatula held almost vertically (Fig. 4-124). Excessive stropping with the spatula can increase the entrapment of air in the mix. After about 30 seconds no streaks of unmixed base and catalyst paste should be visible and final homogenisation of the mix should be done on a separate pad

to avoid picking up unmixed material. The total time of mixing should not exceed 1 minute. Fill the tray with this mix, taking care to cover the tray so that no air bubbles are left between paste and the tray adhesive. The mixing and filling of the tray will always take longer than the preparation of the syringe mix, therefore the latter should be prepared after the heavy body mix. In addition, most heavy body materials will set a little more slowly than syringe mixes so an increased setting time is advantageous.

5. Mix the light or regular body paste in the same way as above and on completion of the mix, set the timer clock for ten minutes. (In the case of polyether materials the setting time is shorter.)

Choice of syringe

There are many ways of loading syringes but the one the author has found most convenient is the "Impregum Syringe"* made for use with polyether impression materials. This syringe is supplied with a small plastic loader and plunger (Fig. 4-125). The paste is pressed into the plastic ring and the plunger then pushes it into the barrel of the syringe. Loading can easily be accomplished in 15 seconds (Fig. 4-126). If the paste is mixed in 30 seconds, the whole operation can be completed in less than one minute. It is for this reason that the author prefers to mix the tray material first since, if the syringe mix is placed too early in the mouth, polymerisation will already have become well advanced at the time of insertion of the tray mix. The syringe mix may easily have reached a level of viscosity higher than the heavy body tray mix which completely defeats the purpose of using this mix as an "hydraulic plunger". Failure to pressurise the syringe mix around the teeth is a frequent cause of creasing in

* ESPE, Seefeld, West Germany.

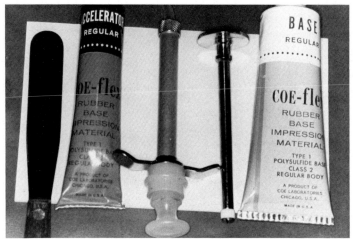

Fig. 4-123a and b (a) Complete kit for taking a rubber base impression. Regular body polysulphide, Impregum syringe, mixing pad and broad, flat-bladed spatula. (b) Impression pastes dispensed in equal lengths on mixing pad.

Figure 4-123a

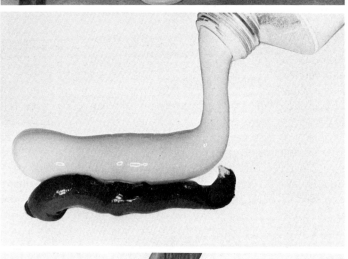

Figure 4-123b

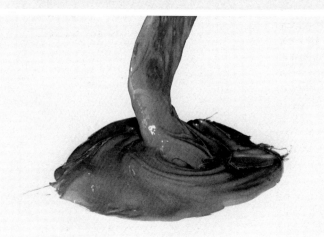

Fig. 4-124 Mixing of heavy body paste using a stirring motion. Mix has now been transferred to a second mixing pad and is now free from streaks.

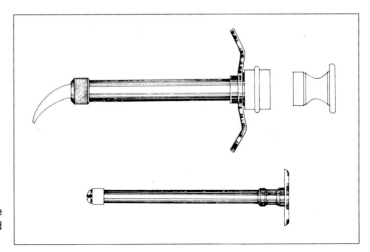

Fig. 4-125 "Impregum" syringe showing loading cylinder and plunger applied to open barrel.

the impression or for areas to collapse because the tray mix is not in intimate contact due to air entrapment. It must also be appreciated that unless some pressure is exerted, it is difficult to be sure whether material is in intimate contact with the tooth in the gingival crevice.

6. Whilst the nurse is filling the syringe, the secondary cords should be removed and all subgingival areas checked for cleanliness. A small pledget of cotton-wool soaked in hydrogen peroxide may be used to wipe away any debris and at this stage, if atomised water spray is used, great care must be taken not to displace the primary cords. Many operators prefer to remove the secondary cord prior to mixing the impression pastes and this a matter of choice. The author has found that the quicker the syringe mix is placed in the crevice once the secondary cord is removed, then the greater the chances of success.

If the primary cords are also removed the preparation can be cleaned with a light atomised water spray.

When the cleanliness of the preparations has been secured and each one dried lightly with cotton-wool or a very light air spray, the syringe mix should be injected around the teeth, taking great care to run evenly and closely around each shoulder area. A gentle air stream may assist in spreading the material but if used too strongly can trap air bubbles. The main object of the technique should be to cover all the teeth with a thin and even layer of impression material (Fig. 4-127). Where four or more teeth are being prepared, it is useful to use multiple syringe mixes to prolong the working time and ensure that one does not run out of material at a critical moment.

7. Insert the tray with a gentle rocking movement and then press firmly home until the stops are engaged. The setting time for the tray mix will be around 12 minutes since the timer clock was set at 10 minutes at the time of mixing the syringe mix. Under no circumstances should the operator be tempted to reduce this setting period since the polysulphide impression materials will not reach a high degree of elastic recovery and dimensional stability until at least ten minutes after mixing.

8. After completion of set, insert two fingers under each side of tray and break suction. remove tray with a steady but rapid pull. Rinse the impression in water, dry and ex-

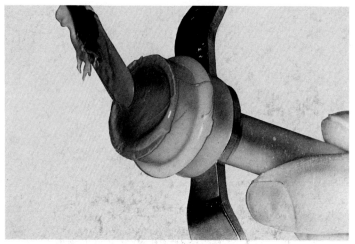

Fig. 4-126a to c   (a) Loading "Impregum" syringe with elastic impression material. (b) Plunger depressed to inject rubber base into syringe barrel. (c) Plastic loading ring is now slid off and metal plunger inserted.

Figure 4-126a

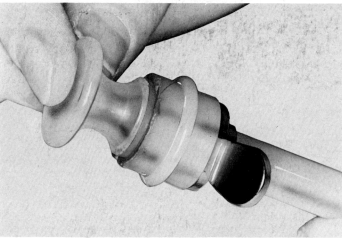

Figure 4-126b

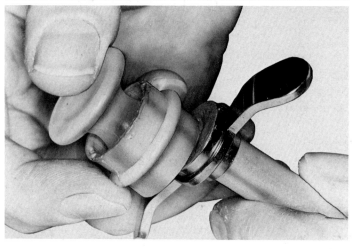

Figure 4-126c

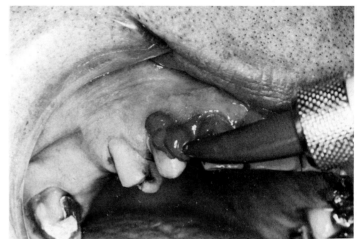

Fig. 4-127 Syringe mix injected around teeth prior to insertion of tray mix. Note the healthy condition of the gingival tissue making impression taking much easier.

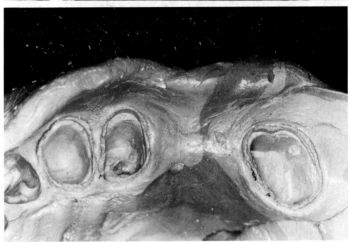

Fig. 4-128 Completed polysulphide elastomeric impression, showing all the margins clearly defined.

amine it for accuracy of reproduction (Fig. 4-128).

9. Remove any primary retraction cords that may not have been removed in the impression and check that no set rubber material has been left in the gingival crevice.

10. Examine the impression for any imperfections such as blow holes, creases, imperfect adaptation (shiny, concave surfaces often indicate this), contamination with blood, tears, or distortion in approximal spaces. If there are imperfections on just one or two tooth preparations in an arch, it may be possible to retake these in a sectional tray and construct transfer copings. However, any major discrepancies are far better dealt with by taking a new impression. If the tray is immersed in hot water and the adhesive softened, the rubber impression can be easily stripped off the tray.

The author does not recommend correcting imperfections by rebasing the faulty area with a fresh mix. Such a procedure could distort the whole impression.

Alternative methods

The various alternative techniques discussed for other materials on page 305 will not be described in this monograph since, in the author's hands none of them have performed as consistently as the polysulphide or polyether elastomers. The student or clinician interested in ceramics is therefore advised to use the techniques described above until he is completely familiar with all procedures in ceramic crown and bridgework. Only then should he start to evaluate other impression techniques since, in this way, he will have a firm base from which to compare his results. As explained earlier, the author does not favour rebase techniques, particularly with high shrinking silicone materials. However, if the newer putty-like tray materials are used with a polysulphide impression system*, then it is likely that the rate of clinical success will be much higher.

Common Causes of Failure in Elastomeric Impression Materials

Surface Defects

1. *Rough surfaces*

   a) Incomplete polymerisation caused by faulty setting. May be due to faulty batch control by manufacturer or improper dispensing of catalyst paste or too early removal from mouth.

   b) Inadequate wetting of tooth because material was setting too quickly when applied to tooth. Caused by too much catalyst paste, humidity, or high temperature.

2. *Voids*

   a) Bubbles entrapped at time of mixing or produced by blood, saliva etc, during syringing of mix. Large bubbles may be produced by failure to pressurise syringe mix during seating of tray.

   b) Irregular smooth voids are caused by failure to wet the tooth and will show as shiny, concave surfaces lacking detail. Caused by improper syringing of mix, particularly on distal aspects of teeth, or failure to pressurise the mix with the heavy body tray mix, i.e. viscosity of syringe mix rising too rapidly.

   c) Irregular rough voids. Caused by contamination with debris or congealed blood etc. Failure to clean tooth surface prior to applying syringe mix.

Dimensional Instability

1. *Shrinkage*

   Caused by too great a bulk of material in tray, faulty base paste to catalyst paste concentra-

---

* Kerr's Accralastic. Kerr Co. Detroit. U.S.A.

tion or the use of highly volatile liquid catalysts.

2. *Swelling*

Caused by water absorption due to molecular structure of elastomer taking up water. Materials subject to this, e.g. polyether, must not be stored in water or high humidity.

3. *Distortion*

a) Inadequate polymerisation is the commonest cause and is generally due to incorrect catalyst paste concentration or too short a setting time. Occasionally batches of elastomeric impression materials can be faulty.

b) Lack of adhesion of impression material to tray. Often due to too thick a coat of rubber adhesive.

c) Premature removal from mouth.

d) Non-rigid trays.

e) Failure to keep tray seated in mouth during setting.

f) Inserting tray mix when material is already setting, i.e. it is developing an elastic memory which can cause distortion.

Cementation of Porcelain and Metal-Ceramic Crowns

The ideal properties required in a dental luting cement are:

1. Production of minimal tissue reaction (minimal pulpal or gingival damage).

2. Adhesion to tooth structure and to the restorative materials, e.g. gold or porcelain.

3. High strength to resist both tensile and compressive forces or a combination of both (i.e. shear).

4. Resistance to plastic deformation (creep resistance).

5. Low film thickness of around 25 μm.

6. Easy manipulative properties in which the powder/liquid ratio is not too critical.

7. Slow rise in viscosity but with rapid hardening at the end of the working time.

8. Resistance to solution in acid media, for example, plaque acid.

9. Possess anticariogenic properties, e.g. liberation of fluoride ions.

10. Translucency.

There are six types of cement available today and their properties are given in Table 4-1.

The phosphate bonded cements are well established materials. The zinc phosphate cements have good manipulative characteristics and are comparatively strong materials with good resistance to plastic deformation. The silico-phosphate cements are even stronger and possess the added advantage of being translucent and containing leachable fluoride. Both types of cement are acidic and can cause pulpal damage, particularly in the case of silico-phosphate. The phosphate bonded cements are non-adhesive to tooth structure and when exposed to plaque acid the phosphate bonding is rapidly broken down, causing solution and erosion of the cement.

Table 4-1

	Properties of Luting Cements							
	Glass-Ionomer (Aspa IV A)		Silico-phosphate (a)	(b)	Zinc Carboxy-late	Zinc Phos-phate	ZOE	EBA
Powder/Liquid Ratio (g/ml)	1.67	2.0	3.0	3.0	1.5	2.6	2.0	6.2
Consistency (mm, 220 g at 2 min)	29	25	28	27	33	30[1])	31	−[2])
Film thickness (μm 2 min)	24	26	33	28	22	32[3])	25	45
Maximum effective particle size (μm)	19	19	20	20	10	15	15	30
Setting time (min)	4.5	4.25	6	−	6.75	7	7.5	6
Compressive strength (N/mm², l d)	128	150	153	104	79	83	39.4	91
Tensile strength (N/mm², l d)	8.2	9.3	9.3	−	12.5	4.9	4.0	7.6
Solubility (per cent m/m, l d)	0.86	0.64	1.1	0.8	0.1	0.08	0.05	0.06
Opacity (CO. 70)	0.69	0.69	0.73	−	1.0	1.0	1.0	1.0

[1]) Determined under 120 g load at 3 min.
[2]) Not applicable.
[3]) Measured at 3 min.

From *Wilson, A. D., Crisp, S., Lewis, B. G.,* and *McLean, J. W.* (1977). Experimental luting agents based on the glass-ionomer cements. Brit. Dent. J. 142: 117−122.

The zinc-oxide-eugenol cements are very bland materials and have excellent sealing properties, which may be due to actual chemical bonding to the tooth surface through a chelation reaction. However, the ZOE cements are weak materials.

The EBA cements, when fortified with alumina, are stronger but both materials are highly sol-uble in mouth fluids where eugenol is extracted over long periods to leave the soluble zinc hydroxide. The chemical reaction may be illustrated as follows:

$$ZnO + 2HE = ZnE_2 + H_2O$$
$$ZnE_2 + 2H_2O = Zn(OH)_2 + 2HE$$

The resistance of both ZOE and EBA cements

to plastic deformation is poor and they are not suitable for cementing bridgework.

The polycarboxylate cements developed by *Smith* (1968) have solved many of the problems associated with the phosphate bonded cements. These new cements show improved adhesion to tooth structure and are less injurious to the tooth pulp. This is probably due to the large molecular size of the polyacrylic acid molecule combined with its ability to complex with proteins. This may limit diffusion through the tissues and down the dentinal tubules.

The polycarboxylate cements are similar in strength to zinc phosphate cements but have less resistance to plastic deformation (creep resistance). They are therefore more prone to "movement" under occlusal stress. The polycarboxylate cements are also more difficult to mix than the zinc phosphate cements. The high viscosity of the polyacrylic acid liquid can deceive the operator as to the actual consistency of the mix and it is easy to add either too much or too little powder. The carboxylate cements also tend to form "cobwebs" during mixing, due to the formation of transient elastomers. Mixing of these cements is therefore better done using measuring devices such as scoops for the powder and syringes for the liquid.

The glass-ionomer cements developed by *Wilson* and *Kent* (1969) are only just becoming available commercially. (De Treys* and Caulk** Chem-Bond and Fuji-Ionomer***). In their present form they are composed of fine calcium aluminosilicate glass powders prepared with a fluoride flux similar to dental silicate powder. The liquid is an aqueous solution of poly(acrylic acid) which is modified by the addition of low

---

* De Trey's Chem-Bond. A.D. International, London, W.1.
** Caulk Chem-Bond. L. D. Caulk Co., Milford, Delaware.
*** Fuji-Ionomer. G. C. Dental Industr. Co., Japan.

molecular weight chelating agents such as tartaric acid which sharpens the setting reaction. The powder and liquid, when mixed together, set in a similar way to silicate cements. Firstly, when the acid is mixed with the powder, a paste is formed which rapidly hardens into a solid mass bound by a polysalt gel. *Wilson* (1977) regards cement formation as an acid-base reaction between polymeric substances.

Glass (base)
Powder
+
Polyacid
Liquid
=
Polysalt gel
Matrix
+
Silica Gel
Particle coating

Thus, an acid (the liquid) reacts with a base (the powder) to form a salt which, because of its polymeric nature, acts as a binding matrix. This matrix binds unreacted glass particles together to form the cement.

Barry et al. (1973) have shown that the matrix of the glass-ionomer cement contains sheathed droplets of calcium fluoride which confers the ability to leach fluoride ions into the surrounding enamel. A study by *Maldonado* et al. (1978) has shown that the glass-ionomer cement should be as effective as silicate cement with respect to inhibition of secondary caries.

Glass-ionomer cements adhere to enamel and dentine in a similar way to carboxylate cements. When these cements are in the form of a fluid paste, many free acid carboxyl ($-COOH$) groups are present. These acid groups promote wetting of polar surfaces because the acid hydrogen has a propensity to form a hydrogen bridge between the polyacid and the substrate. If the cement paste has wetted the surface of the tooth, then during the course of the cement reaction, the hydrogen bridges formed between cement and substrate will be progressively converted to stronger ionic bonds as the hydrogens are displaced by calcium or zinc ions from the carboxylate cement or tooth, or in the case of the glass-ionomer cements by calcium, aluminium or other metal ions.

Recent work has shown that when precious metals such as gold or platinum are electroplated with approximately 1–2 μm of tin, the glass-ionomer cement will adhere to the tin oxide surface via polar and ionic bonds (*Hotz* et al., 1977; *McLean,* 1977).

In addition to the good adhesion, the glass-ionomer cements produce similar pulpal reaction to the polycarboxylate cements (*Tobias* et al., 1978). They are also more resistant to plaque acid attack than the phosphate bonded cements.

The physical properties of the glass-ionomer cements are good. They have greater compressive strength than the zinc phosphate cements and good resistance to plastic deformation. In addition, they are mixed more easily than the carboxylates and have good working properties. The main criticism of these new cements is that they are easily weakened by water contamination in the early stages of set.

Recommended clinical use for dental cements

The zinc phosphate cements still set a high standard for luting materials. They are easy to mix, have good strength and resistance to plastic deformation and are well tried clinically. The main reasons for wishing to replace them are their lack of adhesion to tooth structure, rather acid reaction on the pulp and lack of anticariogenic properties.

The carboxylate cements have excellent adhesion to tooth structure and biocompatibility. However, they are less resistant to plastic deformation than zinc phosphate cements, so that their use on crown preparations with high taper angles can be risky in bridgework.

The glass-ionomer cements will probably overcome these problems since they possess higher strengths than zinc phosphate and are fluoride leachable glasses and give some anticariogenic properties.

In view of the high solubility of the ZOE and EBA cements, they cannot be considered suitable for cementation of bridgework and have limited use in the single crown restoration except where biological compatibility is essential, e.g. a near-exposure of the pulp.

In the light of current research and production of cements both new and conventional, the following recommendations can be made for the cementation of porcelain or metal-ceramic crowns, in order of preference.

Cementation of crowns with good retentive form and where pulpal damage may occur

1. Polycarboxylate or glass-ionomer cement.
2. Zinc phosphate with varnish.

Cementation of crowns with moderate retentive form and where pulpal damage may occur

1. Zinc phosphate with varnish or glass-ionomer cement.
2. Polycarboxylate.

Cementation of crowns where no possible damage to the pulp can occur

1. Zinc phosphate or glass-ionomer.
2. Silicophosphate (fine grain).
3. Polycarboxylate.

Cementation of complete porcelain crowns

1. Glass-ionomer for translucency.
2. Polycarboxylate or zinc phosphate with varnish.

Cementation of post crowns, facings or crowns on metal substructures

1. Zinc phosphate.
2. Possibly silicophosphate or glass-ionomer.

Cementation of fixed splints or bridgework

1. Zinc phosphate with varnish or glass-ionomer.
2. Polycarboxylate.

Clinical Manipulation

The manipulation of the phosphate-based cements is well-known and should not require repetition. In the case of the newer polycarboxylate and glass-ionomer cements, certain recommendations can be made which may not be entirely familiar to the clinician.

1. All mixing should be done on a refrigerated glass slab to prolong working time. Refrigeration of the liquid will decrease its shelf-life due to formation of a gel.
2. An ideal powder-liquid ratio for the glass-ionomer cements is 1.67 g/ml and for the polycarboxylates 1.5 g/ml. The liquid should be dispensed in a syringe with a measuring scoop for the powder to ensure best results. Exposure of the dispensed liquid for more than 60 seconds can result in loss of water by evaporation and concentration of the liquid will produce a more viscous material.
3. The tooth should present as high a surface finish as possible. Smooth dentine surfaces are more easily cleaned of debris which can inhibit chemical bonding. A high finish can be produced on dentine surfaces by using sintered diamond finishing tools* and then polishing with silicon carbide rubber bonded cups (Aaba cups**).
4. Avoid contaminating the surface of the dentine with wax, oil, varnishes or any protein material which can inhibit chemical bonding.
5. Tooth surfaces should be cleaned with hydrogen peroxide (10 vol.) or a similar bland cleanser such as "Cavilax" (Espe, West Germany). Never use citric acid or similar materials which can damage the tooth pulp under cut dentine surfaces.
6. Noble-metal surfaces should be lightly blasted with 30 μm aluminium oxide grit and then plated with 1−2 μm of tin which is lightly oxidised. This tin oxide surface will provide the means for chemical bonding to the carboxyl group in the polyacrylic acid based cements.
7. Porcelain crowns may be lightly etched with a 37 % solution of phosphoric acid to provide a clean surface for the cement. Polyacrylic acid cements will not bond to porcelain crowns by molecular attachment.
8. Tooth surface should be clean but not dehydrated when the cement is applied. Excessive drying can concentrate any protein debris and prevent efficient wetting of the tooth surface.
9. Never use varnishes to protect the tooth if polyacrylic acid type cements are used, since this will prevent chemical bonding to tooth structure.
10. The margins of the cement should be protected with varnish after the initial set (5 to 6 minutes). Under no circumstances should saliva come into direct contact with the unset cement.

* Sintered diamond tools. A.D. International. London W.I.
** Aaba rubber cups. Identoflex AG, Buchs/SG, Switzerland.

Monograph IV

References

Baker, D. L., and *Curson, I.* (1974). A high-speed method for finishing cavity margins. Brit. Dent. J. 137, 391.

Barnes, I. E. (1974). The production of inlay cavity bevels. Brit. dent. J. 137, 379.

Barry, T. I., Miller, R. P., and *Wilson, A. D.* (1973). Dental cements based on ion leachable glasses. XI Conference on the Silicate Industry, Budapest (pp 881 – 893).

Boyde, A. (1973). Finishing Techniques for the Exit Margin of the Approximal Portion of Class II Cavities. Brit. Dent. J. 134:319.

Braden, M. (1974). Selection and Properties of Some New Dental Materials. Dent. Update 1:489.

Braden, M. (1975). Impression Materials. In: Scientific Aspects of Dental Materials. Ed. J. A. von Fraunhofer, pp. 371 – 400. Butterworths, London and Boston.

Braden, M., and *Elliot, J. C.* (1966). Characterization of the Setting Process of Silicone Dental Rubbers. J. Dent. Res. 45:1016.

Braden, M., Causton, B. E., and *Clarke, R. L.* (1972). A Polyether Impression Rubber. J. Dent. Res. 51:889.

Brown, M. H. (1967). Impression Procedures for Restorative Dentistry. D. Clin. North America, March. pp. 147 – 167.

Clayton, J. A., and *Greene, E.* (1970). Roughness of Pontic Materials and Plaque. J. Pros. Dent. 23: 407.

Conod, H. (1937). Etude sur la Statique de la Couronne Jaquette. Rev. Mensuette Suisse d'Ontol. 47:485.

Craig, R. C., El-Ebrashi, M. K., and *Peyton, F. A.* (1967). Experimental Stress Analysis of Dental Restorations. Part II: Two-Dimensional Photo-Elastic Stress Analysis of Crowns. J. Pros. Dent. 17:292.

Derand, T. (1974). Analysis of Stresses in the Porcelain Crown. Odontologisk Revy. 25. Supplement 27.

El-Ebrashi, M. K., Craig, R. G., and *Peyton, F. A.* (1969). Experimental Stress Analysis of Dental Restorations. Part III: The Concept of the Geometry of Proximal Margins. J. Pros. Dent. 22:333.

El-Ebrashi, M. K., Craig, R. G., and *Peyton, F. A.* (1969). Experimental Stress Analysis of Dental Restorations. Part IV: The Concept of Parallelism of Axial Walls. J. Pros. Dent. 22:346.

Fraser, F. (1969). Precision Porcelain Jacket Crowns. Anglo-Cont. Dent. Soc. 21:17.

Heywood, R. B. (1952). Designing by Photoelasticity, pp. 314 – 365. Chapman and Hall Ltd., London.

Hosoda, H., and *Fusayama, T.* (1959). Surface Reproduction of Elastic Impressions. J. Dent. Res. 38:932.

Hotz, P., McLean, J. W., Sced, I. R., and *Wilson, A. D.* (1977). The bonding of glass-ionomer cements to metal and tooth substrates. Brit. dent. J., 142, 41.

Huffman, R. W., Regenos, J. W., and *Taylor, R. R.* (1969). Principles of Occlusion. Ohio State University.

Johnson, J. F., Mumford, G., and *Dykema, R. W.* (1967). Modern Practice in Dental Ceramics. W. B. Saunders & C., Philadelphia and London.

Jørgensen, K. D. (1955). The Relationship Between Retention and Convergence Angle in Cemented Veneer Crowns. Acta Odont. Scandinav. 13:35.

Jørgensen, K. D., and *Holst, K.* (1967). The Relationship Between the Retention of Cemented Veneer Crowns and the Crushing Strength of the Cements. Acta Odont. Scandinav. 25:355.

Kahn, A. E. (1965). Considerations in the Use of Partial and Full Coverage in Periodontal Prosthesis. J. Pros. Dent. 15:83.

Kaqueler, J. C., and Weiss, M. B. (1970). Plaque Accumulation on Dental Restorative Materials. I. A. D. R. Abstract No 615.

Lehman, M. L., and Hampson, E. L. (1962). A Study of Strain Patterns in Jacket Crowns Resulting from Different Tooth Preparations. Brit. Dent. J. 113: 337.

Lewis, R. M., and Owen, M. M. (1959). Mathematical Solution of a Problem in Full Crown Construction. J. Am. Dent. Assoc. 59:943.

Löe, H., Heilande, E., and Jensen, S. B. (1965). Experimental Gingivitis in Man. J. Periodont. 36:177.

Maldonado, A., Swartz, M. L., and Phillips, R. W. (1978). An in vitro study of certain properties of a glass-ionomer cement. J. A. D. A. 96, 785.

McLean, J. W. (1958). Silicone Impression Materials. A research Report. Dent. Pract. 9:56.

McLean, J. W. (1962). An Evaluation of Elastic Impression Materials. In: Modern Trends in Dental Surgery. Ed. G. Morrant. Butterworths (London), pp. 223–231.

McLean, J. W. (1966). The Development of Ceramic Oxide Reinforced Dental Porcelains with an Appraisal of their Physical and Clinical Properties. M.D.S. Thesis, University of London.

McLean, J. W. (1970). Alumina Reinforced Ceramics. In: Tylman, S.: Theory and Practice of Crown and Fixed Partial Prosthodontics (Bridge). C. V. Mosby and Co., St. Louis. Chapt. 36.

McLean, J. W. (1974). Materials Used in Restorative Dentistry. In: Restorative Procedures for the Practising Dentist. Ed. F. J. Harty and D. M. Roberts. John Wright and Sons Ltd., Bristol.

McLean, J. W. (1977). A new method of bonding dental cements and porcelains to metal surfaces. Operat. Dent. 2, 130.

McLean, J. W., and von Fraunhofer, A. (1971). The Estimation of Cement Film Thickness by an In Vivo Technique. Brit. Dent. J. 131:107.

McLean, J. W., Kedge, M. I., and Hubbard, J. R. (1976). The Bonded Alumina Crown. Part II: Construction Using the Twin Foil Technique. Aust. Dent. J. 21:262.

McLean, J. W., and Sced, I, R. (1976). The Bonded Alumina Crown. Part I: The Bonding of Platinum to Aluminous Dental Porcelain Using Tin Oxide Coatings. Austr. Dent. J. 21:119.

McLean, J. W., and Wilson, A. D. (1976). The Clinical Development of the Glass-Ionomer Cements. Austr. Dent. J. 22:31.

McLean, J. W., and Wilson, A. D. (1978). The butt joint versus bevelled gold margin in metal-ceramic crowns (unpublished data).

Moon, P. C., Modjeski, P. J. (1976). The burnishability of dental casting alloys. J. Pros. Dent. 36, 401.

Morrant, G. A. (1963). The Effect of Operative Procedures on the Pulp. In: Modern Trends in Dental Surgery. pp. 81–110. Butterworths, London.

Newcomb, G. (1974). The Relationship Between the Location of Subgingival Crown Margins and Gingival Inflammation. J. Periodontol. 45:151.

Nuttall, E. B. (1961). Factors Influencing Success of Porcelain Jacket Restorations. J. Pros. Dent. 11:743.

Payne, E. (1970). Personal Communication.

Pettrow, J. N. (1961). Practical Factors in Building and Firing Characteristics of Dental Porcelain. J. Pros. Dent. 2:334.

Phillips, R. W. (1973). Skinner's Science of Dental Materials. W. B. Saunders Co., Philadelphia.

Podshadley, A. G. (1968). Gingival Response to Pontics. J. Pros. Dent. 19:51.

Rosenstiel, E. (1957). The Retention of Inlays and Crowns as a Function of Geometrical Form. Brit. Dent. J. 103:388.

Shillingburg, H. T., Hobo, S., and Fisher, D. W. (1973). Preparation Design and Margin Distortion in Porcelain-fused-to-Metal Restorations. J. Pros. Dent. 29:276.

Smith, D. C. (1968). A new dental cement. Brit. dent. J. 125, 381.

Stallard, H., and Stuart, C. E., (1963). Concepts of Occlusion. Dent. Clin. North Amer., S. 591.

Stein, R. S. (1966). Pontic-Residual Ridge Relationship: A Research Report. J. Pros. Dent. 16:251.

Street, E. V. (1953). Effects of Various Instruments on Enamel Walls. J. Am. Dent. Assoc. 46:274.

Stuart, C. E. (1964). Good Occlusion For Natural Teeth. J. Pros. Dent. 14:716.

Swartz, M. L., and Phillips, R. W. (1957). Comparison of Bacterial Accumulations on Rough and Smooth Enamel Surfaces. J. Periodont. 28:304.

Tay, W. M. (1974). Impression Techniques. In: Restorative Procedures for the Practising Dentist. Ed. F. J. Harty and D. H. Robert. John Wright and Sons Ltd., Bristol.

Thomas, P. K. (1976). The Wax-Up Technique in Organic Occlusion. In: Gnathology. Introduction to Theory and Practice. Bauer, A., and Gutowski, A., Quintessence Publishing Co. Berlin. Chicago.

Tobias, R. S., Browne, R. M., Plant, C. G., and *Ingram, D. V.* (1978). Pulpal response to a glass-ionomer cement. Brit. dent. J. 144, 345.

Tylman, S. D. (1970). Theory and Practice of Crown and Bridge Prosthodontics. Ed. 6, The C. V. Mosby Co., St. Lewis.

Walton, C. B., and *Leven, M. M.* (1955). A Preliminary Report of Photoelastic Tests of Strain Patterns within Jacket Crowns. J. Am. Dent. Assoc. 50:44.

Wheeler, R. C. (1969). Dental Anatomy and Physiology. W. B. Saunders Co., Philadelphia and London.

Wilson, A. D. (1977). The development of glass-ionomer cement. Dent. Update, 4:7, 401.

Wilson, W. H., and *Lang, R. L.* (1962). Practical Crown and Bridge Prosthodontics, McGraw Hill, New York. Chapt. 26, page 146.

Wilson, A. D., and *Kent.* (1971). The glass-ionomer cement. A new translucent dental filling material. J. Appl. Chem. Biotech. 21, 313.

Wise, M. D., and *Dykema, R. W.* (1975). The Plaque-Retaining Capacity of Four Dental Materials. J. Pros. Dent. 33:178.

Appendix

Appendix of Conversion Factors to SI Units

Conversion Factors/Equivalent Values

1 inch	=	0.0254 metres
1 lbf	=	0.453 592 kgf
1 kgf	=	9.806 65 N (newtons)
1 Pa (pascal)	=	N/m^2
1 lbf/in^2	=	144 lbf/ft^2 = 6894.76 Pa (or N/m^2)
1 N/mm^2	=	1 MN/m^2 = 1 M Pa
1 kgf/mm^2	=	9.80665 N/mm^2 = 9.80665 M Pa

Prefixes

M	=	mega	=	10^6
k	=	kilo	=	10^3
m	=	milli	=	10^{-3}

To Convert From Force	To	Multiply By
kilograms force (kgf)	pounds	2.2046
kilograms force (kgf)	newtons	9.807
pounds	kilograms force	0.4536
pounds	newtons	4.448
newtons (N)	kilograms force	0.1020
newtons (N)	pounds	0.2248

Force Per Unit Area

lbf/in^2 (p.s.i.)	MN/m^2	0.006895
lbf/in^2 (p.s.i.)	kg/cm^2	0.0703
kg/cm^2	MN/m^2	0.09807
kg/cm^2	llb/in^2	14.2233
MN/m^2	llb/in^2	145.0
MN/m^2	kg/cm^2	10.1968

quintessence books

Shillingburg/Hobo/Whitsett

Fundamentals of fixed prosthodontics

Fixed prosthodontics is an area of restorative dentistry whose successful application requires a combination of many forms of treatment in the broad spectrum of modern dentistry. Patient education and the prevention of further dental disease, thoughtful diagnosis, periodontal therapy, operative skills, occlusion, and on occasion, removable complete or partial prostheses and endodontic treatment must be combined to render successful treatment to the patient requiring fixed prostheses.

"Fundamentals of Fixed Prosthodontics" was written as a basis text for the under-graduated student's introduction to the subject. Because of the scope of the book, the combination of basic principles, background information on recent dental materials, and the detailed descriptions of clinical procedures, it is also an excellent review for the practising clinician. An effort has been made to correlate research findings with practical techniques which will produce a high quality service for the patient. There are over 600 illustrations to assist the reader in understanding the principles and methodes described.

336 pages, 601 illustrations, 17 × 24 cm format, paperback, price: $ 32.50 plus handling and 5 % sales tax in Illinois/USA.

quintessence
books

Axel Bauer/Alexander Gutowski

Gnathology

An Introduction in Theory and Practice

A new textbook which covers all the principle chapters of the gnathological science. This includes: The philosphy, the functions of the stomatognatho system, the positions and movements of the mandible, common concepts of the ideal occlusion. A long chapter covers the determinants of occlusion, Peter K. Thomas wrote the chapter on the wax-up technic in organic occlusion. In another section we have described the simulation of jaw movements by articulators. There is a short chapter about the Whip-Mix-Articulator and a new semiadjustable german articulator. An in depth section is about the use of the Dentatus-Articulator as semiadjustable instrument and a long Step-by-Step chapter about the use of the Stuart-Computer. The oral rehabilitation is covered by using crown and bridgework including remount procedure. There is also a detailed description of the oral rehabilitation by use of combined crowns and partial prosthesis including mucostatic impressions and remount procedures. The last chapter deals with the gnathological aspects of the full denture.

530 pages, more than 1000 illustrations, 500 multi-colored 22.5 × 25.5 cm linen-bound with gold stamping and protective cover, price: $ 150.– plus handling and 5 % sales tax in Illinois/USA.